Understanding Race and Health Inequity in the UK

This timely volume addresses the interpersonal, institutional, and structural factors underpinning inequities in healthcare access, experiences, and outcomes among racialised communities living in the United Kingdom (UK) today.

Bringing together researchers from the UK and Ireland, ranging from established scholars and early-career researchers to those working at the interface of research and community health, this volume assembles their trailblazing work to examine the complex relationship between race, racism, and health. Organised according to the following six themes: Questioning, Research and Data, Maternal Health, Mis/Trust in Services, Chronic Conditions and the Social Determinants of Health, and Beyond Resilience, the chapters uncover how racially unjust systems and practices generate unequal outcomes, while outlining the urgent changes needed to redress these systemic inequities. By examining how racial inequities are produced, sustained, and compounded across key domains of society, healthcare, and health research, the volume offers a critical guide for understanding and, more importantly, addressing racial and ethnic inequities in health in the UK.

This unique and important book is essential reading for educators, students, and policy makers within public health, medical education, public policy, and beyond.

Melanie Etti, Medical Doctor and NIHR Academic Clinical Fellow, University of Oxford, UK.

Julie Botticello, Senior Lecturer and Course Leader, MSc Public Health, University of East London, UK.

'A timely book focusing on health inequities and the importance of taking action to support marginalised and vulnerable communities. The authors expertly articulate key issues in a critical and insightful manner. This is a must-read book for anyone who is interested in developing a greater understanding about the intersections of health, race, inequity, and outcomes'.

– **Professor Marcia Wilson,** *Pro Vice-Chancellor, Birmingham City University*

'This book provides a timely and essential introduction into race and health in the UK, with vitally important case studies. A supportive handbook for those seeking to understand health equity'.

– **Dr Annabel Sowemimo,** *Author of* Divided: Racism, Medicine and Why We Need to Decolonise Healthcare, *Community Sexual & Reproductive Health Consultant, Harold Moody Scholar at King's College London*

'Etti and Botticello's edited volume is a perceptive inquiry into the underpinnings of racial inequity in health in the UK. The authors seamlessly integrate evidence, lived experience and policy insights to create a powerful narrative that exposes systemic gaps, while offering credible paths forward. This book presents invaluable learning and belongs on the desk of healthcare professionals, policymakers, educators, and anyone committed to building fairer, healthier communities in the UK'.

– **Professor Habib Naqvi,** *Chief Executive, NHS Race and Health Observatory*

'This important volume is based on five important truths: "Race" is not biology. "Racial"/ethnic differences in health outcomes are not normal. There is a system of structuring opportunity and assigning value based on "race" which is foundational to the history and wealth of the United Kingdom. That system, racism, continues to manifest in our structures, policies, practices, norms, and values today. Racism saps the strength of our whole society. Congratulations, Drs. Etti and Botticello, on convening this urgent conversation and issuing this call for urgent action within the health sector'.

– **Professor Camara Phyllis Jones,** *Past President, American Public Health Association, Visiting Professor, King's College London*

Understanding Race and Health Inequity in the UK

Edited by
Melanie Etti and Julie Botticello

Routledge
Taylor & Francis Group
LONDON AND NEW YORK

Designed cover image: Getty Images

First published 2027
by Routledge
4 Park Square, Milton Park, Abingdon, Oxon OX14 4RN

and by Routledge
605 Third Avenue, New York, NY 10158

Routledge is an imprint of the Taylor & Francis Group, an informa business

British Library Cataloguing-in-Publication Data
A catalogue record for this book is available from the British Library

ISBN: 978-1-032-73821-5 (hbk)
ISBN: 978-1-032-73820-8 (pbk)
ISBN: 978-1-003-46609-3 (ebk)

DOI: 10.4324/9781003466093

Typeset in Sabon
by Apex CoVantage, LLC

The following Generative AI tools have been used by some chapter authors for language improvement, idea generation, online search, and literature classification: Open AI GPT-5.2, Claude Sonnet 4.5, and Grammarly.

Contents

Acknowledgements

Many thanks to our wonderful and supportive editors at Routledge, Russell George and Amy Thomson, for believing in this project and in us to deliver it. Thanks also to the anonymous reviewers who assessed the project and its value to academia and healthcare in the UK. Your confirmation of the need for this volume energised us all in producing it.

Thank you to everyone who expressed an interest in contributing to this volume, and especially to the 31 authors who have committed themselves for the past three years to ensuring their area of expertise and communities of focus gain the visibility and recognition deserved.

For Melanie, I would first like to give thanks to my family. To my parents, I hope this work honours the journey you made more than 40 years ago. I am immeasurably grateful for all of the sacrifices you made for us along the way. Tash and Ashley, thank you for being a sounding board for all of my ideas and for your never-ending support despite my constant twists and turns. Your encouragement has given me so much strength, and your presence has always allowed me to feel seen. To MyMai and Jesse, I owe so much of my awakening to you both. Thank you for the endless discussions, thought-provoking conversations, and illuminating book and article recommendations. You have both empowered me to see health and medicine through a different lens and enabled me to sharpen my worldview. I am grateful to call you both colleagues and friends. And finally, to Julie. I owe so much of this to you. I am beyond grateful for your unwavering support over the years and your ability to inspire and challenge me when needed. It is the greatest fortune that we were brought together.

For Julie, I wish to express my gratitude to my students on the Public Health BSc and MSc programmes at the University of East London, for your criticality, openness, and willingness to engage deeply with questions of race, racism, and health inequity in the UK. Working with you has been both foundational and transformative; reorienting me as a person and my practice as a teacher. I thank you, Mel, for trusting me as your mentor and for sharing so openly throughout your journey at Harvard and since your return to the UK. I have grown enormously through our relationship, and together we make a formidable pair. To all those with whom I have worked, researched, learned, and taught – across your intersecting roles as parents, carers, healthcare practitioners, and colleagues in decolonisation and anti-racism – I dedicate this volume.

Abbreviations

AI	Artificial intelligence
BAME	Black, Asian, and Minority Ethnic
BHIVA	British HIV Association
BMI	Body mass index
BP	Blood pressure
CAHMS	Child and Adolescent Mental Health Services
CAHN	Caribbean and African Health Network
CESA	Caribbean Elders Support Alliance
CF	Cystic fibrosis
COPD	Chronic obstructive pulmonary disease
COVID-19	Coronavirus disease 2019
CRT	Critical Race Theory
CRISPR	Clustered regularly interspaced short palindromic repeats
CTO	Community Treatment Order
CYP	Children and young people
DHSC	Department of Health and Social Care
eGFR	Estimated Glomerular Filtration Rate
ENAR	European Network Against Racism
EU	European Union
F	Female
GDPR	General Data Protection Regulation
GP	General practitioner
HSC	Health and Social Care
HES	Hospital Episode Statistics
HESA	Higher Education Statistics Agency
HEXI	Health Experience Insights

IOM	International Organization for Migration
IPA	Interpretative Phenomenological Analysis
JSNA	Joint Strategic Needs Assessment
JCWI	Joint Council for the Welfare of Immigrants
LGBT+	Lesbian, Gay, Bisexual, and Transgender Plus
M	Male
MBRRACE-UK	Mothers and Babies: Reducing Risk through Audits and Confidential Enquiries across the UK
MFI-AR	Anti-Racism Model for Improvement
MHA	Mental Health Act
MHRA	Medicines and Healthcare products Regulatory Agency
ML	Machine learning
MLTC	Multiple long-term conditions
NHS	National Health Service
NHSE	National Health Service England
NHS RHO	National Health Service Race and Health Observatory
NICE	National Institute for Health and Care Excellence
NIH	National Institutes of Health
NIHR	National Institute for Health and Care Research
OECD	Organisation for Economic Co-operation and Development
OHID	Office for Health Improvement and Disparities
ONS	Office for National Statistics
PPI	Patient and Public Involvement
PTS	Post-traumatic stress
RCT	Randomised controlled trial
SCD	Sickle cell disease
TSF	The Silences Framework
UCL	University College London
UK	United Kingdom
UKOSS	United Kingdom Obstetric Surveillance System
US/USA	United States/United States of America
VCSO	Voluntary and community sector organisation
WHO	World Health Organization

About the editors

Melanie Etti is an NIHR academic clinical fellow and medical doctor specialising in Clinical Infection in Oxford. Her research career spans four continents, having conducted research in the UK, US, Uganda, and Brazil. In addition to her academic endeavours, which are primarily rooted in health equity and improving health outcomes for underserved and underrepresented communities, she is also deeply committed to widening participation, in both health research delivery and participation.

Julie Botticello is an interdisciplinary scholar and senior lecturer at the University of East London, UK. Her current research foregrounds the economies of care and repair that sustain every ethical daily life in post-colonial and plural contexts. Alongside her scholarly work, she has pioneered university initiatives to foster belonging among students from racialised communities. She has developed antiracist intervention programmes nationally and internationally to support educators in addressing racism pedagogically, practically, and personally.

Contributor biographies

Fiona Alderdice is the senior social scientist at the National Perinatal Epidemiology Unit (NPEU) and co-director of the NIHR Policy Research Unit in Maternal and Neonatal Health and Care based in the University of Oxford. She is also a senior research fellow at Harris Manchester College, University of Oxford, and an honorary professor in the School of Nursing and Midwifery at Queen's University Belfast. Her research focuses on (1) assessing maternal/infant need and experience by developing population surveys that can be used to benchmark perinatal health and well-being and (2) promoting mental health and well-being in the perinatal period.

Megan Armstrong is an associate professor of primary care research and a deputy director of the Centre for Ageing Population Studies at UCL. She leads NIHR-funded work co-designing and testing a digital self-management toolkit for individuals experiencing socioeconomic deprivation with multiple long-term conditions (MLTCs). Her research explores how deprivation impacts MLTC self-management, primary care support, and the implementation of digital health interventions. Megan also co-investigates efforts addressing frailty among people experiencing homelessness. Coming from a working-class background herself, she brings lived experience of socioeconomic disadvantage to her research, ensuring that the voices of underserved communities shape solutions to reduce health inequalities.

Karl Atkin is a professor of sociology at the University of York. He is a medical sociologist, with a particular interest in qualitative approaches, whose research focuses on health and social care in multicultural societies. This includes understanding the social consequences of various long-standing, chronic illnesses (https://www.york.ac.uk/sociology/our-staff/academic/karl-atkin/). He has an interest in understanding inequality and social inclusion. Professor Atkin has received significant funding from a variety of different funding panels, including the Economic and Social Research Council, National Institute for Health Research and NHS England. He has over 140 peer-reviewed papers and authored six books. He is an elected fellow of the Academy of the Social Sciences.

Sarah Akhtar Baz is a qualitative research fellow in the School of Health Sciences, University of Manchester, UK. She was previously a research fellow at the University of York and completed her PhD at the University of Sheffield. Sarah's research interests are at the intersection of ethnicity, family, and health studies. She employs a variety of qualitative methods in her work, including interviewing, ethnographic, and longitudinal methods. Sarah is particularly interested in exploring ethnic minority women's experiences in relation to family studies and health inequalities.

Fouad Berrahou is a retired academic and practitioner in health leadership and management with extensive experience in public health systems and postgraduate education. He joined Birmingham City University in 2014 as subject lead in Health Leadership and management and programme director for the online MBA in Health and continues to contribute to teaching in this field. His research demonstrates the enduring importance of leadership and management competence in achieving effective and efficient service improvement, with a particular focus on how different leadership styles support different types of quality improvement within healthcare systems such as the NHS. Previously, he held senior leadership roles within the Texas Department of Health, securing competitive government funding to improve maternal and child health services.

Claire Carson is an associate professor at the National Perinatal Epidemiology Unit (NPEU) and a deputy director of the National Institute for Health and Care Research (NIHR) Policy Research Unit in Maternal and Neonatal Health and Care (PRU-MNHC), based at the University of Oxford. She is a statistical epidemiologist who specialises in the analysis of observational and routine data in pregnancy and postpartum. Her research interests include maternal morbidity, infertility and fertility treatment, and breastfeeding. Prior to joining the University of Oxford, Claire was a research fellow at the London School of Hygiene and Tropical Medicine, where she also completed an MSc and then a PhD in Epidemiology.

Corina Cheeks is based in Oxford and serves on Biomedical Research Centre steering committees, as a grant reviewer for the National Institute for Health and Care Research, and as a patient reviewer. She is currently a co-applicant on a grant examining in-patient care. Her family's experience with cancer and neurological conditions has made her passionate about addressing health inequalities in clinical research. She is particularly committed to improving the representation of Caribbean and other minoritised communities in research settings, challenging the assumption that proximity to medical excellence guarantees equitable outcomes. Through her various roles, she advocates for meaningful patient and public involvement as essential to achieving health equity.

Savanna M. Daquila is based at the School of Psychology, Trinity College Dublin, Dublin, Ireland. Savanna identifies as a white, cisgender woman conducting her PhD at

Trinity College Dublin. Her degree is in psychology, and her research focuses on health outcomes, challenges, and barriers faced by informal caregivers, addressing intersectionality and equity within healthcare contexts.

Allison Felker is a senior researcher with MBRRACE-UK at the National Perinatal Epidemiology Unit (NPEU) and part of the National Institute for Health and Care Research (NIHR) Policy Research Unit in Maternal and Neonatal Health and Care (PRU-MNHC), based at the University of Oxford. Her research focuses on preventing severe pregnancy-related complications and improving maternal health through the use of high-quality data to inform evidence-based care. Prior to joining the University of Oxford, Allison worked at the Society of Obstetricians and Gynaecologists of Canada (SOGC), and she holds a PhD in Reproductive Immunology from Queen's University, Canada.

Linda Gibson is an emerita professor in Global Public Health at Nottingham Trent University. She is deeply committed to the promotion of health and to upstream interventions that address health challenges at individual, community, and global levels. Linda is actively involved in a range of international research projects across Europe and several African countries, including Uganda, Kenya, Malawi, Burkina Faso, and Nigeria, as well as within the UK. Her research interests centre on health promotion, health systems and services, and community development and engagement. She also has a strong focus on patient safety and the prevention and management of non-communicable diseases. Linda's work is underpinned by a strong emphasis on the social determinants of health and informed by a socio-ecological approach. Her current research is funded by a range of major bodies, including the UK Department for International Development through the Tropical Health Education Trust, the UK Department of Health and Social Care, and the European Commission's Horizon 2020 programme.

Siân Harrison is a social scientist at the National Perinatal Epidemiology Unit (NPEU) and part of the National Institute for Health and Care Research (NIHR) Policy Research Unit in Maternal and Neonatal Health and Care (PRU-MNHC), based at the University of Oxford. Siân's research interests are in perinatal mental health and survey methodology, with a focus on collecting high-quality data on maternal health and maternity experiences to inform policy and improve care and outcomes for women and families. Prior to joining the University of Oxford, Siân worked as a clinical psychologist in the NHS and has a PhD in Clinical Psychology.

Anna M. Hood, Division of Psychology and Mental Health, University of Manchester, Manchester, UK. Anna is a senior lecturer in psychology in the Division of Psychology and Mental Health at the University of Manchester. A dual British and American citizen, her grandparents emigrated from Jamaica to the UK as part of the Windrush generation. She is a clinical health psychologist, and her research examines the biopsychosocial challenges faced by people living with pain, with a particular focus on children and young adults living with sickle cell. Her work seeks to understand pain from structural perspectives, develop mechanisms for restoration, and create pathways for justice to eliminate pain inequities.

Helen Jones is a lived experience leader, having grown up in poverty, family breakdown and abuse. For 20 years, Helen has worked in the charity sector, primarily in her role as a founder employee and CEO at Leeds Gypsy and Traveller Exchange. Whilst there, Helen was heavily involved in promoting solidarity among groups experiencing health inequalities and launched the negotiated stopping programme of work, aiming to secure better treatment of nomadic people in the UK. As part of this, Helen co-founded the Moving for Change network, bringing together disparate groups across the UK around a shared purpose. This project 'broke the glass ceiling' for Romany and Traveller projects by securing £2 million in National Lottery Heritage funding.

Marian Knight is Professor of Maternal and Child Population Health at the National Perinatal Epidemiology Unit (NEPU), University of Oxford, NIHR Scientific Director for Research Infrastructure, and Programme Director for the NIHR Programme Grants for Applied Research Scheme. She is a public health physician and applied health researcher whose research focuses on the care and prevention of severe complications of pregnancy and early life and addressing disparities in outcomes for women and babies from different population groups. She established the UK Obstetric Surveillance System (UKOSS) in 2005 to conduct national studies of severe morbidities in pregnancy and leads the MBRRACE-UK national programme of maternal and perinatal mortality surveillance and Confidential Enquiries. She is an NIHR Senior Investigator and was elected to the fellowship of the Academy of Medical Sciences in 2021 in recognition of her exceptional contribution to the advancement of medical science. She was awarded an MBE in the 2023 King's New Year Honours for services to maternal and public health.

Angela D. Kumah is a public health and mental health professional with over seven years' experience spanning community psychology and juvenile rehabilitation, and public health practice in Ghana and the UK. She is a teaching fellow at Keele University on the Master of Public Health programme. Her doctoral research at Birmingham City University focused on culturally sensitive mental health promotion among Black African and African-Caribbean communities, using appreciative inquiry to explore resilience and service co-design. She has also worked with Birmingham City Council on community-based mental health initiatives, bridging academic research and applied public health practice. Her interdisciplinary interests span global health, race equity, cultural humility, and inclusive pedagogical practice.

Anne MacFarlane is Foundation Chair and Full Professor of Primary Healthcare Research in the School of Medicine, University of Limerick (UL), Ireland. Anne is Co-director of an interdisciplinary Participatory Health Research Unit at the School of Medicine, UL. She is Director of UL's World Health Organization Collaborating Centre for Participatory Health Research with Refugees and Migrants. Anne has researched cross-cultural communication between migrants and their healthcare providers since 2002 and led national and EU research on this topic. She focuses on involving migrants in research to improve the implementation of trained interpreters in daily practice. Her work has contributed to national training initiatives for healthcare interpreting and policy dialogues in Ireland and with the WHO.

Jennifer MacLellan is a senior qualitative researcher at the National Perinatal Epidemiology Unit, Nuffield Department of Population Health, University of Oxford, England. Jennifer has researched health inequalities in the UK since 2012 with a focus on maternity services since completing her PhD in 2019. Jennifer has a particular interest in working with women in democratic and inclusive ways to improve maternity experiences and outcomes. Jennifer is the chief investigator of the NIHR-funded study 'Optimising the use of professionally trained interpreters in maternity'.

Last Mafuba is a community organiser, public health specialist, and social scientist working to disrupt the structural injustices informing migrant mental health in the UK. Her work is grounded in a commitment to racial justice and collective care. Her recent PhD in Social Science and Social Policy examines how hostile migration regimes, racism, and institutional neglect restrict access to mental health services for Black sub-Saharan African migrant communities. She is the founder and CEO of Inini Initiative Ltd, a grassroots social enterprise delivering culturally grounded peer support groups and community-led interventions. She advocates for culturally sensitive mental health care designed with, not imposed on, migrant communities, treating care itself as a form of resistance and a pathway to systemic transformation. She also holds a number of senior leadership and advisory roles, including Independent Chair of Coventry and Warwickshire REACH Mental Health Alliance, and Chair of the Patient and Carer Race Equality Framework (PCREF) Independent Advisory Group within Coventry and Warwickshire NHS Partnership Trust.

Meiko Makita is a sociologist, with a focus on social gerontology and health research, and a lecturer at the School of Health Sciences, University of Dundee. As a Mexican-Japanese cis-woman, her background adds a valuable perspective to her research work, especially as a BAME individual and an immigrant to the UK. Recently diagnosed with a chronic illness condition herself, Meiko draws upon both her personal journey and academic research to provide insightful reflections on the UK healthcare system. Her dual cultural identity and a first-hand appreciation for the challenges within the system contribute to a nuanced understanding of the intersectionality within healthcare experiences.

Alison McFadden is an academic midwife and health services researcher with a focus on reducing health inequities for women, infants, and families in the UK and globally (https://www.dundee.ac.uk/people/alison-mcfadden). She is particularly interested in health policy, improving access to healthcare and the quality of healthcare for marginalised communities. Alison's research uses qualitative and mixed methods and has been funded by the National Institute for Health Research, Medical Research Council, and the Scottish Government.

Shobhana Nagraj is an assistant professor of primary and community care in the Department of Public Health and Primary Care, University of Cambridge, and an honorary senior clinical researcher in the Nuffield Department of Women's and Reproductive Health, University of Oxford. She leads research on the co-design of complex interventions, including digital health technologies, for low-resource settings both locally and globally, using a health equity lens.

Danielle Nimmons is an Alzheimer's Society-funded clinical research fellow in general practice. Her mixed methods PhD is exploring the identification of anxiety and depression in people living with dementia in primary care. Her research interests are in multiple long-term conditions, with a particular focus on dementia, Parkinson's disease, and frailty. She also has an interest in health inequalities, public engagement, and undergraduate medical education. She studied medicine at the University of Manchester, where she also gained an MRes in Medical Sciences with Distinction. She continues to work as a GP alongside her PhD.

Mathew Nyashanu is a senior lecturer at Nottingham Trent University, contributing to a wide range of undergraduate and postgraduate modules. He is actively involved in supervising undergraduate and postgraduate dissertations across health and social care programmes. Alongside his teaching, Mathew collaborates with community groups working in health and development and undertakes research across a variety of public health issues. Mathew has an extensive professional background spanning teaching, health promotion management, and academia. His early career began in Africa, where he worked with rural and urban communities, gaining valuable experience in community-based health education. He later focused on sexual health initiatives aimed at preventing sexually transmitted infections. In the UK, Mathew played a central role in conducting a sexual health needs assessment for Black sub-Saharan African communities in Birmingham, which led to the establishment of the NHS-led Ubuntu scheme.

Tharin Phenwan is a medical doctor, qualitative researcher, and lecturer at the School of Health Sciences, University of Dundee. His research focuses on palliative and end-of-life care, advance care planning, people living with dementia, gerontology, quality of life, thanatology and global health. His experiences of being a Thai immigrant in the UK and an able-bodied man without life-limiting conditions will be reflexively discussed along with his medical background and his understanding of different healthcare systems between the UK and other countries.

Maria Quigley is a professor of statistical epidemiology at the National Perinatal Epidemiology Unit (NPEU). Her research focuses on infant feeding, preterm birth, perinatal mental health, and survey methodology. She has expertise in the analysis of population-based cohorts and surveys, such as the Millennium Cohort Study, in the design and analysis of the NPEU National Maternity Surveys, and in RCTs. She has also used record linkage of large, routinely collected data to address a range of research questions in the area of maternal and child health.

Tanvi Rai is a health researcher based at the University of Oxford. She has an interdisciplinary and international background that spans across public health and applied social sciences. Tanvi maintains a strong interest in health inequalities, and her research so far has been about social and structural determinants of health, developing inclusive research methods and healthcare implementation practices, as well as studies involving socially sensitive health topics and working with variously marginalised populations.

Mohammad Sharif Razai is a clinician, researcher, and writer. He is an NIHR clinical lecturer at the University of Cambridge, an honorary research fellow at City St

George's, University of London, and a college research associate at Wolfson College, Cambridge. He graduated in medicine from the University of Cambridge in 2014, having previously completed a BSc in Anatomy and Developmental Biology at University College London. He holds an MA with distinction in Applied Medical Humanities from Birkbeck, University of London, and an MD (Res) from City St George's. His work focuses on vaccination, particularly maternal vaccination, and ethnic health inequalities. He has received national recognition for this work, including the international John Maddox Prize from Nature and Sense About Science.

Laura Sheard is a reader in the School of Health Sciences, University of Manchester, UK. She is a qualitative methodologist, health sociologist, and implementation scientist. Her research portfolio lies at the intersection of health inequalities and healthcare improvement. Her core research interests include understanding the quality, safety, and experience of NHS healthcare. She specialises in ethnographic methods, particularly longitudinal embedded ethnographies.

Judith Sixsmith is a white British professor of health research who co-directs the Institute of Social Science Research and the Centre for Educational and Life Transitions at the University of Dundee. She also leads the School of Health Sciences' Healthy Active Ageing Research group. Her areas of interest are health and well-being, specifically how marginalisation processes affect older people who live in underprivileged communities within existing health, social and cultural systems. She has substantial experience leading transdisciplinary, qualitative, and participatory national and international research projects. Her current research includes projects on the inclusion of older people with learning disabilities and those who identify as LGBT+ in their communities, placemaking with older people, age-friendly cities and communities, ageing and technology, and intergenerational design.

Angela Tufte-Hewett is an assistant professor of behavioural science and health psychology at the University of Birmingham. She was also a senior lecturer and researcher in health psychology at Birmingham City University, where she has taught since 2014. Her academic work spans behavioural science, health psychology, and public health, with a strong focus on health promotion and applied practice. Previously, she worked as a health promotion coordinator with Prairie Mountain Health and served as deputy director of the Master of Public Health programme at the University of Liverpool. Her experience bridges teaching, programme leadership, and applied public health practice.

Abi Woodward is a qualitative health researcher based at the Wolfson Institute of Population Health, Queen Mary University of London. Her research focuses on understanding and addressing health inequalities at the intersection of ethnicity, culture, socioeconomic deprivation, and access to care. She has a strong applied interest in community-based and culturally relevant interventions, particularly social prescribing and support for South Asian carers. Drawing on a background in Sociology, her work applies a social and structural lens to health research, with the aim of understanding how inequalities are produced and how they might be reduced in practice.

Preface

In 2021, we met through a mentorship programme for early-career, female, global health professionals sponsored by the University of Global Health Equity, Rwanda. Paired in this supportive relationship, we began speaking regularly over the two years of the programme, most often from two countries (Britain and America) and only recently, from just one, Britain. Despite our shifting locations, we shared a passion for making racial inequity in healthcare opportunities, experiences, and outcomes in the UK visible and for demonstrating what work still needs to be done for its eradication.

For Melanie, her journey towards editing this volume began with the internal work she undertook to unlearn so many of the mistruths that she encountered throughout her medical education. This epistemic awakening fuelled her pursuit of a deeper understanding of the factors that underpin the health inequities that affect racialised communities in the UK. This book is the book she needed while she was at medical school.

For Julie, the need for this book arose in the context of teaching public health undergraduates amid the realisation that there were limited options for core texts that addressed race, ethnicity, and health inequalities in Britain. Drawing on texts that addressed race, ethnicity, and public health in the USA, she supplemented these with key authors, articles, and policies that addressed the same in the British context. While offering an international perspective, the lack of a dedicated volume precluded drawing deeper conclusions about the UK.

When an opportunity arose to propose this much-needed volume, Melanie and Julie excitedly accepted the challenge. Once our editors at Routledge reviewed and commissioned it, we sent out calls on public health, healthcare, race, and ethnicity distribution lists covering England, Northern Ireland, Scotland, Wales, and the Republic of Ireland, and directly asked leading authors to contribute to this important collection. Three years after the start of this project, and together with 31 dedicated authors, situated in England, Scotland, and Ireland, we now present to you the first edition of this

UK-focused volume on race, racism, and health inequity. This book pulls together work from a number of contributors of colour and allies, ranging from established scholars, early-career researchers, and those working at the interface of research and community health, who have conducted trailblazing work examining the relationship between race, racism, and health from across the UK and Ireland.

With undergraduates in mind, each chapter not only details its case but also asks reflective questions after and provides a short list of important texts for further exploration. While being published marks an endpoint in this phase of the volume's journey, its real work begins in earnest with *you*, the reader, and the actions you take in response to each author's elaboration of the dire consequences of ethnic and racial health inequity and their recommendations for meaningful change.

Melanie Etti, Oxford
Julie Botticello, London

Introduction

Understanding race and health inequity in the UK

Julie Botticello and Melanie Etti

A brief note about language.

Throughout this volume, the authors will use different terms to refer to people of ethnic minority heritage. We recognise the challenge in finding a unifying term that respectfully encompasses the varying racial and ethnic identities within these communities without inappropriately homogenising them. As highlighted by Meir (2020), race-related discourse should accurately represent the world and the communities living within it.

In this introduction, we use the term 'racialised communities' to refer to people of ethnic minority heritage when speaking generally. We chose this term in recognition of the fact that our racial identities are constructed within the context of the societies in which we live. Where we speak specifically about a particular racial or ethnic group, we refer to them directly by name. To this end, we follow APA guidelines (2024) and capitalise all racial and ethnic group names, i.e.: Black, White, African, Caribbean, Indian, etc.

Persistent and avoidable health inequities exist between racialised communities and White populations in the United Kingdom (UK). Health inequities are defined by the World Health Organization (WHO, 2018) as 'differences in health status or in the distribution of health resources between different population groups, arising from the social conditions in which people are born, grow, live, work and age'. Crucially, the term implies a moral and ethical dimension (Whitehead, 1992); it asserts that such inequalities are representative of social injustice, often occurring as a result of unjust public policies, unequal access, and unfair differences in opportunities.

Health inequities among different racial and ethnic groups in the UK are present across the life course and embedded within differential health outcomes. Only recently (Sowemimo, 2023; Liverpool, 2024; Marmot et al., 2024) have these inequities been addressed through sustained engagement with racism and its impact on health in the

DOI: 10.4324/9781003466093-1

UK. Dominant explanations for health inequalities have tended to prioritise frameworks such as 'proportionate universalism' (Marmot et al., 2010, p. 15), which examine the nexus between poverty, place, and social position to address population-level disadvantage. By demonstrating that health outcomes correlate with socioeconomic position, social gradient approaches have positively led the shift away from notions of personal responsibility to the social determinants of health (Marmot et al., 2010, 2020a): the social, educational, economic, and environmental landscape in which individual and collective decision-making occur. The application of proportionate universalism that does not adequately account for the effects of racism, however, risks obscuring the persistent inequities experienced by racialised communities through broader accounts of disadvantage, masking the specific effect that racism has on morbidity and mortality. Growing numbers of research studies demonstrate that there are consistent patterns of racial and ethnic health inequity in the UK (Byrne et al., 2020), and that this inequity is the culmination of multiple, compounding and intersecting systemic challenges (Mirza & Warwick, 2022). A specific focus on race, ethnicity, and health in the UK is needed to unmask the invisibility of racial and ethnic disparities and to centre health equity in political agendas.

Race, like socioeconomic status and educational attainment, is a social determinant of health. Race is not biologically determined (Omi & Winant, 2014; Jones, 2000), nor is it a genetic marker for illness; rather, racism is a societal stance, where racialised communities have to confront and manage everyday acts of racial discrimination, whether interpersonal, institutional, or structural (Nazroo et al., 2020). While individuals are often classified into racial groups based on phenotypic traits (what they look like), these categories are socially constructed and bear no correlation to genetic differences between groups. In very few circumstances do biological differences correlate with racial phenotypes in accounting for differences in health outcomes. A prime example is that of sickle cell disease, which is more common among people of African heritage due to the protection that sickle cell trait offers against malaria. The increase in sickle cell disease among people living in Africa was, therefore, an evolutionary advantage driven by environmental pressures rather than an attributable characteristic linked to darker skin. Despite this, when examining differences in healthcare metrics between different races or ethnicities, a biological account risks diverting attention from the social, political and structural processes that reproduce health inequity (Bhopal, 2006).

The COVID-19 pandemic exemplified this, with differences in vitamin D levels being sought as an early explanation as to why members of racialised communities in the UK were dying from the disease at higher rates than their White counterparts (Mariño-Ramírez et al., 2021; *cf.* Nazroo, 2024). Similarly, physiological differences between Black people and other racial groups have been proposed as potential reasons for the reduced effectiveness of certain blood pressure medications among people of African and African-Caribbean heritage, leading to the continued recommendation of race-based treatment algorithms by the National Institute of Health and Care Excellence (NICE, 2019), despite their removal of from treatment guidelines produced by US and European societies. The continued use of self-ascribed race, a perilously heterogeneous metric, as the basis on which to draw firm scientific conclusions about biological differences sits uncomfortably at odds with our understanding of race as an inherently social construct.

This book seeks to dismantle harmful and misguided narratives around the reasons for poorer health outcomes among racialised communities by examining the root causes of these differences in the context of British history and modern-day British society. Britain's colonial history and its continued relationship with former colonies in the form of the Commonwealth are often neglected when discussing such issues. As Botticello (2020) substantiates, the historical subjugation of many members of racialised communities living in the UK today and their not-too-distant relatives serves as a persistent reminder of the cruelty of the British Empire and its aftermath, often manifesting as mistrust in the government and its institutions (Bryan et al., 2018), including the healthcare system. From the colonial exploitation of the Indian subcontinent, to the division of Africa through linguistic and tribal lines, and the mistreatment of the Windrush generation who were invited to rebuild the nation after the Second World War, the legacies of these misdeeds remain alive to this day. Public trust is essential for health systems to function effectively (McKee et al., 2024), yet research has consistently shown low public trust in the healthcare system among racialised communities living in the UK (Kadambari & Vanderslott, 2021; Nagesh, 2023; NHS Race and Health Observatory, 2025). Evidence of this mistrust was particularly apparent during the COVID-19 pandemic, where racial and ethnic differences were seen in COVID-19 vaccine uptake, as well as among participants in COVID-19 research studies, despite the disproportionate impact of this disease among these groups (Paul et al., 2022; Etti et al., 2021).

Health equity is informed not only by who is affected by a disease but also by how diseases that disproportionately impact racialised communities are prioritised within healthcare provision, treatment options and research funding. Approximately 15,000 people live with sickle cell disease in the UK (Reynolds & Naqvi, 2025). Despite comparable numbers of people living with cystic fibrosis, which is also inherited but predominantly affects White populations, there remain measurable differences in provision. There are 75% fewer specialist nurses in sickle cell care, a limited pool of treatment options and less than half the amount of research funding awarded (NHS Race and Health Observatory, 2025). The lack of attention to sickle cell disease demonstrates clearly how situations of genetic inheritance translate into ethnic inequities through unfair resource allocation.

This lack of provision maps onto the description articulated by American physician and epidemiologist, Professor Camara Phyllis Jones (2002), which elaborates how racial inequity in healthcare is produced: through differential access to healthcare, differential care provision, and through the differences in access to opportunities that underpin good health. Even within each of these three levels, there are a multitude of complex interactions between various factors that work synergistically to create the conditions within which these inequalities manifest. The United States (US) has developed a substantial body of scholarship spanning many decades (e.g. James et al., 1983; Geronimus, 1992, 2023; Ford et al., 2019; Jones, 2001, 2002, 2018; Smedley & Smedley, 2005; Smedley, 2019; Williams et al., 2003, 2019) explicitly examining racism as a determinant of health, although informed by different historical, political, and healthcare contexts. Given the persistence of genetic explanations of racial difference within British medical guidelines and that race continues to be conflated with biology, rather than a social construction yielding differential exposures to harm and neglect, it is important to attend to the British context specifically. The British context is underpinned by legacies of colonisation and decolonisation, inflexible systems and hostile laws, such as the Immigration Act 2014 (Legislation.gov.uk), and a pervasive lack of cultural competency attending racially and ethnically diverse customs, languages and religions. The persistence of nativism (Sivanandan, 2006; Kollias, 2024), where Whiteness is equated with Britishness and minoritised communities are considered alien, further entrenches discrimination and mistrust.

The consequences of this disconnect between healthcare providers and recipients are evident in the data. Each year, disparate outcomes in a number of health metrics are published, with racialised communities in the UK often faring the worst. Black and Asian women are more likely to die during pregnancy, childbirth, and the postnatal period than White women [a finding that has been consistent since 2000 (Women and Equalities Committee, 2023)] and stillbirths remain higher among Black and Asian infants (Matthews et al., 2022). Black people living with asthma in the UK are most likely to be admitted to hospital with an exacerbation (Simms-Williams et al., 2024), yet are also more likely to live in an area of air pollution or in a home with damp or mould (Jefferies et al., 2025; GOV.UK, 2025). Black people are least likely to have their cancer diagnosed through national screening pathways (Martins et al., 2022), yet are more likely to die of breast and prostate cancer (Workman et al., 2023; Prostate Cancer UK, 2025). These metrics scream of a system that was never designed to serve these communities at risk. Even where treatment access is improved, outcomes remain disparate. Research by Raleigh (2025) found that while people of South Asian heritage with heart disease had higher rates of prescribing for blood pressure and cholesterol-lowering medications, they still had higher rates of mortality from heart attacks. Addressing these inequities, therefore, requires a holistic appreciation of the multiple interdependent contributing factors to better understand how they come together to produce these poor health outcomes. As stated within the WHO Constitution, health is not merely the absence of disease but a state of complete physical, mental, and social well-being (WHO, 2020). A just and equitable society would, therefore, acknowledge and address the varying physical, social, and psychological needs of those within it to mitigate against avoidable causes of ill health. These inequities represent systemic inadequacies and neglect in multiple societal domains, which will be explored throughout the course of this volume.

The relative lack of historical attention to racism and health inequity in the UK reflects the dominance of universalist frameworks (e.g. Marmot et al., 2010, 2020a), limited ethnicity data collection (Raleigh, 2008; Iqbal et al., 2012) with which to inform particularist approaches, and persistent, deep-seated mistrust of healthcare systems among racially minoritised groups and communities (Nagpaul & Naqvi, 2025). Thus, for the past few decades, the emerging articulation that systemic racism is driving health inequity in the UK finally landed in public consciousness with COVID-19, in which racialised inequities became undeniable.

Towards the elaboration of his framework of proportional universalism, over 20 years ago, Marmot (2004) proposed that persistent social gradients between groups supersede any individual action taken. Furthermore, in a high-income country, these hierarchical positionings more accurately predict poor health outcomes than poverty as a unique measure. Marmot consolidated this analysis in Fair Society, Healthy Lives (Marmot et al., 2010). In this 'Marmot Review', he amplified the link between the social gradient and health outcomes, with those positioned along the lowest ranks of society experiencing the worst outcomes.

Despite its comprehensiveness, the review was criticised for its silence on race or ethnicity (Salway et al., 2010). Latif (2010) describes this omission as an anti-climactic follow-on from an earlier report (Acheson, 1998) that advocated for specific provisioning for different racialised communities. Salway et al. (2010) underscore the neglect of ethnicity, stating that the Marmot Review (2010) failed to identify persistent systemic failures that structure and reproduce the hierarchies leading to inequitable experiences and health outcomes for racialised communities. These failures include poor communication, discriminatory behaviour, lack of cultural sensitivity, institutional mistrust, and lack of funding. Salway et al. (2010) further note that due to uneven ethnicity data collection across commissioning and provision services, understanding or meeting the needs of diverse racialised communities remained limited in scope. Notwithstanding calls to improve ethnic monitoring, progress was slow. A Race Disparity Audit, published by the Cabinet Office (Green, 2017), reported some comparative health statistics, but due to insufficient data, little of substance was reported. A decade after the original review, Marmot's Health Equity in England (Marmot et al., 2020a) acknowledged that the intersection of socioeconomic status, ethnicity and racism amplified health inequity for racialised communities, yet it maintained the social gradient as central to its analysis.

It was not until Build Back Fairer (Marmot et al., 2020b), produced in the midst of the COVID-19 pandemic, that structural racism was identified as a prime determinant for its differential health outcomes (Marmot, 2022). Improved data collection during the pandemic revealed marked disparities in COVID-19 morbidity and mortality among racialised communities. While disproportionate exposure through high-risk occupations, multiple occupancy housing and underlying health conditions accounted for some of this risk, excess mortality among racialised communities persisted even after adjustment for these confounding factors.

Although not the origin, the COVID-19 pandemic served as a watershed moment in making these inequities in life chances publicly visible. Racialised communities have long faced earlier onset, higher rates and more aggressive progression of disease, coupled with poorer rates of survival (Razai et al., 2021a). The pandemic seared these long-standing inequities into everyday consciousness, confirming that while all were weathering the same storm, we were not in the same boat. Razai et al. (2021a) highlighted how inequities in employment, income, and housing intersect with failures in the healthcare system, producing compound disadvantage (Powers & Faden, 2008) through interpersonal, institutional, and structural racism. Razai et al. (2021a) argued that these dynamics operate through implicit bias, discriminatory institutional cultures, and policy environments that systematically expose racialised communities to harm.

In response to the disparities revealed by the COVID-19 pandemic, the Commission on Race and Ethnic Disparities (Sewell, 2021) aimed to reassess the position of racialised communities in the UK. Their report emphasised agency and resilience but was widely criticised (BMA, 2021; Razai et al., 2021b; Runnymede Trust, 2021) for downplaying the contribution of institutional and structural racism in the health and socioeconomic inequalities seen among these groups. An alternative response to the ethnic health inequities revealed by the pandemic was the formation of the NHS Race and Health Observatory by Lord Victor Adebowale CBE in 2021 to investigate the links between ethnicity and health inequality (Rao & Adebowale, 2020). Its *Ethnic*

Inequalities in Healthcare: A Rapid Evidence Review (Kapadia et al., 2022) identified structural, institutional and interpersonal racism as the underlying drivers of ethnic inequalities in access to, experiences of, and outcomes of healthcare. Critical findings include persistent failures in ethnicity data collection, inadequate interpretation services, a profound distrust in healthcare providers, and a lack of high-quality research on specific ethnicities. These challenges echo critiques made over a decade earlier. The King's Fund (Morris & Robertson, 2024) subsequently emphasised the urgent need to 'tackle racism and discrimination in the NHS and cultivate a culture of compassion' among their seven priorities for the NHS in their new 10-year health plan. As highlighted by Etti et al. (2023), such a change will likely require reform at every level of the health system, from decolonising and democratising medical education to structural changes that enable equitable and representative leadership within the NHS.

More recent reports continue to underscore the persistence of these inequalities. In 2024, University College London's (UCL's) Institute of Health Equity found that structural racism was producing avoidable and unfair inequalities between different ethnic groups in London (Marmot et al., 2024). While welcoming the attention to one region, we noted in our response (Etti & Botticello, 2024) that a focus on London obscures additional challenges faced by racialised communities in other regions of the country. As the report affirms, the inequitable distribution of the conditions for good health is a profound injustice (Marmot et al., 2024). Extending this analysis nationally, the Health Foundation and Runnymede Trust's *How Racism Affects Health* report (Walcott & Nightingale, 2025) underscores how interpersonal, institutional, and structural racism affect the wider determinants of health for UK-based racialised communities. The report documents entrenched inequalities in income, housing, employment, and environmental conditions, leading to compound disadvantage. Key findings include discriminatory hiring and progression processes favouring White workers, confinement of racially minoritised households to overcrowded and poor-quality housing, and reduced access to green spaces and clean air, culminating in inequitable life chances (Walcott & Nightingale, 2025). The King's Fund has also been instrumental in linking poor health outcomes to social domains outside of healthcare, including the recently updated 'What are health inequalities?' authored by Jefferies and colleagues (2025), in which disparities in housing, green space access, and work stress were again cited as contributing towards health inequities among racialised communities. These indicators are mutually reinforcing: where one is paid less, then housing becomes less affordable, pushing racialised communities into unhealthy and overcrowded accommodation and their children into poverty. These inequities are not the result of individual failure but of the systemic and pervasive injustice in the distribution of freedom, opportunity, and resources for health. Reports produced by these organisations have consistently centred the need for policy reform to redress the social inequality that racialised communities inordinately experience in order to provide the conditions necessary for good health.

Grassroots organisations such as Five X More (https://fivexmore.org/), NAZ (https://www.naz.org.uk/) and Reproductive Justice Initiative (https://reprojusticeinitiative.org/work/) have also sounded the alarm about the chasm in healthcare outcomes that exists between White people and racialised communities in the UK. Such organisations have proved crucial in not only recognising but also responding to the health needs of marginalised members of these communities. Community health partnerships such as the Caribbean and African Health Network (https://www.cahn.org.uk/), Community African Network (http://canafri.org.uk/), and the South Asian Health Foundation (https://www.sahf.org.uk/) provide tailored engagements for their communities of focus, including counselling, health information, and access to health services, to bridge the gap between these populations and the healthcare system. As stated by MacDonald et al. (2024), community-based action to address health inequalities is particularly effective when it is multicomponent, culturally concordant and tailored to the community's needs. The sustained commitment of many of these organisations has also galvanised communities and leaders towards meaningful change. The inclusion of Five X More in the All Party Parliamentary Group on Black Maternal Health (House of Commons, 2026) is one example of just how impactful such organisations can be.

Overall, the trajectory of increasing public consciousness reflects a gradual recognition of racial inequity and systemic racism as central to health inequities in the UK. This volume builds on these foundational studies to examine how racial and ethnic inequities permeate health and sickness across the life course. Whether in maternal, neonatal, and child health; for those living with multiple and chronic health conditions; for those in need of timely and relevant mental healthcare; or within the research infrastructures underpinning healthcare and policy formulation, inequities are reproduced in a cyclical process of exclusion and invisibility. These are fundamental challenges which no one individual or community can resolve. The need for structural change is urgent.

The chapters in this volume respond to this challenge by uncovering how racially unjust systems and practices generate unequal outcomes, while outlining the changes needed to redress the systematic neglect of racialised communities in the UK. Accordingly, the volume is organised under the following six themes: *Questioning, Research and Data, Maternal Health, Mis/Trust in Services, Chronic Conditions and the Social Determinants of Health, and Beyond Resilience*. By examining how racial inequities are produced, sustained, and compounded across key domains of society, healthcare, and health research, this volume offers a critical guide for understanding and, more importantly, addressing racial and ethnic inequities in health in the UK.

References

Acheson, D. (1998). Independent inquiry into inequalities in health – Report. *The Stationery Office*.

APA. (2024). *Racial and Ethnic Identity*. https://apastyle.apa.org/style-grammar-guidelines/bias-free-language/racial-ethnic-minorities

Bhopal, R. (2006). Race and ethnicity: Responsible use from epidemiological and public health perspectives. *Journal of Law, Medicine & Ethics*, *34*(3), 500–507. https://doi.org/10.1111/j.1748-720X.2006.00062.x

BMA. (2021). A missed opportunity: BMA response to the race report. *British Medical Association*. https://www.bma.org.uk/media/4276/bma-analysis-of-the-race-report-from-the-commission-on-race-and-ethnic-disparities-june-2021.pdf

Botticello, J. (2020). Managing multiplicity: Adult children of post-independence Nigerians and belonging in Britain. *Social Inclusion*, *8*(1), 314–323. https://doi.org/10.17645/si.v8i1.2473

Bryan, B., Dadzie, S., & Scafe, S. (2018). *Heart of the Race, Black Women's Lives in Britain*. Virago Press.

Byrne, B., Alexander, C., Khan, O., Nazroo, J., & Shankley, J. (2020). *Ethnicity, Race and Inequality in the UK: State of the Nation*. Policy Press.

Etti, M., & Botticello, J. (2024). Rapid response to: Racism is exacerbating London's health inequalities, report concludes. *British Medical Journal, 387*, q2138. https://www.bmj.com/content/387/bmj.q2138/rr

Etti, M., Fofie, H., Razai, M., Crawshaw, A., Hargreaves, S., & Goldsmith, L. (2021). Ethnic minority and migrant underrepresentation in Covid-19 research: Causes and solutions. *EClinicalMedicine, 36*. https://doi.org/10.1016/j.eclinm.2021.100903

Etti, M., Yuan, M., & Bump, J. B. (2023). Sun, skin and the deadly politics of medical racism. *BMJ Global Health, 8*(8), e013616. https://doi.org/10.1136/bmjgh-2023-013616

Ford, C., Griffin, D., Bruce, M., & Gilbert, K. (2019). *Racism: Science and Tools for the Public Health Professional*. Washington, DC: American Public Health Association Press.

Geronimus, A. T. (1992). The weathering hypothesis and the health of African-American women and infants: Evidence and speculations. *Ethnicity & Disease*, 2(3), 207–221.

Geronimus, A. T. (2023). *Weathering: The Extraordinary Stress of Ordinary Life in an Unjust Society*. New York: Little Brown Spark.

GOV.UK. (2025). *Housing with Damp Problems*. https://www.ethnicity-facts-figures.service.gov.uk/housing/housing-conditions/housing-with-damp-problems/latest/

Green, D. (2017). *Race Disparity Audit*. Cabinet Office.

House of Commons – Register Of All-Party Parliamentary Groups as at 12 January 2026: Black Maternal Health. (2026). Parliament.UK. https://publications.parliament.uk/pa/cm/cmallparty/260112/black-maternal-health.htm

Iqbal, G., Johnson, M. R., Szczepura, A., Wilson, S., Gumber, A., & Dunn, J. A. (2012). UK ethnicity data collection for healthcare statistics: The South Asian perspective. *BMC Public Health, 12*(1). https://doi.org/10.1186/1471-2458-12-243

James, S. A., Hartnett, S. A., & Kalsbeek, W. D. (1983). John Henryism and blood pressure differences among Black men. *Journal of Behavioral Medicine*, 6(3), 259–278. https://doi.org/10.1007/BF01315113

Jefferies, D., Williams, E., Buck, D., Babalola, G., & Maguire, D. (2025). *What Are Health Inequalities? | The King's Fund*. https://www.kingsfund.org.uk/insight-and-analysis/long-reads/what-are-health-inequalities

Jones, C. P. (2000). Levels of racism: A theoretic framework and a gardener's tale. *American Journal of Public Health, 90*(8), 1212–1215. https://doi.org/10.2105/ajph.90.8.1212

Jones, C. P. (2001). Invited commentary: "Race," racism, and the practice of epidemiology. *American Journal of Epidemiology, 154*(4), 299–304. https://doi.org/10.1093/aje/154.4.299/

Jones, C. P. (2002). Confronting institutionalized racism. *Phylon. 50*, 7–22.

Jones, C. P. (2018). Toward the science and practice of anti-racism: Launching a national campaign against racism. *Ethnicity & Disease, 28*(Suppl 1), 231–234. https://doi.org/10.18865/ed.28.S1.231

Kadambari, S., & Vanderslott, S. (2021). Lessons about COVID-19 vaccine hesitancy among minority ethnic people in the UK. *The Lancet Infectious Diseases, 21*(9), 1204–1206. https://doi.org/10.1016/S1473-3099(21)00404-7

Kapadia, D., Zhang, J., Salway, S., Nazroo, J., Booth, A., Villarroel-Williams, N., Bécares, J., & Esmail, A. (2022). Ethnic inequalities in healthcare: A rapid evidence review. *NHS Race and Health Observatory*.

Kollias, C. (2024). Borders, nativism and the politics of belonging. *The Beacon Digest*. London School of Economics. https://beaconjournal.lse.ac.uk/articles/18/files/674b2f8ad2760.pdf

Latif, S. (2010). Health Inequalities for Black and Minority Ethnic Groups in the UK: What has been done? In *Ethnicity and Race in a Changing World, What Has Been Done?* (pp. 34–39). Manchester University Press.

Legislation.gov.uk. (2014). *Immigration Act 2014*. https://www.legislation.gov.uk/ukpga/2014/22/contents

Liverpool, L. (2024). *Systemic: How Racism Harms Health – and What We Can Do about It*. Bloomsbury Publishing.

MacDonald, H., Martin, M., Clark, E., Dehn Lunn, A., Gkiouleka, A., Harasgama, S., Lamb, D., & Ford, J. (2024). *What Works: Community Engagement and Empowerment to Address Health Inequalities*. https://www.heec.co.uk/resource/what-works-community-engagement-and-empowerment-to-address-health-inequalities/

Mariño-Ramírez, L., Ahmad, M., Rishishwar, L., Nagar, S. D., Lee, K. K., Norris, E. T., & Jordan, I. K. (2021, September 20). Vitamin D and socioeconomic deprivation mediate COVID-19 ethnic health disparities, 21263865. https://doi.org/10.1101/2021.09.20.21263865

Marmot, M. (2004). Social causes of social inequalities in health. In S. Anand, F. Peter, & A. Sen (Eds.), *Public Health, Ethics and Equity* (pp. 21–33). Oxford University Press.

Marmot, M. (2022). *Build Back Fairer: Social Determinants, Ethnicity and Health. NHS – Race and Health Observatory*. https://nhsrho.org/news/build-back-fairer-social-determinants-ethnicity-and-health/

Marmot, M., Allen, J., Boyce, T., Goldblatt, P., & Morrison, J. (2020a). Health equity in England: The Marmot Review 10 years on. *The Health Foundation*. https://www.health.org.uk/funding-and-partnerships/our-partnerships/health-equity-in-england-the-marmot-review-10-years-on

Marmot, M., Allen, J., Goldblatt, P., Boyce, T., McNeish, D., Grady, M., & Geddes, I. (2010). Fair society, healthy lives, "The Marmot Review". *Institute of Health Equity*. https://www.instituteofhealthequity.org/resources-reports/fair-society-healthy-lives-the-marmot-review

Marmot, M., Allen, J., Goldblatt, P., Heard, E., & Morrison, J. (2020b). Build back fairer: The COVID-19 Marmot Review. *Institute of Health Equity*. https://www.instituteofhealthequity.org/resources-reports/build-back-fairer-the-covid-19-marmot-review

Marmot, M., Allen, J., Goldblatt, P., Willis, S., Noferini, J., & Callaghan, O. (2024). Structural racism, ethnicity and health inequalities in London. *Institute of Health Equity*. https://www.instituteofhealthequity.org/resources-reports/structural-racism-ethnicity-and-health-inequalities

Martins, T., Abel, G., Ukoumunne, O. C., Mounce, L. T. A., Price, S., Lyratzopoulos, G., Chinegwundoh, F., & Hamilton, W. (2022). Ethnic inequalities in routes to diagnosis of cancer: A population-based UK cohort study. *British Journal of Cancer*, *127*(5), 863. https://doi.org/10.1038/s41416-022-01847-x

Matthews, R. J., Draper, E. S., Manktelow, B. N., Kurinczuk, J. J., Fenton, A. C., Dunkley-Bent, J., Gallimore, I., Smith, L. K., & MBRRACE-UK Collaboration. (2022). Understanding ethnic inequalities in stillbirth rates: A UK population-based cohort study. *BMJ Open*, *12*(2), e057412. https://doi.org/10.1136/bmjopen-2021-057412

McKee, M., Schalkwyk, M. C. I. van, Greenley, R., & Permanand, G. (2024). Trust: The foundation of health systems. *European Observatory on Health Systems and Policies, WHO Regional Office for Europe*.

Meir, N. (2020). Why we will lowercase white. *The Associated Press*. https://www.ap.org/the-definitive-source/announcements/why-we-will-lowercase-white/

Mirza, H., & Warwick, R. (2022). Race and ethnicity. *IFS Deaton Review of Inequalities*.

Morris, L., & Robertson, R. (2024). *Tackling Health Inequalities | Seven Priorities for the NHS | The King's Fund*. https://www.kingsfund.org.uk/insight-and-analysis/long-reads/tackling-health-inequalities-seven-priorities-nhs#seven-priorities-for-the-new-10-year-health-plan

Nagesh, A. (2023). *Covid: Lack of Trust in Government Adversely Affected Minorities – Badenoch – BBC News*. https://www.bbc.co.uk/news/health-67515290

Nagpaul, C., & Naqvi, H. (2025). Patient experience and trust in NHS primary care. *NHS: Race and Health Observatory*. https://nhsrho.org/news/patients-report-alarming-lack-of-trust-in-nhs-primary-care-providers/

Nazroo, J. Y. (2024). Race/ethnic inequalities in health: Moving beyond confusion to focus on fundamental causes, *Oxford Open Economics*, *3*, i563–i576. https://doi.org/10.1093/ooec/odad020

Nazroo, J. Y., Bhui, K. S., & Rhodes, J. (2020). Where next for understanding race/ethnic inequalities in severe mental illness? Structural, interpersonal and institutional racism. *Sociology of Health and Illness*, *42*(2), 262–276. https://doi.org/10.1111/1467-9566.13001

NHS Race and Health Observatory. (2025). *Patient Experience and Trust in NHS Primary Care*. https://nhsrho.org/wp-content/uploads/2025/03/TRUST-IN-PRIMARY-CARE-REPORT.pdf

NICE. (2019). *Recommendations | Hypertension in Adults: Diagnosis and Management | Guidance | NICE*. https://www.nice.org.uk/guidance/ng136/chapter/recommendations

Omi, M., & Winant, H. (2014). *Racial Formation in the United States* (3rd ed.). Routledge. https://doi.org/10.4324/9780203076804

Paul, E., Fancourt, D., & Razai, M. (2022). Racial discrimination, low trust in the health system and COVID-19 vaccine uptake: A longitudinal observational study of 633 UK adults from ethnic minority groups. *Journal of the Royal Society of Medicine*, *115*(11), 439. https://doi.org/10.1177/01410768221095241

Powers, M., & Faden, R. (2008). *Social Justice: The Moral Foundations of Public Health and Health Policy*. Oxford University Press.

Prostate Cancer UK. (2025). *Inequalities in Prostate Cancer Mortality in England*. http://prostatecanceruk.org/for-health-professionals/data-and-evidence/inequalities-in-prostate-cancer-mortality-in-england

Raleigh, V. S. (2008, August 21). Collection of data on ethnic origin in England. *BMJ*, *337*(1), a1107. https://doi.org/10.1136/bmj.a1107

Raleigh, V. S. (2025). *The Health of Women from Ethnic Minority Groups in England | The King's Fund*. https://www.kingsfund.org.uk/insight-and-analysis/long-reads/the-health-of-women-from-ethnic-minority-groups-england

Rao, M., & Adebowale, V. (2020, June 17). The NHS race and health observatory – Its time has come. *BMJ Opinion*. https://blogs.bmj.com/bmj/2020/06/17/the-nhs-race-and-health-observatory-its-time-has-come/

Razai, M., Kankam, H., Majeed, A., Esmail, A., & Williams, D. (2021b). Mitigating ethnic disparities in covid-19 and beyond. *British Medical Journal*, *372*, m4921. https://doi.org/10.1136/bmj.m4921

Razai, M., Majeed, A., & Esmail, A. (2021a). Structural racism is a fundamental cause and driver of ethnic disparities in health. *British Medical Journal*, *373*, n938. https://doi.org/10.1136/bmj.n938

Reynolds, C., & Naqvi, H. (2025). Sickle cell comparative review to inform policy report. *NHS Race and Health Observatory and Sickle Cell Society*. https://nhsrho.org/wp-content/uploads/2025/06/SICKLE-CELL-COMPARATIVE-REPORT-.pdf

Runnymede Trust. (2021). *Statement Regarding the Report from the Commission on Race and Ethnic Disparities*. https://www.runnymedetrust.org/news/statement-regarding-the-cred-report-2021

Salway, S., et al. (2010). Rapid response: Fair society, healthy lives: A missed opportunity to address ethnic inequalities in health. *British Medical Journal*, *340*, c684. https://doi.org/10.1136/bmj.c684

Sewell, T. (2021). Commission on race and ethnic disparities: The report. *GOV.UK*. https://www.gov.uk/government/publications/the-report-of-the-commission-on-race-and-ethnic-disparities

Simms-Williams, N., Nagakumar, P., Thayakaran, R., Adderley, N. J., Hotham, R., Mansur, A. H., Nirantharakumar, K., & Haroon, S. (2024). Risk factors for asthma-related hospital and intensive care admissions in children, adolescents and adults: A cohort study using primary and secondary care data. *BMJ Open Respiratory Research*, *11*(1), e001746. https://doi.org/10.1136/bmjresp-2023-001746

Sivanandan, A. (2006). Britain's shame: From multiculturalism to nativism. *Institute of Race Relations*. https://irr.org.uk/article/britains-shame-from-multiculturalism-to-nativism/

Smedley, A., & Smedley, B. D. (2005). Race as biology is fiction, racism as a social problem is real: Anthropological and historical perspectives on the social construction of race. *American Psychologist*, *60*(1), 16–26. https://doi.org/10.1037/0003-066X.60.1.16

Smedley, B. (2019). Multilevel interventions to undo the health consequences of racism: The need for comprehensive approaches. *Cultural Diversity & Ethnic Minority Psychology*, *25*, 123–125. https://doi.org/10.1037/cdp0000263

Sowemimo, A. (2023). *Divided: Racism, Medicine and Why We Need to Decolonise Healthcare*. Wellcome Collection.

Walcott, S., & Nightingale, G. (2025). How racism affects health. *The Runnymede Trust and the Health Foundation*. www.health.org.uk/reports-and-analysis/reports/how-racism-affects-health

Whitehead, M. (1992). The concepts and principles of equity and health. *International Journal of Health Services*, *22*(3), 429–445. http://www.jstor.org/stable/45131055

Williams, D. R., Lawrence, J. A., Davis, B. A., & Vu, C. (2019). Understanding how discrimination can affect health. *Health Services Research*, *54*(S2), 1374–1388. https://doi.org/10.1111/1475-6773.13222

Williams, D. R., Neighbors, H. W., & Jackson, J. S. (2003). Racial/ethnic discrimination and health: Findings from community studies. *American Journal of Public Health*, *93*(2), 200–208. https://doi.org/10.2105/ajph.93.2.200

Women and Equalities Committee. (2023). *Black Maternal Health*. https://publications.parliament.uk/pa/cm5803/cmselect/cmwomeq/94/report.html

Workman, S. C., Thompson, M. C., & Lau, L. (2023). Decolonising medical knowledge – The case of breast cancer and ethnicity in the UK. *Journal of Cancer Policy*, *36*, 100365. https://doi.org/10.1016/j.jcpo.2022.100365

WHO. (2018). *Health Inequities and Their Causes*. World Health Organization. https://www.who.int/news-room/facts-in-pictures/detail/health-inequities-and-their-causes

WHO. (2020). *Basic Documents: Forty-Ninth Edition* (49th ed.). World Health Organization.

SECTION 1

Questioning

In the opening theme of this volume, the authors attend to the healthcare systems in England and Scotland, questioning the role of race and ethnicity as barriers to receiving quality healthcare and achieving positive health outcomes. Drawing on biographical perspectives, both chapters trace their authors' dawning awareness of the intersection of racism with other characteristics. Chapter 1 focuses on wealth, education, language, gender, and age, while Chapter 2 adds geography to further complicate the landscape in which inequities overlap.

In Chapter 1, Makita, Phenwan and Sixsmith model their discussion as an email exchange, delving into race and ethnicity through the lens of their own experiences as individuals representing different ethnic heritages. Their chapter reveals how, despite holding other forms of privilege (wealth, education, language, gender normativity), race remains an independent barrier to accessing timely diagnoses and appropriate care. Within their chapter, they discuss the colliding effects of structural inequality that result from the failure of the healthcare system to account for the intersectional identities of members of racialised communities. The challenges faced by the authors while seeking healthcare in the UK highlight the shortcomings of a universalist approach to healthcare provision and the harm it can cause to racialised individuals attempting to navigate the healthcare system. To avert these inadequacies, Makita et al. propose a system that prioritises cultural humility and decolonialism in the pursuit of a more equitable healthcare provision model. The sum of their experiences emphasises the need for policies which integrate community-based knowledge and other diverse perspectives into health education and healthcare systems, allowing for more culturally responsive models of healthcare to emerge.

In Chapter 2, Cheeks adds a geographic layer to the questioning theme, asking why, in Oxford, a city renowned for its centres of excellence in healthcare and health research, her family and other members of the Caribbean community have not been equal beneficiaries of these advantages. Drawing on her memories of Caribbean community elders and of her grandfather's journey through cancer, she relates narratives

DOI: 10.4324/9781003466093-2

of indifference, reserve, and a deep mistrust between her community and healthcare professionals. These experiences were foundational in her shift from an unquestioning approach to proactive advocacy for better care. Working in Patient and Public Involvement (PPI), Cheeks navigates her insider/outsider status as she bridges local communities with health research, helping to shift mistrust and avoidance by facilitating community collaboration from inception to implementation. She offers that further efforts are needed, particularly in cultural competency training for healthcare staff and increased representation of diverse populations in research studies, to increase trust and reduce the gap in access to Oxford's excellence.

CHAPTER 1

Access and barriers to health and healthcare

E-mail conversations about underserved BAME populations and health inequity in the UK

Meiko Makita, Tharin Phenwan, and Judith Sixsmith

Introduction

This chapter discusses inequitable access to healthcare and poorer health outcomes in underserved Black, Asian and Minority Ethnic (BAME) groups in the United Kingdom (UK) and identifies barriers to appropriate healthcare. We use the term 'underserved' to refer to people associated with a specific demographic group who have no, inappropriate or limited access to resources, including healthcare, which often leads to inequitable healthcare provision (Mitchell et al., 2023). We also use the term 'BAME' here because it remains common in UK health policy discourse; however, we acknowledge its limitations as an umbrella label that risks obscuring important differences between racially minoritised communities and may reinforce a sense of 'otherness' (see DaCosta et al., 2021).[1] We argue that the disadvantaged positionality of BAME people within health service contexts can be exacerbated by intersections of age, disability, and diverse (including non-heteronormative) gender identities. These intersections create invisible and intransigent barriers to healthcare (Chouhan & Nazroo, 2020). The complexities of interconnected social and personal identities place BAME people at risk of stigma and discrimination that go beyond language barriers or a lack of understanding of healthcare systems and processes (Kapadia et al., 2022). Instead, the normalising of their absence and pathologisation of their presence in healthcare contexts can create conditions in which they are not just underserved but substantially invisible or treated as a problem to be solved, rather than as people deserving of support towards better health outcomes (see Phoenix, 1987; Sixsmith et al., 2012).

Our discussion focuses on the experience of being part of a BAME group and an immigrant in the UK with the experience of being older and part of the white majority in healthcare contexts. We explore access constraints and barriers arising from financial restrictions, a lack of understanding regarding service entitlements, the attitudes and actions of healthcare professionals (including unconscious bias) and expectations of the UK health system. We address the issues of mistrust and lack of confidence in being understood or treated fairly. These issues often lead to an avoidance of healthcare

DOI: 10.4324/9781003466093-3

services, resulting in sub-optimal care, misdiagnoses, delayed treatment, or failure to follow medical advice, which contribute to poor health outcomes (Bhui et al., 2018; Chouhan & Nazroo, 2020). We also discuss the concepts of cultural competence and cultural humility in relation to inequitable healthcare provision, emphasising the importance of awareness and training in these areas to better understand and address the needs of underserved communities (Lekas et al., 2020).

These issues are unpacked from the personal, professional and research-informed perspectives of three academics from a UK-based university, each working in health sciences research. We present the chapter as an email-thread conversation among ourselves, each representing different ethnicities, sexual orientations, gender identities, professional roles, disciplinary backgrounds, and age groups. Our conversation focuses on healthcare access and barriers through the lens of being BAME immigrants in a predominantly White context, being older and living with disability, living with a chronic condition, and identifying as part of the lesbian, gay, bisexual, transgender plus (LGBT+) community.

We conclude the chapter with recommendations to mitigate the interdependent, systemic, and structural factors that affect health equity and well-being for underserved people of BAME heritage, older people and those who occupy positionalities different from the majority context.

[Opening email]

Dear Tharin and Judith,

I hope this email finds you well. As we progress on writing our chapter contribution to *Understanding Race and Health Inequity in the UK*, I wanted to take a moment to reflect on the issues involved by sharing my own personal experience in trying to access healthcare.

As someone living with an autoimmune rheumatic condition, I have experienced firsthand the frustration of navigating a healthcare system that fails to meet the needs of ethnic minoritised communities. Despite seeking answers and support within the UK, I still find myself facing access barriers, with my condition remaining undiagnosed and untreated – or worse; being told to take paracetamol! My general practitioner (GP), although well-intentioned, is limited by systemic constraints (e.g. lack of resources, long-waiting times for referrals) and the persistent scepticism of specialist rheumatologists who have dismissed my symptoms for over 4 years.

It wasn't until I spent 4 months in Mexico, my country of origin, that I was able to access the medical care and support I needed. Over there, I received assessments and treatments from healthcare providers who took my symptoms seriously and provided a diagnosis. However, going back and forth to my country of origin for medical care is not a sustainable solution in the long term. The logistical, financial, and emotional toll of such an arrangement is considerable.

My personal experience is further complicated by the intersection of my health challenges with my identity as a member of the BAME community. To add to this, I'm one of those people who doesn't have a box to tick on forms about ethnicity. As a Mexican-Japanese, I'll either tick 'Mixed' or 'Other', both of which fail to fully capture my identity and are inherently non-inclusive, but that is a whole other topic (see Sohanpal et al., 2025). Initially, I was hesitant to attribute my difficulties solely to my ethnicity or my gender, or both. However, conversations with non-BAME friends, colleagues and acquaintances of similar age who are living with autoimmune diseases or chronic conditions have made it clear that my experiences are not entirely universal. They report facing fewer obstacles in accessing specialist care and being taken more seriously by healthcare providers. This disparity suggests that being part of a BAME community does indeed place one at a disadvantage regarding healthcare access.

Obviously, it does not escape me that I am privileged to have been able to seek care abroad and finally be diagnosed. This privilege, however, underscores the systemic failures of the UK healthcare system in addressing the needs of its diverse population. For many, such an option is simply not available! I am also in a 'privileged' position as I am university educated, fluent in English and working in a university – contributing to the formation of future nurses – which should ideally facilitate my interactions with healthcare providers. Yet, despite these advantages, in my experience my health issues are not taken seriously. This situation highlights the systemic issues that exist within the NHS, as even those with significant educational and linguistic advantages face considerable challenges in receiving adequate healthcare. If someone in my position struggles this much, the barriers for those with fewer resources must be even more overwhelming.

Despite the so-called universal right to healthcare, access to quality services remains unequal, with BAME individuals being underserved: often experiencing systemic inequalities and structural barriers; and as you know the COVID-19 pandemic has further highlighted these inequalities (see Otu et al., 2020; Ajayi Sotubo, 2021, who are themselves BAME authors). A recent review, by the NHS Race & Health Observatory (Kapadia et al., 2022), highlighted the long-standing reality of healthcare disparities faced by BAME communities across the UK. The review concluded that the health of ethnic minority individuals has suffered due to several issues within the NHS, including: the lack of appropriate treatment for health problems; poor quality care or discriminatory treatment from healthcare staff, insufficient high-quality ethnic monitoring data in NHS systems, and a lack of appropriate interpreting services for those not fluent in English. Additionally, delays in or avoidance of seeking medical help due to fear of racist treatment from NHS healthcare professionals have further exacerbated the problem (Kapadia et al., 2022). Similarly, other studies within the UK healthcare context, have shown that BAME individuals often experience longer wait times, less thorough examinations, and dismissive attitudes from healthcare providers (Bhui et al., 2018), all of which might be due to structural racism and can negatively impact their life experience and health outcomes over time (see Marmot et al., 2024).

So this is so far my experience trying to access appropriate treatment for my autoimmune condition through the NHS and a brief overview of the issues BAME individuals face within the UK system. Now, to kick off our discussion, perhaps you could reflect on what you think are the main causes for such healthcare disparities, and how can these be addressed . . . Or maybe you'd want to share your own personal experiences? I look forward to hearing from you.

Best wishes,
Meiko

[e-mail reply 1]

Dear Meiko,

I would like to resonate with you around the inequitable access to healthcare for the BAME community in the UK, specifically the dismissive attitudes towards BAME people. I am a Thai living in the UK and consider myself healthy and rarely need to see a doctor. This stems from my background as a GP since I am aware of urgent conditions that need further assessment by healthcare professionals and the mild ones that will improve over time. However, last month, I needed to access healthcare, and my condition was not taken seriously. The receptionist brushed me off. I am not going into details here, but I am not convinced that a non-trained person will be able to fully assess a condition over a quick phone call. This experience contrasts with my spouse (who is a White British male) who got to see the GP after one phone call; the differences of our experience cannot be more evident. Of course, he might get fast-tracked due to our different health history and age. But that still does not explain the way I was brushed off easily.

I would like to add that non-native English speakers can also face an inherent challenge when they are navigating the healthcare in the UK via telephone calls due to language barrier and the lack of non-verbal cues. Most of my colleagues and students who are BAME and came from overseas consistently mention that they find it incredibly stressful to talk with staff over the phone. Specifically, those who are not fluent in English find the experience intimidating when they cannot see the person at the other side of the call, yet that person starts to raise their tone for whatever reason. This form of exchange goes against natural communication since both verbal and non-verbal cues are very important for effective interactions (Vogel et al., 2018). Limiting communication to 'voice only' risks stripping away important information and, because the healthcare system is structured in this way, BAME people may be denied adequate access to healthcare and critical health issues can be missed. To compound this issue, and in relation to the ever increasing introduction of technology, particularly artificial intelligence (AI) into health systems, I am concerned that non-native English speakers may face further (un)intentional alienation when forced to rely on the use of apps or chatbots powered by AI, given almost all of these tools were developed by and for native English speakers (Myers, 2023). The lack of digital literacy that leads to the 'digital divide' between different populations and age groups may even make this situation worse (Fang et al., 2019).

My suggestions are around the way in which patients can access most healthcare services in the UK: via a telephone. Is it absolutely essential to do that? Can we move away from that approach to a more personal approach? I think we should because this form of communication implies that both parties can converse fully in English without seeing each other. It further implies that the person has a luxury of time to make constant phone calls in the morning; I do not and assume that most people do not either.

We can also create more cultural competency for the healthcare staff as well, given that the population in the UK has become increasingly diverse. We also have more people coming from all over the world, hence it is essential for us to understand people's experience regarding the way in which they access healthcare and how that aligns with the system in the UK. What I experienced in the UK would be considered unacceptable in my country: Thailand. If I needed to seek out a medical service, I could just go to a primary healthcare unit which is integrated anywhere in the country. I would be assessed by a trained professional who can provide more informed opinions about my health. I must admit that this contrasting experience makes me feel sceptical of the UK health system and how much I can put my trust in it.

The discussion so far makes me ponder another point around the healthcare system in the UK, compared to the world. I think there is an assumption and a discourse that the NHS is 'the best' in the world thus there is no need to alter anything; it is not. The latest report shows that we are falling rapidly. There are several indices that people use to assess the quality of healthcare, but my point remains. Based on The Health Care Index (CEOWorld Magazine, 2024), UK is ranked 27th in the world, and if we were to use the Legatum Prosperity Index Health Score (Legatum Institute, 2023) the UK's health score is 78.31 which is even lower than Thailand (78.92). There is a need to change.

Do you have further ideas why we are failing systematically? And how can we improve that?

Best wishes
Tharin

[e-mail reply 2]

Dear Tharin,

Thank you for sharing your experience. It's deeply concerning to hear about the dismissive attitudes you've encountered and the evident disparity in the healthcare experiences between you and your spouse. In fact, it resonates with my own experience, as my spouse is also a White British male: although he rarely sees the GP, when he does, he usually has no trouble getting an appointment on the same day and his ailment is taken care of right away! I understand that there could be various factors at play, such as our GP practice itself (in a rural location), gender, age or the nature of my illness, and not simply ethnicity, so it's important to recognise the complexity of these experiences and avoid oversimplifying the underlying causes. Yet, my experience so far, still raises questions for me.

In your case, your medical background likely makes the inadequacy of the receptionist's treatment even more troubling. I actually never have much trouble when speaking to my GP's receptionist on the phone or in-person. My issue however is when discussing my chronic condition and trying to get a proper treatment from my GP. In addition to the typical challenges of navigating the healthcare system, I am concerned that stereotypes (regarding age, gender, race/ethnicity) held by some GPs or healthcare professionals – whether intentional or unintentional – may influence the quality of care they provide (Hall et al., 2015; Iacobucci, 2022). Definitely, I think our experiences highlight a significant issue within the healthcare system, where biases and inequities can lead to differential treatment for members of the BAME community.

I agree with you about the problems of a system that relies heavily on non-clinical staff to make initial assessments in person or over the phone. While such a system is designed to manage demand and ensure efficiency, this can inadvertently contribute to inequitable care if not properly overseen or staff are not adequately trained to recognise and address potential biases. Such is the case when interacting with people for whom English is not their first language (see Showstack et al., 2019; Slade & Sergent, 2023), especially over the phone. I can see this also being an issue for people with learning disabilities or speech impairments. There is a push now for online appointment booking and online consultations, and that also eventually would bring further inequalities due to digital exclusion (e.g. limited internet access, lack of digital skills), but that probably is a whole other topic, that we won't get into now (see AI chapter in this collection).

Regardless of the appointment booking media, there needs to be a robust mechanism for patients to report and address instances of discrimination and unfair treatment in healthcare settings. Although I'm aware of some options to file complaints, I'm honestly afraid of potential repercussions.

Addressing these issues requires a multifaceted approach, including better training for all healthcare staff on both systemic and implicit bias, the importance of equitable treatment, and cultural humility. Interestingly, even though the concept of cultural humility was introduced in the late 1990s by Tervalon and Murray-García (1998), it is still not as widely known about or practiced in healthcare as perhaps it should be. In fact, it was only last year, while I was updating some teaching material, that I learned that 'cultural competence' awareness and training is no longer, or probably never was, effective to address health disparities based on ethnicity and race. Apparently, this approach can reinforce racial and ethnic stereotypes and perpetuates racism, increasing the risk of *othering* patients, thereby intensifying the 'us' versus 'them' mentality (see Kirmayer, 2012). Instead, the shift is now on cultural humility, that is on promoting healthcare professionals to 'reflect on their own beliefs, values and biases . . . thus revealing their own culture's impact on patients' (Agner, 2020, as cited in Lekas et al., 2020 p. 2). I want to believe that this could be a promising approach that the NHS could offer widely.

I agree that there is an assumption that the NHS is the best healthcare system in the world; this is inaccurate, and I think complacency is actually part of the problem. Thanks for sharing the ranking systems – they clearly show that the UK is far from leading in healthcare quality. This misconception can prevent necessary improvements and hinder innovation. Acknowledging and learning from the strengths of other countries' healthcare systems, even those with fewer resources, such as yours and mine for instance, can provide valuable insights.

Perhaps, a decolonial approach, similar to what we see in equitable Global South-Global North research collaborations, where we [Tharin, Judith and myself] and other Global health researchers are actively trying to shift from a Western-centric view of health research, could lead to significant improvements in the UK healthcare education and healthcare provision systems (see Lokugamage et al., 2023). By valuing and integrating diverse perspectives and experiences, particularly those from historically marginalised or less resourced regions, the UK could benefit from innovative practices and insights that are often overlooked. This aligns with Sowemimo's (2023) critique of the British healthcare system, which argues that this approach should include decolonising the curriculum in health sciences and medical schools by incorporating global healthcare traditions, histories and perspectives. Sowemimo's decolonising vision also advocates for moving beyond cultural competence training to cultural humility and for integrating anti-racist frameworks into healthcare practice, particularly to identify and eliminate racial biases in clinical settings, treatment protocols and healthcare policies (2023).

@JudithSixsmith I wonder what your take is on this. Your insights could add a different perspective to our ongoing discussion on healthcare inequities among BAME communities.

Best wishes,
Meiko

[e-mail reply 3]

Hi both,

From my perspective as an older, white, British female and academic working in the area of health sciences, I feel that some of the issues you raise in accessing healthcare are, as you say, systemic in nature but also relational as well. Relationality (Camargo-Borges & Moscheta, 2016) or *relationality-communality* as discussed by Ajei and Myles (2019), is involved in how such systems operate in practice, whereby relationships between reception staff, healthcare professionals and patients are embedded within health system structures. In my past and early experiences with healthcare, family doctors were the norm. As a family, you would always see the same GP and so that GP would have a strong sense of you as a person and of your family as a unit. In both senses (person and family), the GP-person relationships formed were based on intimate knowledge and understanding of health in a meaningful family-health context. While such relationships were effective in lots of ways to make discussions about health conditions more holistic and effective, they could also constrain discussion around more sensitive health matters for example when sexual health or mental health issues arose.

Family GPs are pretty much a thing of the past now and my current connection with primary healthcare is hampered by a lack of relational understanding. Despite having a long term condition, I see different GPs each time at my doctors' surgery. I am not known as a person (with a lived medical history) but only as the patient presenting in front of the healthcare professional. Consultation times are shorter and rarely discursive, and this makes me feel that I have not made my situation fully understood. This lack of understanding makes me think treatment regimens based on this lack of comprehensive knowledge can be inappropriate.

While the lack of relational understanding in healthcare communications is difficult for many people, I wonder how this translates across different intersectional positionalities and protected characteristics (Silverio et al., 2023). In my case, my ethnicity (white British) is not a concern of mine when thinking about or accessing healthcare in the UK, however I feel my age and gender intersect in ways which are problematic for optimal healthcare treatment. Ill health which might be taken seriously in younger people can be, and has been, written off for myself as 'just' an outcome of ageing, particularly as an older women. The autoimmune condition which affects my skin (and is most often associated with women) surfaced as I grew older. This was not diagnosed for several years because skin changes are the norm as you age. Seeing different GPs at each outbreak meant that no one healthcare professional had a strong sense of the progression of the condition, and all treated it as an isolated health event until a dentist, who had just been to a conference where my condition was discussed, saw, interpreted and conducted a biopsy which confirmed his diagnosis.

Thinking about this in relation to social class adds a further dimension of difficulty when trying to get good healthcare. Deriving from a working-class family background meant that accessing the GP was frowned upon unless for the most serious of issues. The idea was not to be a burden on healthcare resources unless absolutely necessary. There was, in my family, little sense of 'entitlement' to healthcare and soldiering on and waiting to see if time would heal was the first form of healthcare thinking. I have brought this way of thinking with me from these working-class, family roots. In this context, accessing healthcare becomes problematic for me, requiring me to 'screw up my courage' even to phone the surgery reception. Consequently, I did and still do 'wait to see' if a flare up will go away on its own. Our past experiences, cultural assumptions and expectations are strong motivators of healthcare contact as Lakin and Kane (2022) and Vaughn et al. (2009) have suggested.

You mention, Tharin, the protective and sometimes off-putting and (almost) diagnostic role of receptionists, an issue that is evident in the health sciences literature (Litchfield et al., 2023). Communication and interpersonal skills are clearly important mediators of accessibility in this relationship. For me, as an academic who 'knows' the healthcare system from ethnic, experiential as well as academic knowledge bases, I think that important accessibility barriers operate in terms of the psychological, age-related and social class dimensions I have drawn attention to above. How these intersect with BAME identities is important to dissect.

In terms of healthcare 'change' as progress, I am sceptical. Certainly, we have had huge change in the rhetoric around and practice of healthcare, especially concerning 'who is deserving and who is not', responsibilities, how to organise resources effectively, use of technology, staffing levels and so on. I would hesitate to call this 'progress'.

Meiko, your thoughts on cultural competence and its translation into healthcare training certainly reflect research myself and colleagues (Sixsmith et al., 2012) undertook with refugees and asylum seekers in the UK some years ago. That research also highlighted notions of trust and suspicions of authority in healthcare hierarchies; issues which prevent refugees and asylum seekers from seeking healthcare access in the first place. This means that the best and most effective healthcare professional training on understanding inequity in healthcare is not sufficient. A community-based approach is required to enable a grassroots voice in the process and organisation of change in community and health settings to support people to reach the doctor's door in the first place, especially as they grow older (Adja et al., 2020). Also, the standing of community based approaches to enabling, encouraging and supporting health is important to acknowledge here. Health is only partially lived through a health service but is more embedded in our everyday social and community structures. Finally, there is the notion of community 'workers' who can, and currently do, embed aspects of health practice and knowledge and who can stand in for the GP where appropriate. This shifts some of the responsibility for health out of the hands of dominant health service practitioners and into the hands of community folks. I think we need more research on this to properly understand and make positive change happen.

In conclusion of my response here, I guess I am saying that we need to explore not only BAME healthcare inequities, but also more on the intersections of different protected characteristics, identities and positionalities within and across BAME communities to understand equity in healthcare. Thoughts?

Judith

[e-mail reply 4]

Dear both

Judith, you raised important points, particularly around the systemic and relational issues within healthcare. I completely agree that the loss of relational continuity in healthcare is affecting how many people in the UK experience care today. The evidence that continuity of care improves outcomes is strong. A recent study (Kajaria-Montag et al., 2024) underscores how familiarity between patients and GPs contributes to better communication, trust, and ultimately more accurate diagnoses and treatment plans.

In contrast, as you, and many others, have experienced, the shift towards seeing different doctors each time hinders relational continuity and leads to fragmented and inadequate care (see Murphy & Salisbury, 2020).

This lack of continuity is even more problematic for people like us with long-term or complex conditions. Without a relational understanding of the patient's history, GPs may struggle to piece together symptoms over time. You've also highlighted the issue of age and gender intersecting in ways that lead to the dismissal of symptoms as 'just ageing'. This is unfortunately a common experience for many women, particularly older women, where gendered ageism (see HelpAge, 2023) comes into play, leading to diagnostic overshadowing. Research indicates that older women's symptoms are often attributed to ageing rather than being properly investigated (see Tuohy & Cooney, 2019). The experience is rather universal, as it is something I also have encountered in my own research with older Mexican women (Makita, 2014).

On the topic of intersectionality, your experience speaks to how these layers – age, gender, ethnicity, race and social class – interact in healthcare access and outcomes. Research on health inequalities reinforces this idea, showing how socioeconomic background affects not only access to care but the way people interact with healthcare systems (Institute of Health Equity, 2020). We all carry assumptions linked to multiple positional axes (e.g. gender, age, race/ethnicity, class, sexuality, disability) that impact how often we seek care, and these positions can shape both the quality of care received and the health outcomes.

I agree that cultural humility and competency in healthcare are necessary, but these alone cannot resolve the deeper issues of trust and systemic inequality. For instance, cultural training needs to be paired with the practice of self-reflection and a broader intersectional approach that examines how multiple marginalities affect people's access to and experiences within healthcare systems. I would argue that without considering the wider socio-political and historical contexts of marginalisation, cultural humility and/or competence training may only scratch the surface (see Lekas et al., 2020).

An intersectional approach is crucial for tackling healthcare inequalities, as it can allow us to see the full picture of how different identities intersect to create unique healthcare challenges. I agree with your point about grassroots change being essential. To create sustainable progress, we must engage with communities directly to understand their unique challenges and develop trust in the healthcare system from the ground up. Training and learning that takes place in community-based settings (e.g. patients' homes, care homes, clinics, schools, and hospices), such as those provided by existing community health services in the UK (see Charles & Wickens, 2024), may help healthcare providers to engage with and learn from specific populations themselves and better understand the sources of health inequalities and provide an opportunity to tailor care to meet the unique needs of those communities.

Best,
Meiko

[e-mail reply 5]

Dear both,

I think the idea of intersections of health is plausible to help us gain a better understanding of existing health inequities within the BAME community in the UK and beyond. We have examples of how intersectionality helps policymakers gain better insights regarding structural inequality in Scotland (Scottish Government, 2022). The approach may enhance existing strategies within the NHS (NHS England, 2021; NHS Foundation Trust, 2022) that aim to reduce unequal access to care, which is good, since these strategies aim to address intersectionality.

Having said that, we need to be cautious of intersectionality as well. Some academics critique that intersectionality seems to be 'particularised and therefore provisional and incomplete' (Carbado et al., 2013; Nayak, 2023). They mean intersectionality is a work-in-progress that aims to ponder at certain issues constantly. With such a fluid approach, how do we know that we have done 'enough' to address inequality? How do we 'structure' and 'measure' such a fluid concept to ensure that we have fully considered, addressed and mitigated every existing intersection that affects unequal access to care?

Nayak (2023) also posits that intersectionality focuses more on individual experiences rather than the macroeconomic conditions that perpetuate inequity, and as such, it does not sufficiently address the broader systems that shape identities. Moreover, intersectionality focuses on contemporary discrimination but can neglect how power structures have evolved over time. I agree with this critique since we tend to look at the 'now' but not the 'then-now' or the changes that we have achieved so far which could be for better or worse.

Overall, I think intersectionality is critical to help us examine complex human identities as well as the discrimination we are facing. However, it is not as helpful for strategising towards feasible large-scale healthcare reforms.

Warm regards,
Tharin

[e-mail reply 6]

Hi both,

I think we have now identified that it's not only about being BAME, but that intersections of different identities and positionalities with personal and family experiences, sociocultural expectations all play a partial role in access to healthcare and that history and discrimination need to be accounted for as well. This makes achieving good-quality, accessible healthcare for all, a very complex or wicked problem to solve (Boger et al., 2017).

An intersectional lens highlights that it is not just one aspect of a person which fundamentally structures their healthcare access and experiences, but the combination in a more holistic way, of who they are in relation to existing sociocultural norms and systemic disparities. Being an older BAME woman can create very different access issues and experiences of healthcare than being a younger BAME man for instance. By revealing, planning for, and managing healthcare that better fits with a range of different intersectional interdependencies, then there is a greater chance of fit between people and system. That is not to say that this will result in some kind of healthcare utopia; there are so many other problems to solve, including shortage of resources (human and financial), the need to value staff and pay them accordingly, healthcare management, sociocultural and historical factors, ensuring e-health systems are fit for purpose and not exclusionary (Farre et al., 2023) and so on, but may move us towards a more equitable system. As Crisp (2022) has said, if community members were more empowered to speak up when things go wrong for them and have a say over their healthcare management and who bestows this on them, then hopefully more of the needs of diverse people would be met by those who speak like them and look like them and hold the same values as them, not on the phone or via remote conferencing, but face to face, nearby and in community settings through working together.

Judith

Conclusion

While our email exchange has highlighted more challenges than solutions, we believe there are core improvements that could significantly enhance healthcare access and quality for underserved BAME communities. One crucial step is increasing diversity among healthcare staff at every level – from care providers to senior medical specialists – this aligns with Sowemimo's call to decolonise the UK healthcare system. Such diversity would foster greater cultural competence and cultural humility, which can directly improve health outcomes (Greenwood et al., 2020). Another key measure involves translating health information into accessible, culturally appropriate formats for underserved groups, ensuring they can fully understand and engage with available healthcare resources (Randall & Wood, 2023).

We recognise that the challenges presented by health inequities within BAME communities are both diverse and complex. These disparities are not only shaped by varying factors across different groups but also unequal in their distribution and impact, with some communities facing more pronounced and compounded barriers. Certainly, understanding these issues through an intersectional lens can play a critical role in reshaping the healthcare challenges faced by individuals. It is essential to recognise that healthcare needs vary significantly among individuals based on multiple intersecting factors, such as gender, age, disability, sexual orientation, ethnicity, language competency, and mental health. These factors influence not only medical care but also social determinants of health. Factors such as access to culturally competent or cultural humility-trained providers, economic disparities, and systemic biases must all be considered to provide a more comprehensive approach to reducing these health inequities. However, while recognising that diversity of experiences is essential, it is equally important to acknowledge that the British healthcare system, as it currently stands, often fails to address even the most fundamental needs of marginalised communities. In this sense, an excessive focus on intersectional identities – though valuable in academic discourse – may risk detracting from urgent structural reforms needed to improve healthcare access and equity for BAME individuals in the UK. Rather than allowing intersectionality to become a theoretical distraction, we think that the priority should be ensuring that healthcare policies are robust enough to address diversity alongside widespread systemic inequalities.

Acknowledging and addressing these inequalities require more than just awareness; it demands translating that awareness into socially just action with a central focus on the communities themselves. By actively listening to their lived experiences and engaging in collaborative efforts, we can better understand unique healthcare needs and devise strategies that enhance the effectiveness of healthcare. This may involve relocating community-based health knowledge, advice and practice into community settings and into the hands of community members who are trained to deliver upstream and more protective aspects of healthcare, which are socially and culturally grounded. In this way, health becomes something that is lived experientially within our everyday spaces and places, with people that understand who we are in all our complexity and how to best achieve positive health outcomes not for us, but *with* us. Adopting such a community-centred approach can help build more equitable health and community care systems that not only meet these needs but also help bridge the disparities in health outcomes.

In this context, the term 'BAME' itself warrants critical examination, as it groups together a range of people with vastly different ethnicities, healthcare needs, experiences of discrimination and cultural contexts. Breaking down this broad category could lead to more precise, community-specific interventions and practices rather than a one-size-fits-all approach that may not effectively serve all groups. While such a revision of terminology is an important consideration, it must be accompanied by meaningful policy and practice transformation to avoid being a purely semantic exercise. That said, a deeper exploration of this issue may extend beyond the scope of this chapter.

Discussion questions

1. Based on your experiences and background, what factors seem to drive unequal access to healthcare in the UK? Is this issue exclusive to the BAME community, or does it affect other groups as well? Why or why not?
2. How does viewing healthcare through an intersectional lens help you recognise the structural and racial inequalities that influence healthcare access in the UK?
3. How do you think healthcare providers' unconscious biases affect the quality of care for underserved communities, and what steps can be taken to address this?
4. In what ways do policy frameworks and healthcare practices either reinforce or challenge disparities in access to care for people who occupy positionalities different from the majority context?

Note

1 We retain the term BAME for clarity and to situate our discussion in its professional context, but we do so with caution, noting that more precise and inclusive alternatives (e.g. racialised groups, minoritised communities) are increasingly preferred.

Further reading

Bartley, M. (2016). *Health Inequality: An Introduction to Concepts, Theories and Methods* (2nd ed.). Polity Press.

Dougall, D., & Buck, D. (2021). My role in tackling health inequalities. A framework for allied health professionals. *The King's Fund.* Retrieved September 27, 2024, from https://assets.kingsfund.org.uk/f/256914/x/dd211304ca/framework_allied_health_professionals_2021.pdf

Hill Collins, P., & Bilge, S. (2020). *Intersectionality. Key Concepts* (2nd ed.). Polity Press.

Sabik, N. J. (2021). The intersectionality toolbox: A resource for teaching and applying and intersectional lens in public health. *Frontiers in Public Health*, 9, 1904. https://doi.org/10.3389/fpubh.2021.772301

Wilkinson, R. G., & Pickett, K. (2009). *The Spirit Level: Why Equality is Better for Everyone.* Penguin Books.

References

Adja, K. Y. C., Lenzi, J., Sezgin, D., O'Caoimh, R., Morini, M., Damiani, G., Buja, A., & Fantini, M. P. (2020). The importance of taking a patient-centered, community-based approach to preventing and managing frailty: A public health perspective. *Frontiers in Public Health*, *8*, 599170. https://doi.org/10.3389/fpubh.2020.599170

Ajayi Sotubo, O. (2021). A perspective on health inequalities in BAME communities and how to improve access to primary care. *Future Healthcare Journal*, *8*(1), 36–39. https://doi.org/10.7861/fhj.2020-0217

Ajei, M., & Myles, N. O. (2019). Personhood, autonomy and informed consent. In Y. A. Frimpong-Mansoh & C. A. Atuire (Eds.), *Bioethics in Africa: Theories and Praxis* (pp. 77–94). Vernon Press.

Bhui, K., Halvorsrud, K., & Nazroo, J. (2018). Making a difference: Ethnic inequality and severe mental illness. *The British Journal of Psychiatry: The Journal of Mental Science*, *213*(4), 574–578. https://doi.org/10.1192/bjp.2018.148

Boger, J., Jackson, P., Mulvenna, M., Sixsmith, J., Sixsmith, A., Mihailidis, A., Kontos, P., Polgar, J. M., Grigorovich, A., & Martin, S. (2017). Principles for fostering the transdisciplinary development of assistive technologies. *Disability and Rehabilitation: Assistive Technology*, *12*(5), 480–490.

Camargo-Borges, C., & Moscheta, M. S. (2016). Health 2.0: Relational resources for the development of quality in healthcare. *Health Care Analysis: HCA: Journal of Health Philosophy and Policy*, *24*(4), 338–348. https://doi.org/10.1007/s10728-014-0279-2

Carbado, D. W., Crenshaw, K. W., Mays, V. M., & Tomlinson, B. (2013). Intersectionality: Mapping the movements of a theory. *Du Bois Review: Social Science Research on Race*, *10*(2), 303–312. https://doi.org/10.1017/S1742058X13000349

CEOWORLD Magazine. (2024). *Health Care Index by Country*. Retrieved September 9, 2024, from https://ceoworld.biz/2024/04/02/countries-with-the-best-health-care-systems-2024/

Charles, A., & Wickens, C. (2024). Community health services explained. *The King's Fund*. Retrieved March 6, 2025, from https://www.kingsfund.org.uk/insight-and-analysis/long-reads/community-health-services-explained#what-next

Chouhan, K., & Nazroo, J. (2020). 4: Health inequalities. In *Ethnicity, Race and Inequality in the UK* (pp. 73–92). Bristol, UK: Policy Press. https://doi.org/10.51952/9781447351269.ch004

Crisp, N. (2022). *Turning the World Upside Down again: Global Health in a Time of Pandemics, Climate Change and Political Turmoil*. CRC Press.

DaCosta, C., Dixon-Smith, S., & Singh, G. (2021). *Beyond BAME: Rethinking the Politics, Construction, Application, and Efficacy of Ethnic Categorisation*. Retrieved August 28, 2025, from https://pure.coventry.ac.uk/ws/portalfiles/portal/41898015/Beyond_BAME_final_report.pdf

Fang, M. L., Canham, S. L., Battersby, L., Sixsmith, J., Wada, M., & Sixsmith, A. (2019). Exploring privilege in the digital divide: Implications for theory, policy, and practice. *The Gerontologist*, *59*(1), e1–e15. https://doi.org/10.1093/geront/gny037

Farre, A., Fang, M., Hannah, B., Makita, M., McFadden, A., Menezes, D., Rodriguez, A., Sixsmith, J., & Gray, N. (2023). Exploring the use of digital technology to deliver healthcare services with explicit consideration of health inequalities in UK settings: A scoping review. *Digital Health*, *9*, 20552076231185442. https://doi.org/10.1177/20552076231185442

Greenwood, B. N., Hardeman, R. R., Huang, L., & Sojourner, A. (2020). Physician–patient racial concordance and disparities in birthing mortality for newborns. *Proceedings of the National Academy of Sciences of the United States of America*, *117*(35), 21194–21200. https://doi.org/10.1073/pnas.1913405117

Hall, W. J., Chapman, M. V., Lee, K. M., Merino, Y. M., Thomas, T. W., Payne, B. K., Eng, E., Day, S. H., & Coyne-Beasley, T. (2015). Implicit racial/ethnic bias among health care professionals and its influence on health care outcomes: A systematic review. *American Journal of Public Health*, *105*(12), e60–e76. https://doi.org/10.2105/AJPH.2015.302903

HelpAge. (2023). Older women's lived experiences of gendered ageism. *HelpAge Briefing*. Retrieved September 6, 2024, from https://www.helpage.org/silo/files/older-womens-lived-experiences-of-gendered-ageism.pdf

Iacobucci, G. (2022). Most Black people in the UK face discrimination from healthcare staff, survey finds. *BMJ*, *378*, o2337. https://doi.org/10.1136/bmj.o2337

Institute of Health Equity. (2020). *Health Equity in England: The Marmot Review 10 Years On*. London. Retrieved September 11, 2024, from http://www.instituteofhealthequity.org/the-marmot-review-10-years-on

Kajaria-Montag, H., Freeman, M., & Scholtes, S. (2024). Continuity of care increases physician productivity in primary care. *Management Science*, *0*(0). https://doi.org/10.1287/mnsc.2021.02015

Kapadia, D., Zhang, J., Salway, S., Nazroo, J., Booth, A., Villarroel-Williams, N., Becares, L., & Esmail, A. (2022). Ethnic inequalities in healthcare: A rapid review. *NHS Race & Health Observatory*. https://www.nhsrho.org/wp-content/uploads/2022/02/RHO-Rapid-Review-Final-Report_v.7.pdf

Kirmayer, L. J. (2012). Rethinking cultural competence. *Transcultural Psychiatry*, *49*(2), 149–164. https://doi.org/10.1177/1363461512444673

Lakin, K., & Kane, S. (2022). Peoples' expectations of healthcare: A conceptual review and proposed analytical framework. *Social Science & Medicine*, *292*, 114636.

Legatum Institute. (2023). *The Legatum Prosperity Index 2023*. Retrieved September 19, 2024, from https://www.prosperity.com/rankings

Lekas, H. M., Pahl, K., & Fuller Lewis, C. (2020). Rethinking cultural competence: Shifting to cultural humility. *Health Services Insights*, *13*, 1178632920970580. https://doi.org/10.1177/1178632920970580

Litchfield, I., Gale, N., Burrows, M., & Greenfield, S. (2023). "You're only a receptionist, what do you want to know for?": Street-level bureaucracy on the front line of primary care in the United Kingdom. *Heliyon*, *9*(11), e21298. https://doi.org/10.1016/j.heliyon.2023.e21298

Lokugamage, A. U., Rix, E. L., Fleming, T., Khetan, T., Meredith, A., & Hastie, C. R. (2023). Translating cultural safety to the UK. *Journal of Medical Ethics*, *49*(4), 244–251. https://doi.org/10.1136/medethics-2020-107017

Makita, M. (2014). Health and everyday bodily experiences of Old Mexican women. In U. Kriebernegg, R. Maierhofer, & B. Ratzenböck (Eds.), *Alive and Kicking at All Ages: Cultural Constructions of Health and Life Course Identity* (pp. 65–80). (Aging Studies Series; Vol. V). Transcript Verlag.

Marmot, M., Allen, J., Goldblatt, P., Willis, S., Noferini, J., & Callaghan, O. (2024). Structural racism, ethnicity and health inequalities in London. *Institute of Health Equity*. Retrieved March 6, 2025, from https://www.instituteofhealthequity.org/resources-reports/structural-racism-ethnicity-and-health-inequalities/main-report

Mitchell, C., Fryer, K., Guess, N., Aminu, H., Jackson, B., Gordon, A., Reynolds, J., Huang, Q., Jayasooriya, S., Mawson, R., Lawy, T., Linton, E., & Brown, J. (2023). Underserved 'Deep End' populations: A critical analysis addressing the power imbalance in research. *British Journal of General Practice*, *73*(732), 326–329. https://doi.org/10.3399/bjgp23X733461

Murphy, M., & Salisbury, C. (2020). Relational continuity and patients' perception of GP trust and respect: A qualitative study. *The British Journal of General Practice: The Journal of the Royal College of General Practitioners*, *70*(698), e676–e683. https://doi.org/10.3399/bjgp20X712349

Myers, A. (2023). AI-detectors biased against non-native English writers. *Human-Centered Artificial Intelligence, HAI*. Stanford University. Retrieved March 6, 2025, from https://hai.stanford.edu/news/ai-detectors-biased-against-non-native-english-writers

Nayak, B. S. (2023). Limits of intersectionality as a theoretical framework. In B. S. Nayak (Ed.), *Intersectionality and Creative Business Education*. Cham: Palgrave Macmillan. https://doi.org/10.1007/978-3-031-29952-0_10

NHS England. (2021). 2021/22 priorities and operational planning guidance: Implementation guidance. *NHS England and NHS Improvement*. Retrieved September 19, 2024, from https://www.england.nhs.uk/wp-content/uploads/2021/03/B0468-implementation-guidance-21-22-priorities-and-operational-planning-guidance.pdf

NHS Foundation Trust. (2022). Inclusion and health inequalities strategy 2022–2027. *Wirral Community Health and Care, NHS Foundation Trust*. Retrieved September 19, 2024, from https://www.wchc.nhs.uk/wp-content/uploads/2022/05/InclusionStrategy-2022-27.pdf

Otu, A., Ahinkorah, B. O., Ameyaw, E. K., Seidu, A. A., & Yaya, S. (2020). One country, two crises: What Covid-19 reveals about health inequalities among BAME communities in the United Kingdom and the sustainability of its health system? *International Journal for Equity in Health*, *19*(1), 189. https://doi.org/10.1186/s12939-020-01307-z

Phoenix, A. (1987). Theories of gender and Black families. In G. Weinger & M. Arnot (Eds.), *Gender under Scrutiny: New Inquiries in Education* (pp. 123–145). Open University Press.

Randall, S., & Wood, A. (2023). *Translated Health Information Is Essential to Tackling Health Inequality* [Blog post]. Retrieved March 12, 2025, from https://www.nationalvoices.org.uk/blogpost/translated-health-information-is-essential-to-tackling-health-inequality/

Scottish Government. (2022). Using intersectionality to understand structural inequality in Scotland: Evidence synthesis. *Social Research Series*. Retrieved September 11, 2024, from https://www.gov.scot/publications/using-intersectionality-understand-structural-inequality-scotland-evidence-synthesis/documents/

Showstack, R., Santos, M. G., Feuerherm, E., Jacobson, H., & Martínez, G. (2019). Language as social determinant of health: An applied linguistics perspective on health equity. *PAEC Briefs*. American Association for Applied Linguistics. https://www.aaal.org/news/language-as-a-social-determinant-of-health-an-applied-linguistics-perspective-on-health-equity

Silverio, M., Montalvo-Liendo, N., & Carrizales, T. (2023). Intersectionality and healthcare management: The case of crisis and COVID-19. In H. J. Knepper, M. D. Evans, & T. F. Henley (Eds.), *Intersectionality and Crisis Management* (1st ed., pp. 38–58). Routledge.

Sixsmith, J., Lawthom, R., & Fang, M. L. (2012, May 10–11). Understanding asylum seeker and refugee health and access to healthcare: Learning from the UK experience. Workshop presented at *Third Annual Critical Inquiries Workshop*, Vancouver, BC, Canada. (Unpublished).

Slade, S., & Sergent, S. R. (2023). Language barrier. In *StatPearls*. StatPearls Publishing.

Sohanpal, R., Newton, S., Akundo, P., Colligan, G., Crosse, A., Durham, C., Green, H., Hopewell, S., Jackson, T., Jayacodi, S., Khan, I., Kwaku Odoi, C., Lam. E., Lancaster, G., Lawton, S., Makita, M., Mistry, K., Mohammed, A., Lacerda Ratton, B., Smith, J., Sunga, R., Thomson, A., Treweek, S., Williams, C., Mistry, M., & Eldridge, S. (2025). *Improving Inclusivity in Trials through Good Practice in the Collection and Use of Ethnicity Data: Recommendations for Discussion*. (Unpublished).

Sowemimo, A. (2023). *Divided: Racism, Medicine and Why We Need to Decolonise Healthcare*. Profile Books.

Tervalon, M., & Murray-García, J. (1998). Cultural humility versus cultural competence: A critical distinction in defining physician training outcomes in multicultural education. *Journal of Health Care for the Poor and Underserved*, *9*(2), 117–125. https://doi.org/10.1353/hpu.2010.0233

Tuohy, D., & Cooney, A. (2019). Older women's experiences of aging and health: An interpretive phenomenological study. *Gerontology & Geriatric Medicine*, *5*, 2333721419834308. https://doi.org/10.1177/2333721419834308

Vaughn, L. M., Jacquez, F., & Bakar, R. C. (2009). Cultural health attributions, beliefs, and practices: Effects on healthcare and medical education. *The Open Medical Education Journal*, *2*(1).

Vogel, D., Meyer, M., & Harendza, S. (2018). Verbal and non-verbal communication skills including empathy during history taking of undergraduate medical students. *BMC Medical Education*, *18*(1), 157. https://doi.org/10.1186/s12909-018-1260-9

CHAPTER 2

Unpacking the paradox

Excluded communities within geographic centres of medical excellence

Corina Cheeks

Introduction

Van Zyl-Smit's (2018) assertion that 'ignorance is never bliss when it comes to patient care' encapsulates a fundamental challenge facing healthcare systems in the Global North. Ignorance in healthcare manifests at multiple levels: institutional blindness to systemic inequities, lack of awareness of cultural competency requirements in clinical settings, and the broader societal failure to acknowledge how racism permeates healthcare delivery. This is compounded by exhaustion from repeatedly explaining racism to those who benefit from it, creating additional hurdles to addressing these systemic failures (Eddo-Lodge, 2017).

Understanding healthcare disparities requires both empirical evidence and recognition of the lived experiences of service users to do justice to the complex interplay between individual encounters and systemic failures. As highlighted by Merriam and Clark (1993), learning from experience becomes significant when it challenges existing assumptions and creates a new understanding of social phenomena. As such, the intersection of personal narratives with academic analysis provides crucial insights into how healthcare inequalities operate in practice, particularly in spaces where medical excellence, in its presumption of guaranteeing equitable care, silences voices suggesting otherwise.

This chapter examines healthcare inequalities through both experiential and academic lenses, focusing particularly on the underrepresentation of minoritised communities in clinical research and the perpetuation of health disparities in settings where medical excellence is assumed. This analysis demonstrates how medical institutions can perpetuate racial disparities in healthcare outcomes. The persistence of these disparities in centres of medical excellence reveals fundamental contradictions between how healthcare systems are designed and how they operate in reality. Despite significant investments in medical research, advances in technology, and professional training, outcomes remain starkly different among diverse ethnic population groups. This paradox suggests that technical excellence alone cannot address health inequalities

DOI: 10.4324/9781003466093-4

without continuous and dedicated attention to structural racism, the social determinants of health, and systemic practices that perpetuate exclusion. The chapter will also highlight areas where Patient and Public Involvement (PPI) can play a significant role in establishing health equity.

Part I: The paradox of place

Oxford's two faces

Growing up in Oxford, a city renowned for its medical excellence and academic prestige, I experienced a striking paradox. Behind the glossy exterior of world-class healthcare research lay complex inequalities that I felt deeply but struggled to articulate as a child. I occasionally felt a vague unease when visiting the doctor or the dentist, beyond the sense of unfamiliarity which others feel, although I lacked the vocabulary and context to fully express this sentiment. It wasn't until I embarked on a journey of discovery and research that I could finally put words to these long-held feelings and fully analyse the issues at play. After observing and speaking with friends and family, I realised the feeling was that of difference; feeling 'othered' in these spaces.

Oxford, you quickly learn, is a city of stark contrasts. First, there's the familiar Oxford we see to represent the archetypal small British city used in backdrops to film sets, on glossy brochures and tourist snapshots, locally referred to as the 'gown'. Occupied by the universities, colleges, and historical sites, here, in the centre of the city, locals enjoy not only proximity to world-class medical facilities but also the health benefits that come with affluence and education. This is the Oxford often seen by fleeting visitors and tourists.

Then there's the other side of Oxford, for whom the majority of the city's residents are more acquainted, the 'town' side. This is the Oxford of sprawling busy estates and rural outskirts, where access to healthcare isn't always just a matter of walking down the street to the nearest GP surgery. It's the version of Oxford where, depending on your postcode, waiting times can stretch into weeks, where getting a specialist referral may feel like winning the lottery, and where the journey to the hospital can be a logistical nightmare involving multiple bus changes or expensive taxi journeys.

This disparity between these two worlds is a phenomenon observed and experienced by many in the city, including myself. The statistics paint a gloomy picture. In the latest report by the Institute of Health Equity, University College London (2024), they highlight that the life expectancy between the most and least deprived in Oxford is currently 10.3 years, an increase from 8.5 years, which is no change from the previous year. More than a decade of life, gone because of where residents happen to live in a city that's at the forefront of medical advancement. These geographical disparities within relatively small areas demonstrate that proximity to medical excellence does not equate to equitable access or comparable health outcomes. Whilst such healthcare outcomes are complex and linked to a variety of inequalities within healthcare and elsewhere, these gaps are wide, and they continue to increase.

Juxtapositions

Oxford's reputation as a bastion of medical knowledge and innovation is well-deserved. The city boasts world-class institutions, colleges, and numerous research centres dedicated to advancing healthcare. This environment can foster a sense of pride and security in the quality of healthcare available to residents. However, as I delved deeper into the realities of health outcomes across different communities in the city, I uncovered a more complex and troubling picture. This journey began with a sobering realisation: despite Oxford's overall affluence and medical expertise, significant health disparities exist within the city. The Oxfordshire Joint Strategic Needs Assessment (Oxfordshire County Council, 2023) revealed that males living in the most deprived areas of Oxfordshire can expect to live around 11 years less than those in the most affluent areas, with this gap widening to 12 years for females. This stark contrast in life expectancy within a relatively small geographical area was my first confirmation that all was not as it seemed in my local healthcare landscape.

As I dug deeper, I uncovered more unsettling statistics. Oxford's diverse population, which consists of about 16% coming from ethnically diverse backgrounds, faces unique challenges in accessing and experiencing healthcare. Research has shown that ethnic minorities, particularly those who are Black, face higher rates of compulsory admission to psychiatric wards and often receive harsher treatment in inpatient settings. One of the NHS Race and Health Observatory's (2022) key findings is that Black children are ten times more likely to be referred to Child and Adolescent Mental Health Services (CAMHS) via social services than via a GP. This disparity in mental healthcare is particularly shocking given the UK's reputation for trailblazing research and treatment.

Upon learning about these health inequalities, I was struck by a profound sense of disappointment and frustration. The stark disparities I had observed were not just a local anomaly but a reflection of a much larger, systemic issue afflicting our entire nation. The numbers were staggering and, frankly, difficult to stomach. An eight-year life expectancy gap between the most and least deprived areas in England? A difference of 11 years for men between Westminster and Glasgow? These weren't just statistics; they represented real lives, real families, real communities being short-changed.

As a Black woman from a Caribbean background, I've felt the sting of this inequality keenly. The poorer areas of Oxford, where healthcare outcomes are at their worst, are often the most ethnically diverse. It's a cruel irony that those who could benefit most from Oxford's medical expertise (minorities who are statistically more likely to suffer from certain health conditions) are often the least able to access it. The harsh reality of health inequalities hit home. It wasn't just about how long people lived but about the quality of their lives. Learning that someone, who happened to be Black or Brown and born in a 'deprived' area, might spend more of their years in poor health felt deeply unjust. This revelation shook my core beliefs about fairness in our society and the principles underpinning our NHS. It is fair to say that inequalities in healthcare for Black and Brown people reflect systemic inequalities and racism in society at large, though this offers no consolation to those of us living the consequences.

The ethnic disparities in health outcomes left me feeling a mix of incredulity and dismay. Learning that Black women were four times more likely to die in childbirth than white women was a gut punch (MBRRACE-UK, 2019, 2025). How could this be happening in 21st-century Britain? It made me question how much progress we'd really made as a society in addressing racial inequalities. As I grappled with these realities, I couldn't help but feel a sense of urgency. The economic costs of these health inequalities were astronomical – £13 billion in lost productivity, £5 billion in excess NHS costs (Munford et al., 2025). But more than the financial implications, I was haunted by the human cost. How many lives could be improved or even saved if we addressed these disparities?

Part II: Inherited wisdom and generational experiences

A grandparent's legacy

My grandfather, like much of the Windrush generation, had a complex relationship with healthcare in Britain. A proud and self-reliant man, he would only visit the GP when illness had completely overwhelmed him. At first, I thought this reluctance stemmed purely from an independent spirit. But as I grew older, I began to understand that this may not be the only reason. Factors that echoed throughout our community may have played more than a small part in this reluctance.

The stories passed down through our networks painted a troubling picture. In waiting rooms, the weight of unwelcoming stares and uncomfortable silences spoke volumes. When people did seek care, their concerns were often dismissed or minimised. The simple act of being understood could become a barrier; accents are sometimes met with impatience or confusion. These were part of a pattern that made seeking healthcare feel like navigating a fraught environment rather than accessing a basic right.

This collective experience bred a deep-seated mistrust that passed from friends, family, and in some cases, from one generation to the next. The message was clear though unspoken: this system wasn't built with us in mind. What makes this particularly confusing is that many in the Black community helped build the NHS. They worked long hours in its hospitals and clinics, their dedication helping to establish it as one of Britain's most cherished institutions. We grew up hearing stories of their contribution, which instilled in us both pride in the NHS and faith in its principles.

Yet this pride sits uneasily alongside our lived experience of healthcare inequalities. How do we reconcile our community's role in building and sustaining the NHS with the discrimination many of us still face within it? This question has pushed me to develop a more nuanced understanding of healthcare delivery and social equity. The NHS remains a vital and valuable institution, but one that still struggles to serve all communities equally.

This paradox, of being both builders and outsiders, has shaped my own journey of discovery. While the scale of healthcare inequalities sometimes can feel overwhelming, it also strengthens my resolve to work toward change. Our community's complex relationship with healthcare isn't just about past injustices; it's about the ongoing struggle to transform an institution we helped build into one that truly serves everyone.

Respectful indifference

Over time, my grandparents' relationship with the NHS evolved into what I've come to think of as 'respectful indifference' – a careful distance maintained on both sides. The healthcare system offered professional courtesy when doctors and nurses addressed them properly, followed protocols, and provided basic care. My grandparents, in return, developed their own careful approach: they attended essential appointments and followed critical medical advice but kept their engagement minimal and measured.

This dynamic was different from the outright mistrust many in our community felt. Instead, it was a kind of practised neutrality. When my grandad was having investigations before his cancer diagnosis, I remember sitting with him, imagining this subtle interplay. Healthcare providers went through the motions efficiently, while he responded with equal restraint – answering questions just enough to get by, volunteering no more information than necessary. He had learned to navigate the system without fully embracing it, finding a middle ground between rejection and acceptance.

This mutual reserve had its costs. Each visit remained superficial, with no building of rapport or true continuity of care over time. Important details about his life and health history had to be repeated, partly because the system didn't retain them effectively but also because he shared them sparingly. As his health needs became more complex in his later years, this distance became more problematic, though neither side seemed to know how to bridge it.

The pattern was familiar throughout our community. While some, like my grandfather, found this careful balance, others maintained a greater distance born of deeper mistrust. It reflected the complex reality of being part of a generation that helped build the NHS while never feeling fully at home within it. They contributed to the system through their work and respected its importance, yet remained guarded in their personal interactions with it.

Understanding this nuanced relationship has been crucial to my work in healthcare advocacy. It's helped me see how patterns of interaction between healthcare systems and minoritised communities are shaped by both historical experiences and daily realities. The challenge isn't just to address overt barriers to care but to transform these deeply ingrained patterns of mutual reserve into relationships of genuine trust and engagement.

Turning point?

I realised that my experiences in Oxford were just the beginning of a much larger story, one that needed to be told, understood, and acted upon nationally. A poignant example is my grandfather's case, where cancer was initially missed, leading to delayed treatment, unnecessary suffering, and ultimately, a shortened life. This oversight shook our faith in the infallibility of medical expertise and the good standard of care for all, as you would expect in the UK. The consequences were profound – not just a late diagnosis but a reminder of how medical negligence can devastate families. This experience opened our eyes to the harsh realities of healthcare inequalities. We couldn't help but wonder: Would my grandfather's concerns have been dismissed so readily if we lived in a more affluent part of Oxford? If his accent had been different, or his skin a different colour? These questions haunted us, forcing us to confront the uncomfortable truths about race, class, and healthcare in the UK.

Our story, sadly, is not unique. Research has shown that people from ethnic minority backgrounds often face delays in cancer diagnosis and treatment. A study by Cancer Research UK (2023) found that Black women are more likely to be diagnosed with late-stage cancer, at which point treatment options are limited and outcomes are poorer. The issue of missed or delayed diagnoses extends beyond cancer. The NHS England's Learning from Deaths programme has highlighted how diagnostic errors contribute significantly to preventable deaths, with certain groups, including ethnic minorities and those from deprived areas, being disproportionately affected.

My grandfather's case became a turning point for our family. It transformed our relationship with the healthcare system from one of unquestioning trust to cautious advocacy. We learned the importance of being persistent, of seeking second opinions, and of trusting our instincts when something feels wrong. As I continue my journey in understanding and addressing health disparities, I carry with me the memory of my grandfather – his strength, his resolve, and the lessons his experience taught us. It's a constant reminder of why this work is so crucial, and why we must strive for a healthcare system that truly serves all, regardless of postcode, ethnicity, or social status.

Part III: Personal encounters with the system

Contrasting care

My journey through Oxford's healthcare system reads like a tale of two halves, each offering starkly different visions of what medical care can be, but both offering profound opportunities for learning. Some experiences have rendered me dumbfounded, while others have presented glimpses of what truly inclusive healthcare could look like.

Harmful or poor communication has been shown to adversely impact the experiences of Black patients in a variety of healthcare settings. For Black women accessing maternity services, Rayment-Jones et al. (2023) found that they are 'subjected to embedded, structural and systemic discrimination throughout the healthcare service' during their maternity care experience. Their research, which entailed interviewing minority ethnic women with recent experience of UK maternity care, reveals how race and ethnicity shape experiences throughout pregnancy, childbirth, and postnatal care. They specifically found that during labour and delivery, pain management decisions, intervention timing, and emergency response protocols were influenced by racial bias. Postnatal care revealed similar patterns, with their participants reporting feelings of dismissal when raising concerns about their recovery or their infants' well-being. Additionally, their research demonstrates that Black women's awareness of the effects of racial disparities creates additional psychological burdens during pregnancy. Healthcare systems have historically failed women who share their racial identity, inevitably negatively influencing the approaches taken by women of colour in care-seeking and in their perceptions of safety in clinical settings.

The challenging encounters still feel vivid in my memory. I've sat in sterile rooms where routine appointments transformed into uncomfortable interrogations; each question tinged with scepticism about my experiences. As both a mother and a patient, I found myself constantly on edge, feeling the need to present a perfect façade; articulate, composed, and carefully non-threatening, just to be taken seriously. This performance, this constant self-monitoring, added an exhausting layer of stress to already difficult medical situations. After these interactions, all that was left was a feeling of powerlessness and alienation.

Clinicians, though often technically proficient, sometimes displayed a rushed, detached manner that created invisible but formidable barriers to effective care. Their lack of cultural understanding manifested in subtle ways, a dismissive tone, an impatient gesture, or assumptions made without asking, all contributing to a sense that I didn't quite belong in these spaces.

The role of cultural competency

As I was close to losing faith in the system, I encountered healthcare providers who were patient, well-informed about more than just clinical treatment, and knowledgeable about social and cultural differences. They showed true understanding of the importance culture pays to openness in patient care and clinical research. These clinicians exemplified what culturally competent care truly means. They took time to listen, not just to symptoms but to my lived experience. They understood that my cultural background wasn't just a demographic detail but an essential part of a health journey. Their approach went beyond mere politeness; they showed genuine empathy and awareness of the historical and systemic factors that influence health outcomes for people from ethnic minority backgrounds.

As Blake (2024) notes, cultural competency puts the patient and their customs or traditions at the forefront of care. Whether this is the understanding from a clinician that some rashes will present differently on different skin tones, or that redness may not be visible on darker skin, or even the acknowledgement that a patient from a particular faith or cultural background may request that certain healthcare complaints were dealt with in line with their cultural beliefs. These are the seemingly small but incredibly impactful factors that can make patients feel included, considered, and respected.

The impact of encountering healthcare providers from similar cultural backgrounds was particularly profound for me. Often, these interactions carried an unspoken understanding, an immediate ease that made difficult conversations simpler, understanding unspoken and trust implicit. Even more encouraging were the culturally competent providers from different backgrounds who had clearly done the work to understand the unique health concerns and experiences of our community. They proved that cultural competency isn't about matching ethnicities, it's about developing genuine understanding and respect. These positive experiences weren't just personally comforting; they were revolutionary in showing me what healthcare could be. When providers combined medical expertise with cultural understanding and genuine kindness, the entire dynamic of care transformed. Appointments became collaborative rather than confrontational. Questions felt like genuine inquiry rather than cross-examination. Most importantly, I felt seen as a whole person, not just a collection of symptoms or a problematic patient.

This contrast in care has deeply influenced my understanding of what systemic change in healthcare must look like. It's not enough to simply open doors; we must transform what happens once people walk through them. True healthcare equity demands more than access – it requires a fundamental shift in how care is delivered, how providers are trained, and how cultural competency is woven into the very fabric of medical practice. The stark contrast between healthcare providers in Oxford, those who practice cultural competency and those who don't, vividly demonstrates the crucial importance of proper training and awareness in medical care. My personal experiences, as well as those of my family and community members, have highlighted how transformative culturally competent care can be.

Patient and public participation

Patient and Public Involvement (PPI) initiatives have emerged as potential mechanisms for improving research inclusivity and relevance. Beames et al. (2021) argue that integrating lived experience into scientific data synthesis can transform research quality and relevance, particularly when community voices are genuinely centred rather than tokenistically consulted.

In my advisory roles as a public representative, I have been required to present at conferences, contribute to medical journal articles, review research proposals, and sit on steering committees. But, as I began to engage with community organisations working with widening diversity groups in Oxford, I realised that the healthcare challenges my family faced were not isolated incidents. The stories I heard from individuals living just a few miles away revealed a stark disparity in healthcare experiences, often exacerbated by racial and socioeconomic factors. As my awareness of healthcare inequalities grew, I found myself drawn to actively participate in addressing these systemic challenges. My journey led me to engage with various research initiatives and widening participation programmes, both academic and community-led.

This journey has deepened my understanding of systemic issues within our healthcare system and ignited a passionate commitment to addressing these profound inequalities. This role has not been without its challenges. The effectiveness of PPI relies on genuine partnership rather than tokenistic consultation. Happell et al. (2015) explore issues of fear and power when including lived experience in healthcare education, findings that extend to research settings. They identify how power imbalances can silence community voices even within supposedly participatory frameworks, especially when institutional cultures remain unchanged.

In my position as a research co-applicant and public patient, I have felt the weight of being one of the few voices representing my community in these academic research spaces. I have had to navigate the delicate balance of being both an insider and an outsider in various contexts, as well as the subtle yet significant distinction between speaking for and speaking on behalf of others. Effective PPI must recognise that community representatives often carry the burden of speaking for entire ethnic groups whilst navigating complex dynamics of insider/outsider status within academic institutions. This multiple positionality creates particular challenges here, as minoritised community members, such as myself, must often code-switch between community and academic contexts, managing different languages, expectations, and power dynamics.

Relating to the insider/outsider status, one of my first experiences was joining a PPI group for a study on widening participation of Black and Brown communities in research. This opportunity allowed me to contribute my lived experience and community insights to shape the research questions and methodology. It was eye-opening to see how researchers valued our input and how it could potentially improve the relevance and impact of their work.

I became involved in a widening participation programme aimed at encouraging more students from diverse backgrounds to consider careers in healthcare and medical research. Speaking at local events and community centres, I shared my own story and the importance of representation in the medical field. The enthusiasm and curiosity of people I met reinforced my belief in the power of diversity to drive innovation and improve patient care.

Working with researchers, I learned about the challenges they face in making their studies more inclusive. Oftentimes, many were genuinely committed to integrating more diversity and inclusion into their research but struggled with practical issues like recruiting from underrepresented communities who are understandably wary, due to negative media coverage about medical care for those in their community, or adapting their communication styles to be more in more plain English and culturally sensitive, as noted by Pardhan et al. (2025). I found myself in a unique position to support bridging the gap between the academic world and my community, with a view to building trust and facilitating meaningful engagement.

Subsequently, I was involved in a particularly rewarding project in which I collaborated with a team developing a culturally adapted mental health intervention for Caribbean elders. My role included reviewing materials for cultural appropriateness, suggesting modifications to make the intervention more relatable, and facilitating focus groups to gather community feedback. This experience highlighted the importance of co-creation in developing effective healthcare solutions for diverse populations. Too often, community members are invited to participate only after research questions have been determined and methodologies finalised, limiting their ability to influence fundamental aspects of research design. My experience demonstrated that early involvement across the entire research process leads to meaningful community engagement.

Through these various engagements, I have witnessed a growing recognition within the research community of the need for more inclusive practices. I have seen first-hand how involving people from diverse backgrounds throughout the research process can lead to more relevant, impactful, and equitable outcomes. As I continue on this path, I'm inspired by the potential for collaborative, community-engaged research to drive meaningful change in healthcare. My journey of understanding has evolved into a journey of action, fuelled by the belief that by working together – researchers, healthcare professionals, and communities – we can create a more equitable and effective healthcare system for all. The contrast between Oxford's image as a centre of medical advancement and the reality of healthcare experiences in our community highlights how racial inequalities can persist even in supposedly progressive environments. Better serving ignored communities within centres of excellence requires thoughtful action and concerted effort to consistently engage communities through modes of communication that are relatable and trusted.

Conclusion

Understanding and navigating healthcare disparities require looking beyond surface-level prestige and reputations. My journey from ignorance to cognisance as a granddaughter, daughter, mother, and member of the Black British community, to a community advocate, is perhaps unlikely, but one that has allowed me to learn much more about healthcare and health disparities. While positive examples of clinical care and research practices offer hope, the persistence of systemic inequalities demands continued vigilance and advocacy.

The realities of healthcare inequality reveal themselves gradually, through a process of awakening that transforms vague impressions into undeniable patterns. My own journey of understanding began with the dawning realisation that barriers to healthcare and treatment have devastating impacts for families and communities, as seen in my grandfather's delayed cancer diagnosis. This was followed by me positioning myself between the healthcare system and its service users, through years of public engagement in research, with academics, and through community work, and countless conversations with people who had similar experiences of dismissal, misdiagnosis, and systemic oversight.

Contemporary progress in healthcare equity and social awareness presents a complex landscape. While there have been meaningful advances in certain areas, notably in clinical recognition of diagnostic challenges concerning skin conditions in people of colour, and in the broader acknowledgement of diverse lived experiences and their daily impact, such developments, though encouraging, remain disappointingly infrequent. The current pace of change, while moving in the right direction, has yet to achieve the deeper transformation needed to address long-standing disparities in healthcare delivery and social recognition. The impact of racial disparities in healthcare is complex and deeply rooted. From my experience in community work and research engagement, these systemic inequities manifest in countless subtle and overt ways, making them challenging to fully quantify, though the work on the NHS RHO since its inception in 2020 is doing just that. The effects ripple through every level of healthcare delivery, from individual patient-provider interactions to broader institutional policies and outcomes.

The role of medical education cannot be overstated in this evolution. All future healthcare professionals must be trained not only in clinical skills but also in cultural competency, implicit bias recognition, and the historical context of healthcare disparities. This education should become deeply integrated into their core curriculum, shaping how medical professionals understand and approach patient care, the origin and diversity of needs, from the beginning of their training. Equally important is the need for increased representation in medical research and clinical trials. The historical exclusion of ethnically diverse populations from medical research has created significant gaps in our understanding of how different treatments affect various demographic groups. Addressing these gaps requires intentional effort not only to include diverse populations in research studies but also to have them at the decision-making table at the planning stages, to better understand that health conditions that disproportionately affect marginalised communities need to be investigated.

My personal journey, as a patient and as a community advocate, has taught me that change often begins with individual voices speaking up and demanding better. But advocacy must be matched by commitment to change. The path forward requires sustained effort on multiple fronts: continued research, policy changes to address systemic inequities, improved medical education, and increased representation at all levels of healthcare delivery. It also requires something less tangible but equally important: a fundamental shift in how we think about and approach healthcare equity. The stories and statistics presented here represent real lives, experiences, and consequences. The journey from awareness to action is ongoing, and while the challenges ahead are significant, the cost of inaction is far greater. The future of healthcare must be one where equity is not just an aspiration but a fundamental principle guiding all aspects of clinical practice and policy.

Discussion questions

1. How can we make the most out of public and patient involvement to ensure meaningful contributions which effect real change?
2. How can we challenge our own beliefs, biases, and understanding of race in the health context?
3. Where can healthcare professionals in the UK seek opportunities for learning to increase their cultural competency?

Further reading

Sheehan, M., Friesen, P., Balmer, A., Cheeks, C., Davidson, S., Devereux, J., Findlay, D., Keats-Rohan, K., Lawrence, R., & Shafiq, K. (2020). Trust, trustworthiness and sharing patient data for research. *Journal of Medical Ethics, Medethics-2019-106048*. Advance online publication. https://doi.org/10.1136/medethics-2019-106048

Skloot, R. (2011). *The Immortal Life of Henrietta Lacks*. Pan Books.

Sue, D. W. (2023, August 30). How to combat microaggressions, with Derald Wing Sue, PhD [Audio podcast episode]. In K. I. Mills (Host), *Speaking of Psychology*. American Psychological Association. https://www.apa.org/news/podcasts/speaking-of-psychology/microaggressions

Van Zyl-Smit, R. (2018). Ignorance is never bliss when it comes to patient care. *African Journal of Thoracic and Critical Care Medicine*, *24*(3). https://doi.org/10.7196/SARJ.2018.v24i3.226

References

Beames, J. R., Kikas, K., O'Gradey-Lee, M., Gale, N., Werner-Seidler, A., Boydell, K. M., & Hudson, J. L. (2021). A new normal: Integrating lived experience into scientific data syntheses. *Frontiers in Psychiatry*, *12*, Article 763005. https://doi.org/10.3389/fpsyt.2021.763005

Blake, L. (2024). Delivering person-centred care and support for the UK's culturally diverse communities (Frontline Briefing). *Research in Practice, National Children's Bureau*. https://www.researchinpractice.org.uk/media/nlqpcvr3/adults_fb_supportingworkacrosscultures_web.pdf

Cancer Research UK. (2023, January 27). *New Analysis Reveals Black Women in England More Likely to Be Diagnosed with Late-Stage Cancer*. https://news.cancerresearchuk.org/2023/01/27/new-analysis-reveals-black-women-in-england-more-likely-to-be-diagnosed-with-late-stage-cancer/

Eddo-Lodge, R. (2017). *Why I'm No Longer Talking to White People about Race*. Bloomsbury Publishing.

scholarship: How shared values can guide best practices for research integrity, social justice, and principled education. *MetaArXiv*. https://doi.org/10.31222/osf.io/k7a9p

Happell, B., Bennetts, W., Harris, S., Platania-Phung, C., Tohotoa, J., Byrne, L., & Wynaden, D. (2015). Lived experience in teaching mental health nursing: Issues of fear and power. *International Journal of Mental Health Nursing*, *24*(1), 19–27. https://doi.org/10.1111/inm.12091

MBRRACE-UK. (2019). *Saving Lives, Improving Mothers' Care: Lessons Learned to Inform Maternity Care from the UK and Ireland Confidential Enquiries into Maternal Deaths and Morbidity 2015–17*. University of Oxford.

MBRRACE-UK. (2025). *Saving Lives, Improving Mothers' Care: Lessons Learned to Inform Maternity Care from the UK and Ireland Confidential Enquiries into Maternal Deaths and Morbidity 2021–23*. University of Oxford.

Merriam, S. B., & Clark, M. C. (1993). Learning from life experience: What makes it significant? *International Journal of Lifelong Education*, *12*(2), 129–138. https://doi.org/10.1080/0260137930120205

Munford, L. A., Armitage, C. J., Webb, R. T., & Ashcroft, D. M. (2025). Economic case for reducing inequities in patient safety. *BMJ Open Quality*, *14*(1), e003042. https://doi.org/10.1136/bmjoq-2024-003042

National Academy of Sciences of the United States of America, *113*(16), 4296–4301. https://doi.org/10.1073/pnas.1516047113

NHS Race and Health Observatory. (2025, March). *Trust in Primary Care Report*. https://www.nhsrho.org/wp-content/uploads/2025/03/TRUST-IN-PRIMARY-CARE-REPORT.pdf

Oxfordshire County Council. (2023). *Oxfordshire Joint Strategic Needs Assessment*. Oxfordshire County Council.

Pardhan, S., Sehmbi, T., Wijewickrama, R., et al. (2025). Barriers and facilitators for engaging underrepresented ethnic minority populations in healthcare research: An umbrella review. *International Journal for Equity in Health*, *24*, 70. https://doi.org/10.1186/s12939-025-02431-4

Race and Health Observatory. (2022). *Mental Health: Children and Young People of Black African and Black Caribbean Heritage*. Race and Health Observatory.

Rayment-Jones, H., Silverio, S. A., Harris, J., Harden, A., & Sandall, J. (2023). Inside the 'imperfect mosaic': Minority ethnic women's qualitative experiences of race and ethnicity during pregnancy, childbirth, and maternity care in the United Kingdom. *BMC Public Health*, *23*, Article 2542. https://doi.org/10.1186/s12889-023-17505-7

Van Zyl-Smit, R. (2018). Ignorance is never bliss when it comes to patient care. *African Journal of Thoracic and Critical Care Medicine*, *24*(3), 89–90. https://doi.org/10.7196/sarj.2018.v24i3.226

SECTION 2

Research and data

The next two chapters tackle specifically the impact of race and racism on research in the generation and utility of data. Both Chapters 3 and 4 confront the challenges of equitable engagement, fair inclusion, and just representation of ethnic minority priorities in health research. These challenges are methodological and epistemological, whether as interpersonal research encounters or through the large-scale effects of machine learning using racially biased data.

In Chapter 3, Rai addresses the nexus between race and inequity in health research in the UK. She argues that current methodologies continue to exclude and alienate those it claims to include and empower. As Rai identifies, due to past and present harms, racially minoritised populations remain distrustful of the state and are less willing to engage in research to benefit it. Furthermore, methodological and epistemological Whiteness undergird most studies, with assumptions about participant willingness to be questioned about certain topics, in particular ways, amid the consumption of participant time, energy, and goodwill. Without the development of specific structures for information gathering and sharing, both among participants and in the research team, methodological Whiteness precludes equitable inclusion. Rai's chapter raises important questions about the epistemological ground on which health research is constructed and derived. Conscious of this environment, she recommends the development of alternative methodologies and research techniques which protect minoritised participants and minoritised researchers alike, so as not to further entrench the inequities the research intends to ameliorate.

Razai and Nagraj's chapter heralds the artificial intelligence (AI) revolution that will likely infiltrate the British healthcare system over the coming decades. In Chapter 4, they detail the inherent biases present in the data that inform the algorithms powering these new technologies. While the use of machine learning is touted to improve fairness and parity in healthcare provision, Razai and Nagraj highlight the evergrowing risk that these systems could amplify and further entrench negative racial stereotypes and biases within the healthcare system. To mitigate these concerns, they argue for

DOI: 10.4324/9781003466093-5

robust, interdisciplinary governance of AI technology, from initial development to roll out, to ensure that its use does not reduce patient safety by promoting inequitable care. The authors also advocate for inclusive leadership in the research informing the development of these technologies so that cultural blind spots derived from historically biased data can be recognised and revised. Finally, they emphasise the need for continued evaluation of the outputs of these systems to ensure that any inequitable outcomes are promptly identified and addressed.

CHAPTER 3

Race and health research

Challenges for transforming practice

Tanvi Rai

Introduction

In this chapter, we will explore how race and ethnicity feature in the design and production of research into the health of human populations in order to influence actions such as developing clinical guidelines, public health messaging, creating national strategies for treating or preventing different health conditions, and so on. I begin with a brief recounting of how race and ethnicity came to be used as a classification for interpreting variation in population health, and the inherent problems associated with their use. I then explore how health research in the UK is organised, funded, and conducted and how this influences the way race and ethnicity are understood with respect to health. In the final section, I briefly describe two research projects as case studies to illustrate what these problems look like in real life, and in the process, I illustrate some ways in which to adopt a race-conscious approach to research such that our practices avoid reproducing, exacerbating, or entrenching existing racialised health inequities in society.

Race/ethnicity as a way to classify people

Racial categories were created by European imperial empires as part of the wider project to control and subjugate colonised populations. The initial exercise of classifying humans started in the field of genetics by Carl Linnaeus, a botanist from Sweden, regarded as the father of modern taxonomy. In 1735, the first edition of Linnaeus' *Systema Naturae* was published, which presented a detailed classification of animals and plants known at the time, and also included more 'exotic' contributions whose descriptions had been gleaned from the accounts of European travellers returning from faraway places. Within this collection was also presented a system for classifying and ordering human populations, offered as types of 'man', and based upon a combination of skin colour, geographical distribution, and what today would be regarded as overtly racist assumptions.

Despite a number of revisions and expansions of the initial classification of human populations, white Europeans remained at the top of the pyramid, distinct from all the

DOI: 10.4324/9781003466093-6

other groupings, who were variously described as having one or more combinations of inferior appearance, behaviours, intellect, or abilities, compared to the white European group. This initial categorisation is often regarded as the origin of scientific racism, as it gave scientific legitimacy for the continuation and intensification of violence against non-white racialised groups by European colonisers in their extensive plunder and conquest across the world and other eugenics-inspired legacies (Rutherford, 2021a, 2021b; Saini, 2019).

We now know, most significantly since the mapping of the human genome in 2003 (NIH, 2003), that racial groupings, as they are conventionally and routinely used, bear little correspondence to inherited, biological sources of variation. Race and ethnicity are primarily social and relational categories with important historical and political legacies. They are also deeply context-dependent and shift over time. In other words, the same person classified (or racialised) as one race or ethnicity in a particular geopolitical context may be classified in a different racial category in another place. Racial/ethnic categories also shift over time, often due to international political developments that can impact how differently minoritised populations are viewed by the majority population of that region (Haney Lopez, 1994; Omi & Winant, 2014). It is for these reasons that nowadays the terms' racially or ethnically 'minoritised' rather than 'minority' are preferred. The term 'minoritised', originally coined by anthropologist Yasmin Gunaratnam (Gunaratnam, 2003), uses a social constructionist approach which calls to attention that there is nothing *natural* or inherent about some people being 'minorities' – it is an *active* and *dynamic* social process determined by the configurations of power that are present in specific contextual settings.

There are some further uncertainties regarding terminology – for example, some people feel uncomfortable using the term 'race' and prefer using 'ethnicity'. This is because the term race implies a 'biological' classification, mainly based on physical appearance, and therefore reminds us of Britain's (and other European imperial powers') violent colonial past. On the other hand, ethnicity implies a 'cultural' grouping of people with shared history, customs, and traditions, an altogether nicer description, and removes most of the malign undercurrent that race has. Ultimately, it is just a superficial difference, and both terms can be (and are) used interchangeably in academic and scientific writing to facilitate discussions of group-level characteristics. What is more important to remember is that when race/ethnicity are used in social and health research findings, these terms are serving as a *proxy* for a complex (and problematic) combination of ancestry and family history alongside relative social, economic, and structural advantage (or disadvantage) faced by different groups of people depending upon how they are racialised in particular contexts (Bécares et al., 2015; Cerdeña et al., 2020; Rai et al., 2022).

Many commentators say, more simply, that it is not *race* (or ethnicity) but *racism* that is a 'fundamental cause' (Phelan & Link, 2015) of health inequalities. As with all white-majority countries with imperialistic pasts, it is a product of the particular political history stemming from Britain's empire-building and traumatic damage inflicted upon societies overseas, the subsequent movement of large groups of people from these colonised regions to the UK (often via other parts of the British empire), and the status afforded to them within British social hierarchical structures. The continuation of racism in modern Britain helps maintain the clustering of resources, socioeconomic assets, and political power such that it stays close to the white majority while excluding racialised minorities (Jones, 2000; Krieger, 2012; Williams, 1997), with measurable negative impacts upon their health (Hackett et al., 2020; Hayanga et al., 2023).

Given the unpleasant history of these categories, it may seem appropriate to decommission their use in academic and scientific narratives. However, race/ethnicity (in its proxy variable usage, as described earlier) has consistently remained one of the strongest determinants of health status, experiences, and outcomes in white-majority countries like the UK, and this is the case across nearly all health conditions, be it heart disease, cancer, mental health, or maternal and child health (Raleigh, 2023). We are therefore compelled to continue using these social categories if we are to truly understand, record, and eventually alleviate these racialised inequalities. But we must do this with extreme care and caution, or else we risk reinforcing, crystallising, and perpetuating racial myths about the superiority of some groups over others.

How mainstream health research reproduces racialised inequities

The data problems – representation and inclusion

There is a strong scientific imperative in medical research to recruit study samples that are representative (i.e. closely resemble the social demographics) of the population affected by the health issue under study. This is to ensure that the results from the research are generalisable, which means the research findings can safely inform the development of new drugs or treatments or medical interventions or national health policies and guidelines, such that they will benefit *everybody* affected by that health condition. In reality, however, there has been a long-standing problem of research studies failing to include people from minoritised racial groups in their study samples, and this is the case even when these groups are disproportionately impacted by the health issue being studied (e.g. in studies of heart disease, stroke, or COVID-19).

Among other effects, this bias in the creation of medical evidence eventually leads to biases and gaps in clinical guidance, knowledge, and support available for minoritised racial groups (Amutah et al., 2021; Fawzy et al., 2022; Vyas et al., 2020). For example, clinicians may hesitate to prescribe a course of treatment for their non-white patients if they find that the evidence of effectiveness just does not exist for that group. Worse still, there are examples where racial bias in medical evidence has created divergent treatment guidelines and care pathways based on how the patient is racialised, for example, as white or Black. As an example, in the UK, up until 2021, the clinical measurement to estimate a person's kidney function, the estimated glomerular filtration rate or eGFR, included a 'race correction'. This means that patients deemed to be of Black ethnicity (and there is a lack of clarity about how this was determined) were set a lower cut-off for diagnosing kidney disease compared to white patients, thereby delaying initiation of their treatment or transplant options until their clinical pathology worsened (Kidney Research UK, 2021). The explanation for this adjustment came from the now discredited belief that Black people have more muscle mass than white people (and this would influence kidney function). It was only in 2021 that an American medical taskforce announced recommendations to remove Black race as a factor in the eGFR calculation, leading to changes in the UK guidelines as well (UK Kidney Association, 2021). Unfortunately, there remain several other race correction algorithms within the medical literature which are used in routine clinical practice (Cerdeña et al., 2020; Vyas et al., 2020).

The reasons for the lack of representation of participants from non-white ethnicity in research are numerous and multifaceted. Health research literature from white majority countries like the UK often reports findings from near-homogenous samples (most participants being white, educated, and middle-class). Sometimes, they have a few lines in the 'Limitations' section of the Discussion, where they rationalise this, for example, by explaining that racially minoritised people 'lack awareness' about science or 'lack trust' in medical research. While not substantiating such claims with actual evidence, these explanations (more often than not) also offer no context for these potential fears, if they do exist.

We have already explored how structural racism in the UK means that non-white racialised groups are more likely to have reduced access to educational, economic, environmental, and cultural resources compared to white people (see also (Finney et al., 2023; Mirza & Warwick, 2022; The Runnymede Trust, 2020). Given this intersection of relative wealth and race/ethnicity, there are often greater practical concerns (such as costs, say for arranging extra childcare or travel) and opportunity costs (e.g. losing a day's wages if working on zero-hours contract jobs) of research participation for racially minoritised people. Furthermore, those who are socially marginalised, facing racism in their day-to-day existence, over lifetimes and generations, have limited experience of being seen as valuable and worthy citizens. Participation in research is based on an unspoken expectation that people feel a sense of belonging and community responsibility. It assumes that they feel valued and cared for by the state, irrespective of who they are and where they live, and therefore will find it entirely ordinary to be invited to shape improvements in healthcare. However, what this possibly naïve approach fails to recognise is how this expectation sits within the wider realities of racialised life in the UK, where racially minoritised groups are disproportionately hurt by national policies and changes such as stop-and-search (Gov.UK., 2024), the 'hostile environment' and anti-immigrant political rhetoric and policies (Jeffery et al., 2024), austerity measures, and the recent resurgence of white nationalist populist movements (Mondon & Winter, 2019; Rhodes & Hall, 2020). Adding to this, there are also historical and more recent episodes of harm caused directly by unethical medical research practices carried out on non-white bodies (in the West and abroad, see for example (Lenzer, 2006; McVean, 2019; Rodriguez & García, 2013), which cast a long shadow on how racially minoritised people view medical research and researchers, no matter how well-intentioned they may be.

Interpretation of race or ethnicity-based difference

Even when studies collect race or ethnicity-based data, the analysis of those data is often shallow and reductive. A standard risk factor analysis may be carried out, looking at associations with the study outcomes in similar ways as would be done for other measures, such as age, body weight, sex, or deprivation index, where the study population is classified into discrete categories and there is no further explanation of what those categories represent. In the absence of any deeper engagement with how different racial categories have been derived and standardised, and what assumptions are enfolded in and thus obscured in this process, this kind of approach and resulting research findings offer 'scientific' legitimacy and strength to the patterning of health by people's race/ethnicity in fixed and immutable ways.

As Dororthy Roberts, Professor of law and sociology, wisely said:

> Race is not a biological category that naturally produces these health disparities because of genetic difference. Race is a social category that has staggering biological consequences . . . . because of the impact of social inequality on people's health.
>
> *(Roberts, 2017)*

If left unchallenged in the creation of mainstream knowledge, such methodological approaches further pathologise racially minoritised groups. They uphold deficit-based explanations; in other words, they focus on what certain kinds of people (who look a certain way) *didn't have* or *didn't do*, which goes straight back to explanations that evoke either a deficient 'biology' or a deficient 'culture' (or a combination of the two) to explain observed disparities. For example, when the COVID-19 pandemic struck the UK, Black, and South Asian people suffered the worst outcomes (ICNARC, 2020). Early scientific reports proposed that they might be 'genetically predisposed' to have a worse health impact from the infection, rather than reflecting on the fact that many such people were employed in inflexible and insecure jobs, which required them to use public transport and/or work in public-facing, busy indoor settings where they were more likely to catch COVID-19. Similarly, another frequent explanation offered for the rapid spread of COVID-19 among South Asian communities was how they were 'culturally' expectated to live in multigenerational households and congregate at large events. Little attention was paid to the possibility that poorer Asian families might not be able to afford separate households due to financial pressures and/or they might have intergenerational dependencies, such as the caring needs of elderly relatives or children (Ansari-Thomas, 2024).

There are increasing moves towards expanding the use of risk prediction models to guide clinical decision making. This means stratifying risk according to patient profiles, in order to determine different treatment or care pathways such that resources are channelled most effectively (Beam & Kohane, 2018; Moons et al., 2009). However, since the algorithms that these models are trained on are informed by clinical and epidemiological databases drawn from predominantly white populations, they risk under- or over-estimating disease risks for minoritised groups (Obermeyer et al., 2019). Ethnicity data are known to be often either missing completely or inappropriately categorised (notwithstanding the issue of its biological validity) (Butt & Cooper Stubbs, 2025). An improperly selected, fitted, and evaluated model that shows lower risk of racially minoritised patients could increase the burden of risk factors that they need in order to meet, say, treatment thresholds. Moreover, if models repeatedly 'demonstrate' reduced risk for particular minoritised groups, it may influence decisions about how data are collected in the future, risking a longer-term 'invisibilisation' of the problem (Chen et al., 2021). It could also permanently reduce funding and provision of healthcare for those groups due to these faulty assumptions (Kass, 2001).

There is therefore a critical need for deeper interrogation on the reported association between race/ethnicity and risks and outcomes, and some tools have recently been developed to support this (Naicker, 2024). If models are based and adjusted purely on 'data signals' of racialised difference in disease risk, they would be subscribing to a purely genetic or biological model of race/ethnicity and health despite well-characterised social factors that are also at play (Vyas et al., 2020). In recent years, there have been widespread calls to reject race-based approaches in favour of a 'race-conscious' one that 'emphasises racism, rather than race, as a key determinant of illness and health, encouraging providers to focus only on the most relevant data to mitigate health inequities' (Cerdeña et al., 2020).

Researcher barriers

The shift that is required in terms of epistemic assumptions and methodological practices requires a fundamental and multi-level change in the way that medical and health research is designed, funded, supported, conducted, and disseminated. For instance, the leadership of academic institutions and funding bodies is what builds and maintains academic and institutional cultures; however, when it lacks racial diversity (Powell et al., 2022), it is drawing from a very narrow breadth of lived experience perspectives, thereby biasing what kinds of research is commissioned and funded. The repeated use of non-ethnically diverse study samples is a consequence of insufficient resourcing, short timelines, and inadequate skillsets of research teams (Rai et al., 2022). All these factors impede the routine inclusion of outreach activities and co-production work in study protocols that could facilitate trust-building and longer-term meaningful partnerships between academic researchers and community groups, such that a wider range of people felt encouraged to participate in research. Furthermore, even if the study sample manages to include sufficient numbers of people from minoritised groups, the metrics of success as measured by funding organisations (e.g. numbers recruited in various ethnicity categories) limit capacity to contextualise racialised findings in ways that actually deepen our understanding of what these top-level associations actually mean. The superficial use of ethnicity data as a single 'variable' with no guiding theory to understand what these classifications mean for that particular research context risks perpetuating ethnic inequalities, not just describing them (Nazroo, 2022). It also ignores the role of intersectionality (Crenshaw, 1991), which is a framework to understand how people's overlapping social and political identities (in terms of ethnicity, gender, age, migration status, etc.) intersect to produce their unique experiences of discrimination and privilege, due to wider, overlapping systems of oppression (racism, sexism, ageism, xenophobia, etc.) (Shannon et al., 2022). When the 2018 MBRRACE-UK report (MBRRACE Collaboration, 2018) found that Black women were five times, and Asian women were twice,[1] more likely to die in the perinatal period than white women, this was followed by the Birthrights Enquiry, which found that 'it is racism, not broken bodies' that were at the root of many of these inequities (Birthrights UK, 2022).

There is also deeper affliction within research orthodoxy and 'standard' practices that is best described by sociologist professor Gurminder Bhambra's term 'methodological whiteness' (Bhambra, 2017), which is:

> a way of reflecting on the world that fails to acknowledge the role played by race in the very structuring of that world, and of the ways in which knowledge is constructed and legitimated within it.

In our research plans, processes, and tools, there is an unwitting tendency to normalise whiteness (Rai et al., 2022) and use it as a vantage point from where to seek and situate other kinds of experiences. Published studies often cast racially-minoritised people as 'hard-to-reach' or 'seldom heard' as if to suggest that these people are somehow hidden away, making themselves quite unreachable, and therefore, the researcher has no choice but to exclude them from their project. Instead, I would encourage readers to engage with the more plausible explanation that it is in fact, researchers and academics who are 'hard-to-trust' (Islam et al., 2021). As mentioned earlier, there is a long and painful history of eugenics and medical experimentation that legitimate the distrust of medical and health research felt among racially minoritised groups. There is also ongoing structural racism within daily life and healthcare seeking (Bécares et al., 2022; Obermeyer et al., 2019; Sowemimo, 2023) so the expectation that a research project would be viewed as something isolated and estranged from these ordinary realities makes little sense.

In order to illustrate this point, we can take an example of the standard documentation routinely used to recruit participants to research studies. Often these are quite official-looking, each page stamped along the top with institutional logos, and the extensive content is written in dense, formal language that is compliant with GDPR (data protection) regulations, giving lots of detail about what participation involves and how the participant data will be handled. The imperative to protect participants and demonstrate clarity of intentions produced these institutional and regulatory requirements, but it also makes these information materials quite difficult to follow. Only people with significant social and cultural capital, fluency in English, and ultimately secure confidence that the research and the institutions that conduct it do indeed have their best interests in mind, would feel encouraged to participate. The methodological whiteness plays out here in researchers' lack of insight that these documents might look too much like other official documentation that is essentially hostile and punitive, say for example, eviction notices or immigration-related warnings (see, for example, activities leading to the Immigration Acts 2014 and 2016, which endowed a wide range of third parties responsibility for operationalising overt hostility towards 'foreigners' (Griffiths & Yeo, 2021, JCWI)). Routinised and institutionalised research processes assume an 'ideal' research participant, usually a reflection of the academic teams who design and conduct the research. Given the whiteness of the academy and funding organisations, this process can become circular and self-affirming, with little hope for change without a conscious and deliberate shift to widen membership of these institutions.

In the final section of the chapter, I give a couple of examples from my own research to illustrate how all these situations and processes become enacted in practice. It often begins with the fundamental epistemological basis of any proposed piece of research, the knowledge assumptions about that topic, which then inform plans going forward, and expectations for what we are going to learn from the work.

Reflections from learning on the job

The BP:Together study

A few years ago, I was the lead researcher on a new project to develop and optimise a health intervention for people who have had a stroke before to manage their blood pressure (poorly controlled high blood pressure is one of the biggest risk factors for repeat strokes). Study participants would be sent a blood pressure monitor and an information booklet, and would download an application (or app) onto a digital device that they owned (a phone or computer). The app was highly interactive: it would send them monthly reminders to check and enter their blood pressure, and the average reading would be sent directly to their GP, enabling medical intervention if necessary. For those without a smartphone or computer, it would work via text messaging. My role was to road test the intervention on a small sample of stroke patients and use their feedback to optimise its design and implementation processes, prior to a large randomised controlled trial (Rai et al., 2021).

Given my background in public health, I searched for the prevalence of stroke in the UK. Compared to white people, Black people are twice as likely to have strokes, and Black and Asian people, particularly those from socially deprived backgrounds, are likely to have recurrent strokes at younger ages and with worse long-term outcomes (The Stroke Association, 2018). I assumed, therefore, that there would be plans in the study protocol to recruit high numbers of Black and Asian participants to inform the intervention development, as this group would potentially have most to gain from the intervention.

However, I was told that this was a desirable but near-impossible dream – accepted wisdom was that Black and Asian people generally do not take part in research and, therefore, trying to recruit them was somewhat pointless. I was then steered to use participant recruitment methods that are used 'normally' in primary care research: GP practices in the study area are 'invited' to participate in the project, and those who express interest would run an algorithm through their patient database (using our study's inclusion/exclusion criteria). Everyone on the generated list would then be posted a study information pack by the GP practice (participant information booklet, consent form), provided by us. Those who wished to participate would then send us their signed consent form via the pre-paid envelopes provided, and we would then arrange to meet them.

Sampling and recruiting in this way yielded a very narrow demographic of participants: very quickly, we learned that almost all were elderly, highly educated, and white, many of whose strokes had occurred since retirement. This outcome emboldened me to propose an alternative set of recruitment practices to the study team, to which they thankfully agreed. I conducted extensive public outreach activities to promote the research; for example, I presented the work at religious congregations at churches and mosques (majority Black and Asian people attending), and at stroke support groups in deprived neighbourhoods. I followed up with those who showed interest through informal phone conversations to clarify the objectives of the research and explain how their input would be valued. This shift in recruitment practice had a powerful impact on securing a much more representative study sample: it now reflected the stroke population in the UK.

We did, however, fail at the larger task, which was to make the research and its outcomes more inclusive and equitable. We managed to get a 'representative' sample, but we were not prepared to truly incorporate (or even fully elicit) their perceptions about the intervention. This was for a number of related reasons – for a start, we were working within a tight timeline and budget. Once I started visiting racially minoritised participants, it became clear that the burden of research participation felt heavier for them, in terms of what they were expected to do, both linguistically and practically.

Congruent with national stroke statistics, they were often sicker, with significant cognitive and physical disability. They were less fluent in reading English and using digital devices, and needed more time to understand the purpose of the study in order to make a contribution. My task was to arrive at people's homes at the time arranged over previous phone conversations. Having exchanged pleasantries and settled down, I was to remind them about the study and show them the patient booklet, blood pressure monitor, and app. I would then invite them to 'think aloud' (part of the 'person-based approach' to intervention development (see Yardley et al., 2015) as they explored each item. After this, I had to ask them to demonstrate before me how they would use the monitor to measure their own blood pressure and enter the readings on the app.

All of the warm and trusting friendliness I had nurtured with them up until that point (through the informal phone calls and chitchat about family life) seemed to be abrasively supplanted by something that was purely transactional and business-like. The data collection processes involved felt like I had come to 'test' them. This was not just because of their post-stroke impairments affecting cognition and/or movement; their multiple intersectional social disadvantages meant that being invited to contribute in these ways to such a project was at significant odds with their lived experiences of exclusion and diminishment in regular British life. Many found the tasks quite laborious and even humiliating, as if they were being asked to perform and prove some version of good citizenship and self-competence by reading aloud the booklet and handling the BP monitor, as instructed. In contrast to the middle-class, white participants who were comfortable giving their opinions on the intervention, for racially minoritised participants living in relative poverty, this process was entirely incongruous within their day-to-day lives, and indeed, may have reminded them of more unpleasant encounters with authoritative and hostile institutional entities.

On later reflection, which we wrote up as a publication (Rai et al., 2022), we described how our study materials, processes, and expectations were steeped in methodological whiteness. It was blind to, and ignorant about, the lived realities of this set of participants and hence had no way of making accommodations for them. The BP:Together intervention did not make sense to many of the participants in the way it was presented, but we had no time to unpack this. Despite building capacity to conduct qualitative research, and even after allowing those alternative recruitment strategies, ultimately our research model was oriented towards the impending large trial, so the only responses we could work with were simple binaries – do you like this? Yes or no. Our plans were to 'optimise' the intervention, and that is as far as we went, even if it excluded the very set of people who had the most to benefit from it (Rai et al., 2022).

The NOURISH-UK study

Building on the example of the BP:Together study, I will now discuss a different qualitative research project, one that I was lucky enough to lead alongside an excellent lead researcher and study team, about how women and birthing parents living with HIV decide how to feed their babies (breast milk or formula). But first, some context: the huge medical advancements in highly effective antiretroviral treatment (ART) for HIV have meant that if people with HIV take their ART medication as prescribed such that they have an undetectable viral load they cannot pass the infection on through sex (Rodger et al., 2016). Unfortunately, the evidence so far shows that risk of vertical transmission of HIV via breast milk is not completely zero (even though it is extremely low) even when the mother/birthing parent is taking ART (Flynn et al., 2018). Low-income countries, including those within Africa and Asia, follow the World Health Organization (WHO) guidance for infant feeding in the context of maternal HIV, which recommends exclusive breastfeeding, as they see the risk from infant malnutrition and diarrhoeal disease (due to unclean water) to be significantly greater than the (small) risk of the baby acquiring HIV (WHO, 2016). By contrast, high-income countries like the UK follow their own guidance (not WHO), which recommends formula feeding as it removes all risk of HIV transmission. Since 2018, under some strict conditions, breastfeeding can be clinically supported, but this is still rare in the UK (BHIVA, 2020).

HIV clinicians in the UK routinely advise women and birthing parents to formula feed their babies. However, two-thirds of new mothers with HIV are from Black African and Caribbean diasporic communities (Peters, 2022), who also simultaneously face a strong cultural expectation to breastfeed. They are aware of the contrasting WHO guidance (due to their own transnational networks) and understand that breastfeeding avoidance within their diasporic groups can signal an HIV-positive status of the mother (McKnight, 2022). As a consequence of all this, many pregnant women and birthing parents living with HIV in the UK are placed in a difficult position regarding infant feeding (Rai et al., 2023), and through our research, we wanted to find out what was going on.

The research findings are reported elsewhere (Kasadha et al., 2024; Rai et al., 2023), but here I focus on how we designed and conducted the research, such that we did not just recruit a representative sample but also actively shaped our approach to enable listening and responding to what they told us (Kasadha et al., 2025). We were inspired by Professor Serrant-Green's Screaming Silences Framework, which examines:

> how an issue, as experienced by the listener, 'screams' out to them in relation to their health, because of its relationship or impact in their reality. Conversely, the same issue may be relatively 'silent' in the consciousness or experience of the greater majority in society, or absent from the available evidence base where it fails to have wider impact on shared aspects of health.
>
> *(Serrant-Green, 2011, p. 349)*

This framework builds on Foucauldian concepts about how knowledge, and what is recognised as knowledge, is socially constructed and shaped powerfully by the identity and positionality of those who seek to present it. It prompts deeper engagement with how the socio-political identity of researchers leading the work fundamentally shapes which (and how) data are collected, considered, interrogated, and presented. Starting from this position, we carefully assembled the core study team and the patient and public involvement (PPI) panel, such that we were an intentionally diverse set: majority non-white women who were academics, clinicians, and/or those with lived experience of HIV, advocacy, and motherhood, and included six Black women living with HIV. Our study team included members from the national committee who develop UK HIV guidelines (the British HIV Association or BHIVA) as well as colleagues with strong links to HIV clinics and third-sector organisations, who helped us recruit a representative group of pregnant and recently postpartum women living with HIV (Kasadha et al., 2024; Rai et al., 2023). Fundamental to our success was our lead researcher, who was herself a young, Black woman with a strong HIV advocacy background.

There is little room to go into detail here (see Kasadha et al. (2025) for a fuller account), but at different stages of the research process, we observed how various aspects of our team members' identities became more or less salient, rising in and out of view at different times. Similar to our participants, our own social and intersectional identities, formed by experiences of migration, minoritisation, HIV, motherhood, breastfeeding, and professional affiliations, clearly affected our contributions to the work differently at different stages. For example, the lead researcher had been a PPI contributor on other research projects, but now that she was conducting the research she wanted to ensure that she did not replicate some of damage and hurt she had experienced from academics she had collaborated with in the past.

> As a research community rep over the years, I've worked with some great people. However, I have also experienced patronising academics . . . Sometimes we [black women with HIV] are not seen as knowledgeable in anything else. In this role, which is my first academic role, I was mindful of not replicating the harms I've experienced.
>
> *(Kasadha et al., 2025, p. 6)*

We kept a keen eye on our privileged status as architects of this particular knowledge project and how that could bias what we are able to hear. For example, while we scheduled joint meetings with the whole team alongside the PPI panel, we also held separate meetings with just the PPI contributors, the researcher and myself, keeping our clinical colleagues out of that space. This meant that our PPI members could voice perspectives that may potentially elicit concern from clinicians. Our approach to participants was similar to the one we used in the BP:Together study – gradually building trust through informal and friendly contacts, taking time to explain the rationale for the study, and letting the participant make choices about how and in what ways they wished to contribute. We also presented study findings (including on a public-facing information and support website (HEXI, 2023)) in ways that signalled the intersectional and richly contextualised backgrounds of our participants, in order to situate their experiences within their living circumstances, their migration histories, their relationships with their HIV status, and familiarity with HIV community and peer-support groups. This was done in partnership with them, with attention paid to protect their anonymity.

Our interdisciplinary co-produced approach led to multiple lay (HEXI, 2023) and academic outputs (Kasadha et al., 2021, 2024a, 2024b, 2025; Rai et al., 2023), an urgent clarification in sub-policy regarding 'mixed' feeding (Gilleece et al., 2022), and contributed significantly to the newly updated national guidelines on HIV and infant feeding released in 2025 (BHIVA, 2025).

Conclusion

Examining and deconstructing historically unjust epistemic practices and methodological processes to replace them with race-conscious and socially just engagement and tools that are attuned to the historical, political, and structural realities of contemporary

British society is key to overcoming inequities in health research. We began this chapter tracing the dubious history of racial categorisation and why they persist today when studying human health. Racialisation of human populations is closely intertwined with colonial and migration histories, and the creation of modern societies where the distribution of wealth, privilege, and health is unequal. The strong association between race/ethnicity and health means that despite the many problems with these categories, they cannot be abandoned, but we need to keep developing more intelligent, theoretically rigorous, and thoughtful ways of working with them. Race/ethnicity often serves as a euphemism for racism, and there is evidence about how racism sustained and accumulated over decades and generations does indeed start to appear as measurable biological changes (Gravlee, 2009).

Structural racism within social and professional elite groups and hierarchies means the funders and leaders of health research, and political forces that shape national priorities, include only those within very narrow social demographics and do not reflect the UK population. Despite recent ideological shifts towards more inclusive attitudes and research planning frameworks (for example, the National Institute of Health and Care Research's INCLUDE frameworks [NIHR-INCLUDE]), limited perspectives about health and healthcare challenges and the epistemological and practical assumptions and choices made thereof introduce racialised biases in priority setting for research and plans for how research should be conducted. The teams, tools, and processes we employ in research suffer from methodological whiteness that may appear benign in day-to-day work (there is usually no overt or interpersonally-expressed racism) but have powerful potential to deepen existing racialised inequities in health. Furthermore, the poor theorisation about racialised patterning of health issues stems from a reductive, 'risk factor' view of race/ethnicity, as if they are discrete, static, and water-tight categories with rigid boundaries that are scientifically meaningful and unaffected by any of the social, environmental, and other stressors that are known to affect human health. The increasing use of artificial intelligence in risk prediction models, which are informed by race-based parameters and may determine future guidance about healthcare pathways and the allocation of scarce resources for different patient profiles, runs the veritable risk of baking in racial inequities in ways that eventually fall completely out of view.

Through my reflections on the BP:Together study, I illustrated how sometimes racial discrimination happens inadvertently due to routinised and normalised research practices which have been developed for an idealised participant who is often a reflection of the research team themselves: highly educated, confident in the English language, well-versed in their rights as a citizen, and white. While we took some steps to redress the effect of these shortcomings in our research materials and plans, the basic epistemological premise of the study and output designs could not accommodate the full spectrum of experiences of stroke patients, ironically excluding the very groups that had the most to benefit from the research, that is, economically poor and/or Black people, who are at greatest risk of strokes at young ages. In the NOURISH-UK study, we took a different approach from the start: by identifying the core study team and PPI team who had appropriate expertise and experience about the research topic, by planning the structure and nature of meetings that created space for marginalised perspectives to be voiced, and by establishing links with community-based organisations with long-standing links with the groups affected. Rather than 'doing diversity' as an afterthought or an add-on to the *real* work, we made it an integral part of the work. We also reflected upon our own intersectional identities and what we would, alone and collectively, bring to the work and what we might miss. The Screaming Silences theory helped us see where we needed to go, as well as acknowledge the limits of our work.

Honesty, integrity, and reflexivity are core values for those doing health research, especially when looking at racialised inequities. There is a fundamental need to name racism and the many forms it takes, both in the people we conduct research on and on the structures of research and academic institutions and funding bodies that control the flow of work and resources. A shared commitment between academics, funders, clinicians, and health policy makers is necessary in order to make long-term, meaningful, and sustainable changes such that health research is truly generative and valuable for all, without replicating or exaggerating existing racialised inequalities.

At the time of writing, the United States is in the process of rolling back multiple important health equity endeavours and investments, both in country and abroad, at breathtaking speed. These are health programmes and collaborations that have taken decades to establish and operationalise and have now been violently uprooted and defunded by a racist and callous government that wishes only to reward and protect the futures of the most privileged. There is no guarantee that this shift in direction would not happen in the UK, with some signs already appearing of increasing xenophobia and white nationalist extremism, which does not tolerate the protection or equal rights granted to those not racialised as white. It is, therefore, more vital and urgent than ever to engage with these issues and demand racially just approaches to be embedded deeply in health research.

Discussion questions

1. In your work (or studies), do you recall any situations where racialised health patterns or behaviours have been observed or commented on? What were the explanations given for why a particular ethnic group demonstrated that behaviour?
2. Think about how you understand the world. We all have our own blind spots – what are yours? Who are the social groupings about whose life experiences you understand very little?

Note

1 These figures have been revised in more recent MBRRACE reports. In the 2024 report, there was a nearly three-fold difference in maternal mortality rates amongst women from Black ethnic backgrounds and an almost two-fold difference amongst women from Asian ethnic backgrounds compared to White Women.

Further reading

Gunaratnam, Y. (2003). *Researching Race and Ethnicity: Methods, Knowledge and Power.* Sage.

Hirsch, A. (2018). *Brit(ish): On Race, Identity and Belonging.* Vintage.

Rutherford, A. (2023). *The Dark History of Genetics.* The Royal Institution Haldane Lecture. https://www.youtube.com/watch?v=Gddkc5Snq3I

Saini, A. (2019). *Superior: The Return of Race Science.* Fourth Estate.

References

Amutah, C., Greenidge, K., Mante, A., Munyikwa, M., Surya, S. L., Higginbotham, E., Jones, D. S., Lavizzo-Mourey, R., Roberts, D., Tsai, J., & Aysola, J. (2021). Misrepresenting Race – The Role of Medical Schools in Propagating Physician Bias. *New England Journal of Medicine*, *384*(9), 872–878. https://doi.org/10.1056/NEJMms2025768

Ansari-Thomas, Z. (2024). Immigration and intergenerational co-residency among working-aged adults in the United Kingdom. *Journal of Family Issues*, *45*(3), 744–769. https://doi.org/10.1177/0192513x231155660

Beam, A. L., & Kohane, I. S. (2018). Big data and machine learning in health care. *JAMA*, *319*(13), 1317–1318. https://doi.org/10.1001/jama.2017.18391

Bécares, L., Nazroo, J., & Kelly, Y. (2015). A longitudinal examination of maternal, family, and area-level experiences of racism on children's socioemotional development: Patterns and possible explanations. *Social Science & Medicine*, *142*, 128–135. https://doi.org/10.1016/j.socscimed.2015.08.025

Bécares, L., Shaw, R. J., Katikireddi, S. V., Irizar, P., Amele, S., Kapadia, D., Nazroo, J., & Taylor, H. (2022). Racism as the fundamental cause of ethnic inequities in COVID-19 vaccine hesitancy: A theoretical framework and empirical exploration using the UK Household longitudinal study. *SSM Popul Health*, *19*, 101150. https://doi.org/10.1016/j.ssmph.2022.101150

Bhambra, G. K. (2017). Brexit, Trump, and 'methodological whiteness': On the misrecognition of race and class. *The British Journal of Sociology*, *68*(S1), S214–S232. https://doi.org/10.1111/1468-4446.12317

BHIVA. (2020). *BHIVA Guidelines for the Management of HIV in Pregnancy and Postpartum 2018 (2020 Third Interim Update) [Online]*. https://www.bhiva.org/pregnancy-guidelines

BHIVA. (2025). *BHIVA Guidelines on the Management of HIV in Pregnancy and the Postpartum Period 2025*. https://bhiva.org/clinical-guideline/pregnancy-guidelines/

Birthrights UK. (2022). *Systemic Racism, Not Broken Bodies: An Inquiry into Racial Injustice and Human Rights in UK Maternity Care*. https://birthrights.org.uk/wp-content/uploads/2022/05/Birthrights-inquiry-systemic-racism_exec-summary_May-22-web.pdf

Butt, J., & Cooper Stubbs, H. (2025). *Exploring Ethnicity Data Use and Gaps in Health Care*. Race Equality Foundation. https://raceequalityfoundation.org.uk/wp-content/uploads/2025/11/Exploring-Ethnicity-Data-Use-and-Gaps-in-Health-Care-2025.pdf

Cerdeña, J. P., Plaisime, M. V., & Tsai, J. (2020). From race-based to race-conscious medicine: How anti-racist uprisings call us to act. *The Lancet*, *396*(10257), 1125–1128. https://doi.org/10.1016/S0140-6736(20)32076-6

Chen, I. Y., Pierson, E., Rose, S., Joshi, S., Ferryman, K., & Ghassemi, M. (2021). Ethical machine learning in healthcare. *Annual Review of Biomedical Data Science*, *4*, 123–144. https://doi.org/10.1146/annurev-biodatasci-092820-114757

Crenshaw, K. (1991). Mapping the margins: Intersectionality, identity politics, and violence against women of color. *Stanford Law Review*, *43*(6), 1241–1299. https://doi.org/10.2307/1229039

Fawzy, A., Wu, T. D., Wang, K., Robinson, M. L., Farha, J., Bradke, A., Golden, S. H., Xu, Y., & Garibaldi, B. T. (2022). Racial and ethnic discrepancy in pulse oximetry and delayed identification of treatment eligibility among patients with COVID-19. *JAMA Internal Medicine*, *182*(7), 730–738. https://doi.org/10.1001/jamainternmed.2022.1906

Finney, N., Nazroo, J., Bécares, L., Kapadia, D., & Shlomo, N. (2023). *Racism and Ethnic Inequality in a Time of Crisis: Findings from the Evidence for Equality National Survey* (1 ed.). Bristol University Press. https://doi.org/10.2307/jj.3279115

Flynn, P. M., Taha, T. E., Cababasay, M., Fowler, M. G., Mofenson, L. M., Owor, M., Fiscus, S., Stranix-Chibanda, L., Coutsoudis, A., Gnanashanmugam, D., Chakhtoura, N., McCarthy, K., Mukuzunga, C., Makanani, B., Moodley, D., Nematadzira, T., Kusakara, B., Patil, S., Vhembo, T., . . . Team, t. P. S. (2018). Prevention of HIV-1 transmission through breastfeeding: Efficacy and safety of maternal antiretroviral therapy versus infant nevirapine prophylaxis for duration of breastfeeding in HIV-1-infected women with high CD4 cell count (IMPAACT PROMISE): A randomized, open-label, clinical trial. *JAIDS Journal of Acquired Immune Deficiency Syndromes*, 77(4), 383–392. https://doi.org/10.1097/qai.0000000000001612

Gilleece, Y., Byrne, L., Bamford, A., Lyall, H., Seery, P., & Tariq, S. (2022). *Interim BHIVA Position Statement on HIV and Mixed Infant Feeding*. https://bhiva.org/wp-content/uploads/2024/10/BHIVA-position-statement-on-HIV-and-mixed-infant-feeding.pdf

Gov.UK. (2024). *Stop and Search*. https://www.ethnicity-facts-figures.service.gov.uk/crime-justice-and-the-law/policing/stop-and-search/latest/

Gravlee, C. C. (2009). How race becomes biology: Embodiment of social inequality. *American Journal of Physical Anthropology*, *139*(1), 47–57. https://doi.org/10.1002/ajpa.20983

Griffiths, M., & Yeo, C. (2021). The UK's hostile environment: Deputising immigration control. *Critical Social Policy*, *41*(4), 521–544. https://doi.org/10.1177/0261018320980653

Gunaratnam, Y. (2003). *Researching Race and Ethnicity: Methods, Knowledge and Power*. Sage.

Hackett, R. A., Ronaldson, A., Bhui, K., Steptoe, A., & Jackson, S. E. (2020). Racial discrimination and health: A prospective study of ethnic minorities in the United Kingdom. *BMC Public Health*, *20*(1), 1652. https://doi.org/10.1186/s12889-020-09792-1

Haney Lopez, I. (1994). The social construction of race: Some observations on illusion, fabrication and choice. *Harvard Civil Rights-Civil Liberties Law Review*, *29*, 1–62.

Hayanga, B., Stafford, M., & Bécares, L. (2023). Ethnic inequalities in multiple long-term health conditions in the United Kingdom: A systematic review and narrative synthesis. *BMC Public Health*, *23*(1), 178. https://doi.org/10.1186/s12889-022-14940-w

HEXI. (2023). *Feeding a Baby While Living with HIV*. University of Oxford. https://hexi.ox.ac.uk/Feeding-a-baby-while-living-with-HIV/overview

ICNARC. (2020). *ICNARC Report on COVID-19 in Critical Care 31 July 2020*. https://www.icnarc.org/DataServices/Attachments/Download/42ceb4d2-3dd3-ea11-9128-00505601089b

Islam, S., Joseph, O., Chaudry, A., Forde, D., Keane, A., Wilson, C., Begum, N., Parsons, S., Grey, T., Holmes, L., & Starling, B. (2021). "We are not hard to reach, but we may find it hard to trust". . . . Involving and engaging 'seldom listened to' community voices in clinical translational health research: A social innovation approach. *Research Involvement and Engagement*, 7(1), 46. https://doi.org/10.1186/s40900-021-00292-z

JCWI. *The Hostile Environment Explained*. The Joint Council for the Welfare of Immigrants. https://jcwi.org.uk/reportsbriefings/the-hostile-environment-explained/

Jeffery, A., Gascoigne, C., Dykxhoorn, J., Blangiardo, M., Geneletti, S., Baio, G., & Kirkbride, J. B. (2024). The effect of immigration policy reform on mental health in people from minoritised ethnic groups in England: An interrupted time series analysis of longitudinal data from the UK Household Longitudinal Study cohort. *The Lancet Psychiatry*, *11*(3), 183–192. https://doi.org/10.1016/S2215-0366(23)00412-1

Jones, C. P. (2000). Levels of racism: A theoretic framework and a gardener's tale. *American Journal of Public Health*, *90*(8), 1212–1215. https://doi.org/10.2105/ajph.90.8.1212

Kasadha, B., Hinton, L., Tariq, S., Nyatsanza, F., Namiba, A., Freeman-Romilly, N., & Rai, T. (2024a). How women living with HIV in the UK manage infant-feeding decisions and vertical transmission risk – a qualitative study. *BMC Public Health*, *24*(1), 2130. https://doi.org/10.1186/s12889-024-19581-9

Kasadha, B., Tariq, S., Freeman-Romilly, N., Pope, C., Namiba, A., Nyatsanza, F., Hinton, L., & Rai, T. (2024b). "We decided together": A qualitative study about women with HIV navigating infant-feeding decisions with the father of their children. *BMC Pregnancy Childbirth*, *24*(1), 41. https://doi.org/10.1186/s12884-023-06198-w

Kasadha, B., Tariq, S., Namiba, A., Freeman-Romilly, N., Moepi, N., Letting, G., & Rai, T. (2025). Hearing the silence and silenced: Co-producing research on infant-feeding experiences and practices with Black women with HIV. *Sociology of Health & Illness*, *47*(1), e13871. https://doi.org/10.1111/1467-9566.13871

Kasadha, B., Tariq, S., Nyatsanza, F., Freeman-Romilly, N., Namiba, A., & Rai, T. (2021). Stakeholder engagement is essential to maximise the impact of research on infant feeding in the context of HIV. *Therapeutic Advances in Infectious Disease*, *8*, 20499361211057970. https://doi.org/10.1177/20499361211057970

Kass, N. E. (2001). An ethics framework for public health. *American Journal of Public Health*, *91*(11), 1776–1782. https://doi.org/10.2105/ajph.91.11.1776

Kidney Research UK. (2021). *Ethnicity Adjustment for Kidney Function Testing Removed from NICE Chronic Kidney Disease Guideline*. Kidney Research UK. https://www.kidneyresearchuk.org/2021/08/25/ethnicity-adjustment-for-kidney-function-testing-removed-from-nice-chronic-kidney-disease-guideline/

Krieger, N. (2012). Methods for the scientific study of discrimination and health: An ecosocial approach. *American Journal of Public Health*, *102*(5), 936–944. https://doi.org/10.2105/ajph.2011.300544

Lenzer, J. (2006). Secret report surfaces showing that Pfizer was at fault in Nigerian drug tests. *BMJ*, *332*(7552), 1233. https://doi.org/10.1136/bmj.332.7552.1233-a

MBRRACE Collaboration. (2018). *Saving Lives, Improving Mothers' Care 2018*. MBRRACE-UK, National Perinatal Epidemiology Unit, University of Oxford. https://www.npeu.ox.ac.uk/assets/downloads/mbrrace-uk/reports/MBRRACE-UK%20Maternal%20Report%202018%20-%20Web%20Version.pdf

McKnight, U. (2022). Replacement feeding and the HIV Diaspora: A case of ontological multiplicity and fluid technologies. *Sociology of Health & Illness*, *44*(1), 169–187. https://doi.org/10.1111/1467-9566.13405

McVean, A. (2019). *40 Years of Human Experimentation in America: The Tuskegee Study*. Office for Science and Society, McGill University, Canada. https://www.mcgill.ca/oss/article/history/40-years-human-experimentation-america-tuskegee-study

Mirza, H., & Warwick, R. (2022). *Race and Ethnicity* (IFS Deaton Review of Inequalities, Issue). https://ifs.org.uk/inequality/wp-content/uploads/2022/11/Race-and-ethnicity-IFS-Deaton-Review-of-Inequalities.pdf

Mondon, A., & Winter, A. (2019). Whiteness, populism and the racialisation of the working class in the United Kingdom and the United States. *Identities*, *26*(5), 510–528. https://doi.org/10.1080/1070289X.2018.1552440

Moons, K. G., Altman, D. G., Vergouwe, Y., & Royston, P. (2009). Prognosis and prognostic research: Application and impact of prognostic models in clinical practice. *BMJ*, *338*, b606. https://doi.org/10.1136/bmj.b606

Naicker, R. (2024). *Critically Appraising for Antiracism*. https://www.criticallyappraisingantiracism.org/

Nazroo, J. (2022). *Race/ethnic Inequalities in Health: Moving beyond Confusion to Focus on Fundamental Causes*' (IFS Deaton Review of Inequalities, Issue). https://ifs.org.uk/inequality/wp-content/uploads/2022/11/Race-health-inequalities-final-IFS-Deaton-Review-Inequality.pdf

NIH. (2003). *The Human Genome Project*. NIH National Human Genome Research Institute. https://www.genome.gov/human-genome-project

NIHR-INCLUDE. https://www.nihr.ac.uk/about-us/who-we-are/research-inclusion/making-research-inclusive

Obermeyer, Z., Powers, B., Vogeli, C., & Mullainathan, S. (2019). Dissecting racial bias in an algorithm used to manage the health of populations. *Science*, *366*(6464), 447–453. https://doi.org/10.1126/science.aax2342

Omi, M., & Winant, H. (2014). *Racial Formation in the United States* (3rd ed.). Routledge.

Peters, H. (2022). *ISOSS Pregnancy Characteristics and Outcomes of Women with Vertically-Acquired HIV in the UK*. BHIVA Spring Conference, Manchester.

Phelan, J. C., & Link, B. G. (2015). Is Racism a Fundamental Cause of Inequalities in Health? *Annual Review of Sociology*, *41*(1), 311–330. https://doi.org/10.1146/annurev-soc-073014-112305

Powell, R. A., Njoku, C., Elangovan, R., Sathyamoorthy, G., Ocloo, J., Thayil, S., & Rao, M. (2022). Tackling racism in UK health research. *BMJ*, *376*, e065574. https://doi.org/10.1136/bmj-2021-065574

Rai, T., Hinton, L., McManus, R. J., & Pope, C. (2022). What would it take to meaningfully attend to ethnicity and race in health research? Learning from a trial intervention development study. *Sociology of Health & Illness*, *44*(S1), 57–72. https://doi.org/10.1111/1467-9566.13431

Rai, T., Kasadha, B., Tariq, S., Keating, S., Hinton, L., Namiba, A., & Pope, C. (2023). Infant feeding as a transgressive practice in the context of HIV in the UK: A qualitative interview study. *Women's Studies International Forum*, *101*, 102834. https://doi.org/10.1016/j.wsif.2023.102834

Rai, T., Morton, K., Roman, C., Doogue, R., Rice, C., Williams, M., Schwartz, C., Velardo, C., Tarassenko, L., Yardley, L., McManus, R. J., & Hinton, L. (2021). Optimizing a digital intervention for managing blood pressure in stroke patients using a diverse sample: Integrating the person-based approach and patient and public involvement. *Health Expect*, *24*(2), 327–340. https://doi.org/10.1111/hex.13173

Raleigh, V. (2023). *The Health of People from Ethnic Minority Groups in England*. The King's Fund. https://www.kingsfund.org.uk/insight-and-analysis/long-reads/health-people-ethnic-minority-groups-england

Rhodes, J., & Hall, N.-A. (2020). Racism, nationalism and the politics of resentment in contemporary England. In *Routledge International Handbook of Contemporary Racisms* (1st ed.). Routledge. https://www.taylorfrancis.com/chapters/edit/10.4324/9781351047326-22/racism-nationalism-politics-resentment-contemporary-england-james-rhodes-natalie-anne-hall

Roberts, D. E. (2017). What's race got to do with medicine? In *TED*. https://www.npr.org/transcripts/514150399

Rodger, A. J., Cambiano, V., Bruun, T., Vernazza, P., Collins, S., van Lunzen, J., Corbelli, G. M., Estrada, V., Geretti, A. M., Beloukas, A., Asboe, D., Viciana, P., Gutiérrez, F., Clotet, B., Pradier, C., Gerstoft, J., Weber, R., Westling, K., Wandeler, G., . . . Group, F. T. P. S. (2016). Sexual activity without condoms and risk of HIV transmission in serodifferent couples when the HIV-positive partner is using suppressive antiretroviral therapy. *JAMA*, *316*(2), 171–181. https://doi.org/10.1001/jama.2016.5148

Rodriguez, M. A., & García, R. (2013). First, do no harm: The US sexually transmitted disease experiments in Guatemala. *American Journal of Public Health*, *103*(12), 2122–2126. https://doi.org/10.2105/ajph.2013.301520

The Runnymede Trust. (2020). *The Colour of Money*. T. R. Trust. https://www.runnymedetrust.org/publications/the-colour-of-money

Rutherford, A. (2021a). *How to Argue with a Racist: History, Science, Race and Reality*. W&N.

Rutherford, A. (2021b). *Race, Genomes & Data: The Bias Built into Science*. Centre for Personalised Medicine, University of Oxford. https://cpm.ox.ac.uk/revisiting-2021-annual-lecture-by-dr-adam-rutherford/

Saini, A. (2019). *Superior: The Return of Race Science*. Fourth Estate.

Serrant-Green, L. (2011). The sound of 'silence': A framework for researching sensitive issues or marginalised perspectives in health. *Journal of Research in Nursing*, *16*(4), 347–360. https://doi.org/10.1177/1744987110387741

Shannon, G., Morgan, R., Zeinali, Z., Brady, L., Couto, M. T., Devakumar, D., Eder, B., Karadag, O., Mukherjee, M., Peres, M. F. T., Ryngelblum, M., Sabharwal, N., Schonfield, A., Silwane, P., Singh, D., Van Ryneveld, M., Vilakati, S., Watego, C., Whyle, E., & Muraya, K. (2022). Intersectional insights into racism and health: Not just a question of identity. *The Lancet*, *400*(10368), 2125–2136. https://doi.org/10.1016/S0140-6736(22)02304-2

Sowemimo, A. (2023). *Divided: Racism, Medicine and Why We Need to Decolonise Healthcare*. Profile Books Ltd.

The Stroke Association. (2018). *State of the Nation: Stroke Statistics*. https://www.stroke.org.uk/sites/default/files/state_of_the_nation_2018.pdf

UK Kidney Association. (2021). *The Rationale for Removing Adjustment for Ethnicity From eGFRcreatinine and Recommendations for Implementation of the Change in Practice*. https://www.ukkidney.org/sites/renal.org/files/guidelines/Rationale_and_recommendations_for_implementation_NICE%20CKD%20Guideline%202021.pdf

Vyas, D. A., Eisenstein, L. G., & Jones, D. S. (2020). Hidden in Plain Sight – Reconsidering the Use of Race Correction in Clinical Algorithms. *New England Journal of Medicine*, *383*(9), 874–882. https://doi.org/10.1056/NEJMms2004740

WHO. (2016). *Infant Feeding for the Prevention of Mother-to-Child Transmission of HIV*. Geneva: World Health Organization.

Williams, D. R. (1997). Race and Health: Basic Questions, Emerging Directions. *Annals of Epidemiology*, *7*(5), 322–333. https://doi.org/10.1016/S1047-2797(97)00051-3

Yardley, L., Ainsworth, B., Arden-Close, E., & Muller, I. (2015). The person-based approach to enhancing the acceptability and feasibility of interventions. *Pilot and Feasibility Studies*, *1*, 37. https://doi.org/10.1186/s40814-015-0033-z

CHAPTER 4

Artificial intelligence (AI) and racial health equity

Promise and peril

Mohammad Sharif Razai and Shobhana Nagraj

Introduction

Leveraging artificial intelligence's (AI's) capacity for vast data analysis, this chapter discusses how AI could improve diagnostic accuracy, streamline treatment decisions, and potentially democratise health access across diverse demographics. However, it also examines ethical concerns associated with AI, such as perpetuating existing biases, infringing on patient privacy, and compromising care quality.

We discuss the importance of developing explainable and transparent AI systems that foster trust among both ethnic minority patients and healthcare professionals. It emphasises the necessity of embedding fairness and inclusivity in AI design to mitigate algorithmic biases that could reinforce health inequalities. We call for the safe deployment of AI with ongoing evaluation to protect patient well-being and uphold ethical principles.

The inclusion of diverse datasets is crucial for preventing systemic biases. Equitable access to AI requires the development of user-friendly technologies and targeted efforts to improve health literacy and digital access across diverse communities. This includes creating culturally sensitive educational programmes tailored to the needs of ethnic minority groups, enabling them to benefit fully from AI advancements in healthcare.

Additionally, we discuss AI's implications for patient data privacy and governance, stressing the importance of secure and ethical data handling practices to maintain patient trust. It explores the balance between AI's efficiency and the autonomy of healthcare professionals, advocating for AI as a tool to augment, rather than replace, human expertise in healthcare.

To navigate these challenges responsibly, we need interdisciplinary collaboration, effective regulatory frameworks, and engagement from patients, the public, healthcare professionals, and other stakeholders. This will ensure that AI can be safely and effectively integrated into healthcare systems.

DOI: 10.4324/9781003466093-7

This chapter provides students, health professionals, and policymakers with an introduction to the role of AI in ethnic health inequalities. By the end, readers will have a better appreciation of the complexities of integrating AI into healthcare systems and the critical need for an ethical approach to its design, evaluation, and implementation.

Health inequalities in the UK

Health inequalities in the UK are long-standing and deeply rooted in the country's social, economic, and political history. Compared to white people, those from ethnic minority groups face a range of disparities throughout their life course in health outcomes as well as access to experiences of and satisfaction with healthcare services (Kapadia et al., 2022). However, the full extent of ethnic health disparities remains unclear due to a lack of high-quality data and a historical failure to record ethnicity consistently within the health service (Razai et al., 2021).

A major contributor to these disparities is socioeconomic deprivation, which disproportionately affects minoritised communities (Ministry of Housing, Communities and Local Government, 2020; UK Government, 2020). Deprivation is intertwined with broader structural issues, such as systemic racism, which manifests in housing, education, employment, and the criminal justice system, further exacerbating health inequalities (Razai et al., 2021). Moreover, evidence shows that racism and discrimination can directly harm the physical and mental health of minorities (Williams et al., 2019). Race is widely regarded as a social construct created by societies to categorise people according to perceived physical characteristics such as skin colour and facial features. These classifications have been used historically to organise social hierarchies and distribute power and resources (Braveman & Parker Dominguez, 2021). The COVID-19 pandemic dramatically revealed these structural disadvantages and likely accelerated and widened health inequalities, with its economic and social impacts continuing to unfold. These factors operate across multiple dimensions – including protected characteristics, socioeconomic status, and geography – and intersect in ways that further intensify health inequities (Robertson et al., 2021).

Tackling entrenched inequalities requires a multidimensional and systemic approach, including integrating novel technological solutions. While digital health innovations (Wadhawan et al., 2023), particularly those driven by AI, hold promise for transforming healthcare, they also bring challenges. AI is defined as 'a cross-disciplinary approach to understanding, modelling, and replicating intelligence and cognitive processes invoking various computational, mathematical, logical, mechanical, and even biological principles and devices' (Frankish & Ramsey, 2014). It has shown potential in several key areas of health, such as improving diagnostic accuracy, streamlining treatment processes, predicting risks, personalising treatments, and democratising access to healthcare by bringing advanced tools to underserved communities (Joshi & Morley, 2019). However, the effectiveness of these technologies is highly dependent on the quality and inclusiveness of the data on which they are based (O'Brien et al., 2022), how these data are generated, coded, and the clinical processes that lead to their use in patient care (Moore, 2022). Without careful consideration of potential challenges, there is a danger that AI could prolong and even amplify health inequalities (Moore, 2022). Therefore, this chapter discusses both the promises and perils of AI in achieving racial health equity in the UK.

AI technologies in healthcare

AI is likely to transform healthcare by leveraging vast amounts of data to increase the accuracy, efficiency, and accessibility of medical services (OECD, 2024). AI systems that use computer algorithms such as machine learning (ML) can learn and improve from data, enabling them to perform complex tasks autonomously. For instance, online shopping platforms analyse browsing and purchase history to suggest products. Banks use ML to detect fraud by identifying unusual spending patterns, such as a sudden large transaction in another country. Navigation apps, including Google Maps, predict traffic and suggest the best routes based on real-time and historical data. This capability can be powerful in healthcare, where AI, combined with big data, can automate disease prevention, diagnosis, and treatment processes, leading to more personalised and effective patient care (Komorowski et al., 2018). However, to perform specific tasks, algorithms are trained on large datasets, tested for accuracy, and fine-tuned to improve performance.

AI in healthcare can be categorised into predictive and generative types based on their functions. Predictive AI forecasts outcomes, detects patterns, and identifies risks using existing data. Generative AI creates new data, mimicking original datasets. In clinical settings, predictive AI is increasingly used in areas such as medical imaging, where it assists in analysing radiological images, histopathology slides, and dermatological scans, as well as in providing cancer risk prediction (Arasu et al., 2023; Hogarty et al., 2020; Hosny et al., 2018; Kumar et al., 2023; Niazi et al., 2019). It is also integrated into clinical decision-support systems to provide healthcare professionals with real-time insights and recommendations based on patient data to enhance the precision of diagnostics and treatment plans (Joshi & Morley, 2019). Operationally, predictive AI contributes to the efficiency of healthcare systems through automated tools that optimise tasks like staff scheduling and patient flow management. These applications could reduce patient waiting times and improve the overall operational efficiency of healthcare facilities (Joshi & Morley, 2019). Emerging evidence shows that generative AI is also used in healthcare. Its primary applications include providing health-related insights, answering questions, and assisting in disease diagnosis and prediction. Benefits include rapid access to information and improved accuracy in prediction and diagnosis. However, these tools also generated inaccurate or fictional content and fake references and had lower accuracy in answering complex questions (Moulaei et al., 2024).

Reflecting the growing role of AI in healthcare, the UK Government made substantial investments, committing £144 million to AI technologies to enhance diagnostics and healthcare outcomes across the UK (Smith et al., 2023; UK Government, 2025). Furthermore, increasing investment in AI research is expected to drive the development of innovative interventions aimed at further improving healthcare delivery (NIHR, 2023).

AI in ethnic minority healthcare: Risk, bias, and inequality

While AI in healthcare presents risks for all, ethnic minorities face increased vulnerabilities due to socioeconomic disparities and historical biases, which can result in AI models reinforcing and amplifying existing inequalities (Eubanks, 2018). For example, a study found that AI algorithms used for chest X-ray pathology classification consistently underdiagnosed underserved populations, with higher rates of underdiagnosis in intersectional subgroups, such as Hispanic women (Seyyed-Kalantari et al., 2021). In addition, a UK study showed that most publicly available datasets for eye conditions originate from Asia, North America, and Europe, underrepresenting some populations. Moreover, diseases such as glaucoma, diabetic retinopathy, and age-related macular degeneration are disproportionately included, while key demographic factors like age, sex, and ethnicity are often poorly reported (Khan et al., 2021).

AI risks for the general population include data privacy concerns, lack of transparency, and the diminution of human oversight in clinical decision-making. As AI systems rely on large datasets, there is a risk of data breaches, misuse, or commercial exploitation of sensitive health information. Given that healthcare data are highly personal, any privacy breach could have severe ethical and legal implications, potentially undermining trust in healthcare providers and systems (House of Commons Science, Innovation and Technology Committee, 2024).

Additionally, the transparency and explainability of AI decisions – or the lack thereof – pose critical risks. Many generative and predictive AI systems, particularly those using deep learning, operate as 'black boxes', where the decision-making process is not easily interpretable by humans. This opacity can make it challenging for healthcare providers to understand, trust, and use AI-driven recommendations (House of Commons Science, Innovation and Technology Committee, 2024). When AI systems make decisions that affect patient care, the inability to explain these decisions undermines accountability and complicates the ethical landscape of medical practice. Furthermore, the increasing reliance on AI in healthcare could reduce the human element of patient care (OECD, 2024). While AI could improve efficiency and support clinical decision-making, over-reliance on AI tools may diminish the role of human judgment and empathy in healthcare. This could negatively impact patient-provider relationships, patient satisfaction, and overall care quality. Additionally, there is a concern that healthcare professionals might lose critical skills as they may become overly dependent on AI for tasks that traditionally require their expertise (Razai et al., 2024).

The economic implications of AI adoption in healthcare must also be considered. While AI promises efficiency gains, it also raises concerns about job displacement, particularly for roles that AI systems might replace. With recent UK Government (2022a) legislation to move the NHS towards net zero targets, AI algorithms can both generate a substantial carbon footprint and have the potential to reduce this footprint (Wolf et al., 2022). The AI's carbon footprint is due to the computational power required for data processing, model training, and deployment. The energy demands of data centres, often reliant on non-renewable energy sources, contribute to these emissions. Conversely, AI can reduce the NHS's carbon footprint by optimising resource allocation, minimising waste, and improving patient flow management. Additionally, the high costs associated with developing, implementing, and maintaining AI technologies could strain healthcare providers, especially in deprived areas, a pattern that became more evident during the COVID-19 pandemic, widening the gap in healthcare access and quality.

A survey of over 1,500 UK households in 2023 revealed that nearly half of families with children lacked the necessary digital skills or access to devices, data, and broadband, with minority ethnic groups particularly disadvantaged. Ethnic minority families were twice as likely to fall below the digital inclusion threshold (Yates et al., 2024). The report highlighted the need for coordinated efforts across public, private, and voluntary sectors to address these disparities and ensure digital equity. Additionally, according to UK Ofcom (2024), 26% of households struggle to afford broadband and other communication services, making digital exclusion a serious barrier to education, employment, and overall well-being, especially for minority ethnic and low-income households. Furthermore, the NHS Race and Health Observatory also noted that while there were few documented ethnic differences in attitudes towards digital health apps, ethnic minorities may use these apps less frequently due to mistrust of how government agencies use data. Older ethnic minorities face additional challenges due to limited access to digital devices, lack of digital literacy, and language barriers (Kapadia et al., 2022).

Ethnic minorities face specific risks at each stage of AI development, from research (problem selection, data collection, and defining outcomes) to algorithm development and AI deployment (integrating AI models into practical applications) (Chen et al., 2021). A critical challenge lies in the prioritisation of research questions, as funding decisions are often influenced by societal biases. For example, in the UK, sickle cell disease (SCD), which primarily affects Black people, receives less than half the funding of cystic fibrosis (CF), which predominantly affects White populations, despite SCD being more common. According to a UK parliamentary report (UK Parliament, 2022), between 2017 and 2022, 130 CF studies were funded, compared to only 54 for SCD. A similar pattern is seen in the USA, where SCD receives 3.5 times less funding than CF (Strouse et al., 2013). This disparity can influence the development of AI technologies, leading to solutions that may not adequately tackle the healthcare needs of minority groups.

The lack of diversity in research teams and leadership roles within healthcare and research institutions further exacerbates these issues. In the UK, ethnic minorities are underrepresented in academia and healthcare leadership. For instance, in 2022, 13% of NHS board members were from ethnic minorities, while 24% of the NHS workforce were from these groups (NHS, 2022). In 2023, out of 22,345 university professors in the UK who declared their ethnicity, only 210 (0.9%) were Black according to Higher Education Statistics Agency (HESA, 2024). This underrepresentation of ethnic minorities in senior and leadership positions, who are typically the key decision-makers in research and development, means that the perspectives and needs of minoritised communities may not be adequately considered. In addition, data from the USA show that diversity in AI researchers and developers remains low. Women account for less than 18% of AI PhD graduates in North America and only 16% of tenure-track computer science faculty worldwide. In 2019, among new US resident AI PhD graduates, 45% were White, 22.4% Asian, 3.2% Hispanic, and only 2.4% African American. Over the past decade, White (non-Hispanic) graduates have consistently made up around 62.7% of computing PhDs, while Black and Hispanic graduates averaged just 3.1% and 3.3%, respectively (AI Index Steering Committee, 2021).

The lack of accurate and consistent ethnicity data in NHS healthcare systems presents further problems. In 2019/20, 87% of inpatient admissions had a valid ethnicity code, but 8.5% were marked as 'not stated' and 8.8% as 'other', making them unsuitable for analysis (NHS Race & Health Observatory, 2021). Records without ethnicity codes were not evenly distributed between ethnic groups, and specific minority ethnic groups were underrepresented in health data compared to national population estimates by ethnicity. In contrast, 'other' ethnicity codes were over-represented, with records of patients from ethnic minorities being less likely to be recorded consistently over time or have a specific code. These inconsistencies, particularly prevalent among minority groups, introduce bias into health data analysis, undermining the reliability of these records (NHS Race & Health Observatory, 2021). Building on this, previous studies have revealed major discrepancies in ethnicity data within NHS databases. In one study, for minority ethnic patients, there was a 20–30% discordance between self-reported ethnicity and that recorded in the NHS Hospital Episode Statistics (HES) database, compared to just 2.2% for White British patients (Saunders et al., 2013). Additionally, another study found discordance between ethnicity coding in the HES and the Clinical Research Practice Datalink for over 50% of ethnic minority patients, highlighting inconsistencies in how ethnicity is recorded across datasets (Mathur et al., 2014).

Training AI models using datasets that include ethnicity as a variable can embed historical biases if the underlying data is biased (O'Brien et al., 2022). A recent investigation by Amnesty International UK raised serious concerns about the London Metropolitan Police's Gangs Matrix, where approximately 80% of individuals listed were Black, despite Black people making up only 13.5% of London's population based on UK government diversity data (2022). Many of these individuals had a 'zero-harm' score, indicating the lowest risk of committing violence. A subsequent review by the Mayor of London's office found that Black people were overrepresented in the Matrix relative to their likelihood of offending or being victims of crime (Densley & Pyrooz, 2020).

The inappropriate inclusion of race as a variable in clinical prediction models is also problematic (Vyas et al., 2020). A notable example is the race-based correction factor previously used in estimating kidney function, which can delay diagnosis and treatment for Black patients (Madhusoodanan, 2020). Such practices risk embedding racial inequities into clinical decision-making, leading to poorer health outcomes for minority groups. However, when used appropriately, ethnic categories can serve as a vital social tool for monitoring, understanding, and tackling health disparities (Williams et al., 2002).

Unrepresentative data is also a major concern in developing and deploying AI systems. AI relies on large datasets to learn and make decisions, but AI models can produce biased results if these datasets are representative of only some of the population. Many AI algorithms in healthcare are developed using data primarily from White patients, leading to errors when applied to minority populations. The AI-powered dermatological algorithm, Skin Image Search, demonstrated the importance of training AI on representative samples. When tested on dark skin (Fitzpatrick 6), the algorithm achieved only 17% accuracy compared to 69% on Caucasian skin (Fitzpatrick 1/2). The poor performance on dark skin types is likely because the AI was primarily trained on datasets from White patients (Kamulegeya et al., 2023).

Another issue arises from the inappropriate inclusion or exclusion of social determinants of health in AI models. Failing to consider factors such as access to healthcare, employment conditions, and housing may produce less accurate predictions for already disadvantaged populations. A case in point is an algorithm developed by Optum that is used in the USA to identify patients with complex medical needs and assign them a 'risk score'. This algorithm was trained to prioritise patients expected to incur higher future healthcare costs as they are at higher risk. However, because it focused on costs rather than actual health needs, the algorithm disproportionately favoured White patients with higher incomes and better insurance coverage while overlooking African American patients who might seek medical care only when symptoms are severe. Consequently, African Americans, who should have comprised 47% of the high-risk group, were underrepresented at just 18%. This bias led to White patients gaining access to critical resources ahead of African American patients with poorer health (Obermeyer et al., 2019). In the UK, where healthcare is publicly funded, similar biases may emerge if AI models favour economic efficiency over clinical need. If algorithms optimise for cost-saving measures, they may overlook ethnic minority patients who often have complex, resource-intensive conditions.

The challenges posed by AI in healthcare for ethnic minorities are both technical and rooted in the socio-political context. The underrepresentation of minority voices in decision-making, the biases present in data, and the problematic use of race in clinical models all contribute to a care environment where AI has the potential to exacerbate existing disparities. As AI continues to evolve and integrate into healthcare systems, it is important to examine and mitigate these risks to ensure that AI technologies contribute to a more equitable system.

Ensuring equity and mitigating bias in AI-driven healthcare: Strategies and challenges

Tackling the risks and challenges associated with AI in healthcare requires visionary leadership, a deep understanding of the key issues, and a steadfast commitment to ethical practices.

One of the challenges in developing data-driven technologies is the risk of inherent bias from unrepresentative data. To mitigate this, collecting and generating data that accurately reflects the broad spectrum of social, demographic, and clinical factors influencing health outcomes across diverse population groups beyond merely recording ethnicity is essential. The quality, breadth, and depth of data are crucial because, while resampling methods like the Synthetic Minority Oversampling Technique can address imbalances by generating synthetic data from existing datasets, these methods are limited by the scope of the original data and may not correct underlying biases (O'Brien et al., 2022). Therefore, additional measures are needed to strengthen data inclusivity, ensuring it captures the diverse social and clinically relevant factors impacting health outcomes.

The NHS AI Lab's Ethics Initiative STANDING Together (2023) has provided recommendations that emphasise the need for thorough documentation and careful selection of datasets to ensure AI health technologies are inclusive and minimise bias. Data users should identify and justify the inclusion of contextualised groups at risk of disparate outcomes, ensuring these groups are adequately represented in the datasets. Performance across all relevant groups must be evaluated to detect and address any biases, with transparency in reporting limitations and discordance between the intended use and dataset suitability. Formal bias and impact assessments are also crucial, and mitigation strategies should be clearly documented to manage risks effectively throughout the AI lifecycle.

To further increase the impartiality of AI in healthcare, there may be a need to preferentially use data sources that better represent the population to which the model will be applied. This involves expanding data collection beyond demographic information.

For example, non-invasive monitoring systems, such as recorded vital signs during surgeries or triage data from emergency departments, provide relatively unbiased data that can mitigate clinical judgment biases (Parikh et al., 2019). Moreover, releasing open datasets representative of the population could help reduce the bias caused by the less diverse datasets that are often privately held (UK House of Lords, 2018). However, there are also concerns about bias in medical devices, with evidence suggesting that pulse oximetry (a small clip-on device for the finger or toe that estimates blood oxygen levels by passing light through the skin) may be less reliable for darker-skinned patients (NHS Race & Health Observatory, 2023).

In 2024, the UK House of Commons recommended that the UK Government and regulators mandate that AI models undergo independent testing and performance analysis before deployment. Developers and deployers must summarise their efforts to mitigate bias in training datasets and report bias levels in AI outputs, similar to company pay gap reporting (House of Commons Science, Innovation and Technology Committee, 2024). In addition, the UK Medicines and Healthcare Products Regulatory Agency now requires that new medical device approval applications explicitly address potential biases, ensure datasets are representative, and increase transparency in the use of data for AI development in healthcare (UK Government, 2024).

Ensuring equity in AI deployment requires careful consideration of the intended use and impact of AI models. Defining the objectives of an algorithm involves thoroughly assessing what the algorithm is designed to predict, the populations it will affect, the data required, and the outcome variables that will be used. AI models in clinical practice aim to maximise predictive accuracy across the population. However, this can lead to varying performance across patient characteristics, such as ethnicity, age, gender, and health status. This discrepancy raises the challenge of balancing overall model accuracy with equitable performance for all groups (O'Brien et al., 2022).

To tackle this, developers can implement sensitivity checks, such as using simulated datasets with omitted variables, to ensure consistent model performance (Parikh et al., 2019). Furthermore, it is suggested that, rather than solely focusing on overall predictive accuracy, models should aim to reduce harmful misclassifications or integrate fairness directly into their objectives (Sagawa et al., 2019; Zink & Rose, 2020). Evidence indicates that enhancing model fairness by up to 98% may result in only a minimal 4% decrease in predictive accuracy, showing that ensuring equity in AI may not have a major impact on overall performance. Statistical methods such as data stratification or sub-population weighting can help prevent AI algorithms from underperforming for minority ethnic groups by addressing the limitations of testing based solely on aggregate outcomes across the entire population. Additionally, out-of-sample testing may help validate an algorithm's performance on data that is different from the training data (O'Brien et al., 2022).

The 'black box' problem in AI development presents a challenge where more accurate algorithms often appear less explainable. This lack of transparency raises both technical and ethical concerns, as AI-driven decisions can directly affect patient care and safety. Healthcare providers must be empowered to better understand and interpret AI decisions and implement effective quality assurance processes. Ethical and regulatory guidelines rightly emphasise the importance of AI explainability and transparency as key to maintaining trust in AI systems (WHO, 2023). However, this emphasis must be more effectively translated into practice to ensure these principles are consistently applied in clinical settings.

There are concerns that AI adoption by digitally advanced care providers in future could leave other centres and patients behind, thereby worsening health inequities. Data from Office for National Statistics (ONS, 2019) showed a regional pattern of digital exclusion. London had the lowest proportion of internet non-users (7.0%), while Northern Ireland had the most (14.2%), followed by the North East (12.1%). Moreover, the outcomes of AI deployment are often unclear; while it might increase economic efficiency or diagnostic accuracy, it could also diminish healthcare quality or patient experiences. Thus, it is essential to define and measure AI deployment, usage, and patient outcomes with a focus on ethnic equity, addressing disparities in access, clinical outcomes, and broader socio-technical impacts on healthcare (O'Brien et al., 2022).

The NHS Race and Health Observatory has provided recommendations for improving healthcare digital app design, data collection, and working methods. These include reviewing existing NHS design frameworks to address systemic inequalities, identifying barriers that prevent minoritised communities from benefiting from digital apps, and ensuring that digital teams collaborate with local partners to meet community-specific needs. Linked data should focus on ethnic health disparities to inform app development. Data collection must cover ethnicity, health outcomes, and digital behaviours, with transparent communication on data use and privacy to build trust. NHS organisations should strengthen data infrastructure and enforce standards for consistent and secure data practices. Building diverse digital teams and offering anti-racism training are critical ways of working. NHS leadership should prioritise ethnic diversity at the top, invest in digital transformation, and foster collaboration to reduce ethnic health disparities (Wadhawan et al., 2023).

Expanding internet access and enhancing technology literacy are urgent needs, particularly as AI is increasingly integrated into healthcare. However, it cannot be assumed that everyone will engage equally in the digital aspects of society, especially given the disparities in digital access and literacy among ethnic minorities, migrants, the elderly and lower-income groups. Patient voices, especially from minority groups, are often overlooked in AI development; qualitative insights and patient engagement are necessary to understanding AI's impact on diverse populations during algorithm development and before implementation (O'Brien et al., 2022).

Policy and regulatory considerations

The World Health Organization's (WHO, 2023) regulatory considerations for AI in healthcare focus on several key areas to ensure the safe, effective, and equitable deployment of AI technologies. These include:

1. Documentation and transparency: Calls for clear documentation of AI systems, detailing their medical purpose, development, and datasets to ensure traceability and accountability.
2. Risk management and lifecycle approach: Advocates a full lifecycle approach, covering development, post-market monitoring, and updates, with a focus on managing risks like cybersecurity threats and algorithmic bias.

3. Intended use and validation: Emphasises defining the AI system's purpose and validating performance using independent datasets that reflect the target population.
4. Data quality: Stresses the need for high-quality data, tackling biases and errors in early evaluations to prevent harm.
5. Privacy and data protection: Recommends integrating privacy measures early, ensuring regulatory compliance and strong cybersecurity protections.
6. Engagement and collaboration: Supports stakeholder collaboration and streamlined regulation to aid innovation and effective AI adoption in healthcare.

WHO highlights the importance of ongoing dialogue among regulators, developers, and other stakeholders to adapt to the rapidly evolving AI landscape, advocating for international cooperation to achieve regulatory convergence and harmonisation.

The Organisation for Economic Co-operation and Development (OECD, 2024) report also emphasises that while AI in health presents considerable opportunities, it also carries substantial risks that must be managed through 'Responsible AI' practices that prioritise trustworthiness, ethics, and the minimisation of risks, all while respecting human rights and democratic values. The report acknowledges key risks associated with AI, including bias, privacy and security issues, discrimination, and a lack of transparency. The report highlights the need for clear accountability, coherent data standards, and improved digital foundations in health systems to deal with these challenges. Collaboration across countries is essential for leveraging diverse data sets, reducing costs, improving regulatory efficiency, and enhancing the safety of AI solutions. The report also stresses the importance of developing health-specific AI guidance to ensure consistent adoption and cross-industry collaboration.

As AI technologies become increasingly integrated into healthcare systems, there is a growing recognition of the need for effective legal and policy frameworks to govern their development and deployment. While aspects such as privacy and discrimination are partly addressed by existing UK and European Union (EU) legislation, these laws provide only a foundation for tackling the broader ethical and legal challenges posed by AI in healthcare. For instance, the UK's equalities legislation prohibits discrimination based on nine protected characteristics, including ethnicity, sex, and age. Moreover, health data, classified as special category data under the EU General Data Protection Regulation (GDPR), which is incorporated into UK law, receives additional protection to safeguard individual privacy and prevent misuse (Information Commissioner's Office, n.d.).

In March 2024, the European Union Parliament passed the Artificial Intelligence Act, marking the world's first binding legislation on AI. The Act seeks to balance innovation with safety, focusing on protecting fundamental rights, democracy, and environmental sustainability. It introduces strict regulations for high-risk AI applications, such as those used in healthcare, law enforcement, and critical infrastructure, requiring stringent transparency, accuracy, and human oversight. The legislation mandates the establishment of regulatory 'sandboxes' (controlled environments for testing new technologies under regulatory supervision) and real-world testing environments at the national level to support start-ups and businesses in developing and refining innovative AI technologies before they are introduced to the market (European Union, 2024).

Complementing this, the UK Government's 2023 AI White Paper introduced a framework centred around five key principles: safety and security, transparency and explainability, fairness, accountability and governance, and contestability. These principles will initially be implemented through existing regulators without statutory enforcement, with the potential for legislative backing if necessary. The framework also includes key support functions such as monitoring and evaluating the effectiveness of the regulatory framework, and assessing AI-related risks across the economy. It involves horizon scanning and gap analysis to respond to emerging AI trends. It also supports testbeds and sandbox initiatives to help innovators bring new technologies to market, while promoting interoperability with international regulatory frameworks (UK Government, 2023).

Finally, the National Institute for Health and Care Excellence (NICE) Evidence Standards Framework (ESF), published in 2022, is designed to support individuals within the health and care system responsible for evaluating, authorising, and assessing digital health technologies. The ESF provides a structured classification system for categorising digital health technologies and sets clear standards for demonstrating their effectiveness and value. For developers, it guides the demonstration of a product's impact and assists in engaging with evaluators. For decision-makers, it facilitates more informed and consistent decisions regarding the commissioning or purchasing of digital health technologies, ultimately promoting the integration of effective digital solutions in healthcare (NICE, 2022).

Conclusion

To harness AI's power for good, it is essential to integrate equity considerations at every stage of its development and deployment, from data collection to algorithm design to clinical application. This involves ensuring that AI tools are trained on diverse, representative datasets and that their performance is rigorously tested across different population groups to avoid reinforcing existing biases.

Diversity within AI developers and technologists is also crucial for ensuring that AI tools are effective and representative of the populations they aim to serve. A lack of diversity in the workforce can lead to AI systems that overlook or misinterpret the needs of underrepresented groups, resulting in inequitable outcomes. Therefore, it is essential to involve diverse perspectives at every stage of AI development – from research and design to deployment – to ensure these technologies are inclusive and beneficial for all.

The impact of AI on clinician performance and the broader healthcare system must be carefully managed. Existing hierarchies and discrimination within healthcare institutions, such as the NHS, can exacerbate the challenges of equitably implementing AI technologies. Addressing these issues requires creating an environment where all staff feel empowered to voice concerns and contribute to the development and application of AI technologies without fear of discrimination or retaliation.

Developing AI algorithms that prioritise marketability over dealing with healthcare inequities can hinder their potential to meet patient needs. To ensure AI technologies are equitable, patient input must be integrated into all stages of AI development – from design and funding to implementation and evaluation – especially for those with limited digital and healthcare experience. Involving patients and the public helps dispel misconceptions and build trust in AI and is essential for meaningful innovation (O'Brien et al., 2022). Patient and Public Involvement and Engagement (PPIE) are essential in AI healthcare development, ensuring systems are tailored to real-world needs, ethically sound, and patient centred. It increases trust, transparency, and adoption by integrating patient and public insights, tackling bias, and aligning AI innovations with public health priorities for more effective, equitable care. However, meaningful engagement is challenging and demands crucial skills and commitment (NIHR, 2019). Furthermore, there is a risk of tokenism (the superficial inclusion of underrepresented groups without genuine engagement or influence), where diversity becomes symbolic rather than a true effort to incorporate a broad range of perspectives, voices, and backgrounds. In light of this, emphasis should be placed on the quality of engagement to ensure meaningful inclusion.

Recent attempts in the UK have tried to move beyond patient and public engagement towards sharing power and responsibility. The approach to participatory co-design and co-production involves active collaboration between researchers, patients, and the public in the development of healthcare solutions. In the context of AI, this approach can create AI tools that are developed with direct input from end-users, making them more relevant, usable, and in line with patient needs. By involving stakeholders from the outset, this method supports the ethical grounding, trustworthiness, and effectiveness of AI systems, leading to innovations that are technically advanced, socially responsible, and widely accepted in healthcare settings (NIHR, 2021).

The evolving nature of AI technologies presents both opportunities and challenges. As AI continues to advance, new issues and gaps in knowledge are likely to emerge, necessitating ongoing research and adaptation. The dynamic nature of AI means that regulations, ethical guidelines, and best practices must continually evolve to keep pace with technological developments. Future directions should focus on bridging these gaps, improving understanding of bias in AI, and developing frameworks that support AI technologies in reducing health disparities rather than exacerbating them.

Achieving equity and fairness in AI-driven healthcare requires a multi-dimensional approach that prioritises diversity, addresses systemic biases, and remains adaptable to the evolving landscape of AI technologies. By fostering inclusive development practices and staying vigilant to emerging challenges, we hope that AI contributes to a healthcare system that is fair, just, and beneficial for all.

Discussion questions

1. How do algorithmic biases in AI technologies drive health inequities among ethnic minority populations in the UK, and what measures can be implemented to mitigate these biases?
2. How can health literacy levels and digital access among minority communities impact the effectiveness of AI-driven health interventions, and how can these challenges be addressed?
3. Discuss the ethical considerations surrounding privacy and consent in using AI in healthcare, particularly for ethnic minorities. How can trust be built between these communities and AI developers?

Further reading

1. World Health Organization. (2023). *Regulatory Considerations on Artificial Intelligence for Health*. World Health Organization. https://iris.who.int/handle/10665/373421. License: CC BY-NC-SA 3.0 IGO

2. Noble, S. U. (2018). *Algorithms of Oppression: How Search Engines Reinforce Racism.* New York University Press. The book explores the impact of algorithmic biases in digital platforms on marginalised communities.
3. Eubanks, V. (2018). *Automating Inequality: How High-Tech Tools Profile, Police, and Punish the Poor.* St. Martin's Press. Eubanks provides insight into how automated systems can exacerbate social inequalities, with implications for healthcare.
4. O'Neil, C. (2016). *Weapons of Math Destruction: How Big Data Increases Inequality and Threatens Democracy.* Crown. The author discusses the negative impacts of poorly regulated big data.
5. Benjamin, R. (2019). *Race after Technology: Abolitionist Tools for the New Jim Code.* Polity Press. Benjamin examines the intersection of race, technology, and justice, offering insights into combating digital racial discrimination.

References

AI Index Steering Committee. (2021). "Diversity in AI." In *Artificial Intelligence Index Report 2021.* Stanford Institute for Human-Centered Artificial Intelligence, Stanford University. https://hai.stanford.edu/ai-index/2021-ai-index-report

Arasu, V. A., Habel, L. A., Achacoso, N. S., Buist, D. S., Cord, J. B., Esserman, L. J., Hylton, N. M., Glymour, M. M., Kornak, J., & Kushi, L. H. (2023). Comparison of mammography AI algorithms with a clinical risk model for 5-year breast cancer risk prediction: An observational study. *Radiology, 307*(5), e222733.

Braveman, P., & Parker Dominguez, T. (2021). Abandon "race." Focus on racism. *Frontiers in Public Health, 9*, 689462.

Chen, I. Y., Pierson, E., Rose, S., Joshi, S., Ferryman, K., & Ghassemi, M. (2021). Ethical machine learning in healthcare. *Annual Review of Biomedical Data Science, 4*(1), 123–144.

Densley, J. A., & Pyrooz, D. C. (2020). The matrix in context: Taking stock of police gang databases in London and beyond. *Youth Justice, 20*(1–2), 11–30.

Eubanks, V. (2018). *Automating Inequality: How High-Tech Tools Profile, Police, and Punish the Poor.* St. Martin's Press.

European Union. (2024). *EU AI Act.* https://artificialintelligenceact.eu/ai-act-explorer/

Frankish, K., & Ramsey, W. M. (2014). *The Cambridge Handbook of Artificial Intelligence.* Cambridge University Press.

Higher Education Statistics Agency (HESA). (2024, January). *Higher Education Staff Statistics: UK, 2022/23.* https://www.hesa.ac.uk/news/16-01-2024/sb267-higher-education-staff-statistics

Hogarty, D. T., Su, J. C., Phan, K., Attia, M., Hossny, M., Nahavandi, S., Lenane, P., Moloney, F. J., & Yazdabadi, A. (2020). Artificial intelligence in dermatology – where we are and the way to the future: A review. *American Journal of Clinical Dermatology, 21*, 41–47.

Hosny, A., Parmar, C., Quackenbush, J., Schwartz, L. H., & Aerts, H. J. (2018). Artificial intelligence in radiology. *Nature Reviews Cancer, 18*(8), 500–510.

House of Commons Science, Innovation and Technology Committee. (2024, May 23). *Governance of Artificial Intelligence (AI). Third Report of Sessions 2023–24.* https://publications.parliament.uk/pa/cm5804/cmselect/cmsctech/38/report.html

Information Commissioner's Office. (n.d). *Data Protection After the End of the Transition Period.* https://ico.org.uk/for-organisations/data-protection-and-the-eu/

Joshi, I., & Morley, J. (2019, January). *Artificial Intelligence: How to Get It Right.* NHSX. https://transform.england.nhs.uk/ai-lab/explore-all-resources/understand-ai/artificial-intelligence-how-get-it-right/

Kamulegeya, L., Bwanika, J., Okello, M., Rusoke, D., Nassiwa, F., Lubega, W., Musinguzi, D., & Börve, A. (2023). Using artificial intelligence on dermatology conditions in Uganda: A case for diversity in training data sets for machine learning. *African Health Sciences*, *23*(2), 753–763.

Kapadia, D., Zhang, J., Salway, S., Nazroo, J., Booth, A., Villarroel Williams, N., Bécares, L., & NHS Race and Health Observatory. (2022, February). *Ethnic Inequalities in Healthcare: A Rapid Evidence Review. NHS Race and Health Observatory.* https://www.nhsrho.org/research/ethnic-inequalities-in-healthcare-a-rapid-evidence-review-3/

Khan, S. M., Liu, X., Nath, S., Korot, E., Faes, L., Wagner, S. K., Keane, P. A., Sebire, N. J., Burton, M. J., & Denniston, A. K. (2021). A global review of publicly available datasets for ophthalmological imaging: Barriers to access, usability, and generalisability. *The Lancet Digital Health*, *3*(1), e51–e66.

Komorowski, M., Celi, L. A., Badawi, O., Gordon, A. C., & Faisal, A. A. (2018). The artificial intelligence clinician learns optimal treatment strategies for sepsis in intensive care. *Nature Medicine*, *24*(11), 1716–1720.

Kumar, Y., Koul, A., Singla, R., & Ijaz, M. F. (2023). Artificial intelligence in disease diagnosis: A systematic literature review, synthesizing framework and future research agenda. *Journal of Ambient Intelligence and Humanized Computing*, *14*(7), 8459–8486.

Madhusoodanan, J. (2020). Is a biased algorithm delaying health care for Black people? *Nature*, *588*(7839), 546–547.

Mathur, R., Bhaskaran, K., Chaturvedi, N., Leon, D. A., vanStaa, T., Grundy, E., & Smeeth, L. (2014). Completeness and usability of ethnicity data in UK-based primary care and hospital databases. *Journal of Public Health*, *36*(4), 684–692.

Ministry of Housing, Communities and Local Government. (2020). *People Living in Deprived Neighbourhoods.* GOV. UK. https://www.ethnicity-facts-figures.service.gov.uk/uk-population-by-ethnicity/demographics/people-living-in-deprived-neighbourhoods/latest/

Moore, C. M. (2022). The challenges of health inequities and AI. *Intelligence-Based Medicine*, 6, 100067.

Moulaei, K., Yadegari, A., Baharestani, M., Farzanbakhsh, S., Sabet, B., & Afrash, M. R. (2024). Generative artificial intelligence in healthcare: A scoping review on benefits, challenges and applications. *International Journal of Medical Informatics*, 105474.

NHS. (2022). *NHS Workforce Race Equality Standard (WRES) 2022 Data Analysis Report for NHS Trusts.* https://www.england.nhs.uk/long-read/nhs-workforce-race-equality-standard-wres2022-data-analysis-report-for-nhs-trusts/#wres-indicator-9

NHS Race & Health Observatory. (2021, June). *Ethnicity Coding in English Health Service Datasets.* https://www.nhsrho.org/research/ethnicity-coding-in-english-health-service-datasets/

NHS Race and Health Observatory. (2023). *Pulse Oximetry and Racial Bias: Recommendations for National Healthcare Regulatory and Research Bodies.* https://www.nhsrho.org/research/pulse-oximetry-and-racial-bias-recommendations-for-national-healthcare-regulatory-and-research-bodies/

Niazi, M. K. K., Parwani, A. V., & Gurcan, M. N. (2019). Digital pathology and artificial intelligence. *The Lancet Oncology*, *20*(5), e253–e261.

NICE. (2022). *Evidence Standards Framework (ESF) for Digital Health Technologies.* https://www.nice.org.uk/about/what-we-do/our-programmes/evidence-standards-framework-for-digital-health-technologies

NIHR. (2019). *UK Standards for Public Involvement: Better Public Involvement for Better Health and Social Care Research.* Supported by the UK Public Involvement Standards Development Partnership London, UK: National Institute of Health and Care Research. https://sites.google.com/nihr.ac.uk/pistandards/home

NIHR. (2021). *NIHR Guidance on Co-Producing a Research Project.* https://www.learningforinvolvement.org.uk/content/resource/nihr-guidance-on-co-producing-a-research-project/

NIHR. (2023, July). *Artificial Intelligence: 10 Promising Interventions for Healthcare.* https://evidence.nihr.ac.uk/collection/artificial-intelligence-10-promising-interventions-for-healthcare/

Obermeyer, Z., Powers, B., Vogeli, C., & Mullainathan, S. (2019). Dissecting racial bias in an algorithm used to manage the health of populations. *Science*, *366*(6464), 447–453.

O'Brien, N., Van Dael, J., Clarke, J., Gardner, C., O'Shaughnessy, J., Darzi, A., & Ghafur, S. (2022). *Addressing Racial and Ethnic Inequities in Data-Driven Health Technologies*. Institute of Global Health Innovation, Imperial College London. https://spiral.imperial.ac.uk/handle/10044/1/94902

OECD. (2024, January). *Collective Action for Responsible AI In Health*. OECD Artificial Intelligence Papers. https://www.oecd.org/en/publications/collective-action-for-responsible-ai-in-health_f2050177-en.html

Ofcom. (2024, February). *Communication Affordability Tracker*. https://www.ofcom.org.uk/phones-and-broadband/saving-money/affordability-tracker

Office for National Statistics (ONS). (2019). *What Is the Pattern of Digital Exclusion across the UK?* https://www.ons.gov.uk/peoplepopulationandcommunity/householdcharacteristics/homeinternetandsocialmediausage/articles/exploringtheuksdigitaldivide/2019-03-04

Parikh, R. B., Teeple, S., & Navathe, A. S. (2019). Addressing bias in artificial intelligence in health care. *Jama*, *322*(24), 2377–2378.

Razai, M. S., Al-Bedaery, R., Bowen, L., Yahia, R., Chandrasekaran, L., & Oakeshott, P. (2024). Implementation challenges of artificial intelligence (AI) in primary care: Perspectives of general practitioners in London UK. *PLoS One*, *19*(11), e0314196.

Razai, M. S., Kankam, H. K., Majeed, A., Esmail, A., & Williams, D. R. (2021). Mitigating ethnic disparities in covid-19 and beyond. *BMJ*, *372*.

Robertson, R., Williams E, et al. (2021, June). *NHS Race & Health Observatory. Ethnic Health Inequalities and the NHS*. https://www.nhsrho.org/research/ethnic-inequalities-in-healthcare-a-rapid-evidence-review-2/

Sagawa, S., Koh, P. W., Hashimoto, T. B., & Liang, P. (2019). Distributionally robust neural networks for group shifts: On the importance of regularization for worst-case generalization. *arXiv preprint arXiv:1911.08731*.

Saunders, C. L., Abel, G. A., El Turabi, A., Ahmed, F., & Lyratzopoulos, G. (2013). Accuracy of routinely recorded ethnic group information compared with self-reported ethnicity: Evidence from the English Cancer Patient Experience survey. *BMJ Open*, *3*(6), e002882.

Seyyed-Kalantari, L., Zhang, H., McDermott, M. B. A., Chen, I. Y., & Ghassemi, M. (2021). Underdiagnosis bias of artificial intelligence algorithms applied to chest radiographs in under-served patient populations. *Nature Medicine*, *27*(12), 2176–2182. https://doi.org/10.1038/s41591-021-01595-0

Smith, C., & Barclay, S. (2023). *£21 Million to Roll Out Artificial Intelligence across the NHS*. Department of Health and Social Care.

STANDING Together. (2023, October 30). *Recommendations for Diversity, Inclusivity, and Generalisability in Artificial Intelligence Health Technologies and Health Datasets*. https://www.datadiversity.org/recommendations

Strouse, J. J., Lobner, K., Lanzkron, S., & Haywood Jr, C. (2013). NIH and national foundation expenditures for sickle cell disease and cystic fibrosis are associated with PubMed publications and FDA approvals. *Blood*, *122*(21), 1739.

UK Government. (2020, October 30). *Ethnicity Facts and Figures*. https://www.ethnicity-facts-figures.service.gov.uk/

UK Government. (2022a). *Health and Care Act 2022*. https://www.legislation.gov.uk/ukpga/2022/31/contents/enacted

UK Government. (2022b, December). *Regional Ethnic Diversity*. https://www.ethnicity-facts-figures.service.gov.uk/uk-population-by-ethnicity/national-and-regional-populations/regional-ethnic-diversity/latest/

UK Government. (2023). *A Pro-Innovation Approach to AI Regulation*. https://www.gov.uk/government/publications/ai-regulation-a-pro-innovation-approach/white-paper#executive-summary

UK Government. (2024, March 12). *New Action to Tackle Ethnic and Other Biases in Medical Devices*. https://www.gov.uk/government/news/new-action-to-tackle-ethnic-and-other-biases-in-medical-devices?

UK Government. (2025). *AI Opportunities Action Plan.* https://www.gov.uk/government/publications/ai-opportunities-action-plan/ai-opportunities-action-plan

UK House of Lords. (2018). *Select Committee on Artificial Intelligence. AI in the UK: Ready, Willing and Able?* https://publications.parliament.uk/pa/ld201719/ldselect/ldai/100/100.pdf

UK Parliament. (2022). *Cystic Fibrosis and Sickle Cell Diseases: Health Services.* https://questions-statements.parliament.uk/written-questions/detail/2022-03-07/135634/

Vyas, D. A., Eisenstein, L. G., & Jones, D. S. (2020). Hidden in plain sight – Reconsidering the use of race correction in clinical algorithms. *The New England Journal of Medicine, 383*(9), 874–882. https://doi.org/10.1056/NEJMms2004740. Epub 2020 June 17. PMID: 32853499.

Wadhawan, M., Nguyen, Z., et al. (2023, January). *Digital Apps and Reducing Ethnic Health Inequalities.* NHS Race & Health Observatory. https://www.nhsrho.org/research/digital-apps-and-reducing-ethnic-health-inequalities/

Williams, D. R. (2002). Ethnicity, race, and health. In *International Encyclopedia of the Social and Behavioral Sciences* (pp. 4831–4838). Oxford, UK: Elsevier.

Williams, D. R., Lawrence, J. A., & Davis, B. A. (2019). Racism and health: Evidence and needed research. *Annual Review of Public Health, 40*(1), 105–125.

Wolf, R. M., Abramoff, M. D., Channa, R., Tava, C., Clarida, W., & Lehmann, H. P. (2022). Potential reduction in healthcare carbon footprint by autonomous artificial intelligence. *NPJ Digital Medicine, 5*(1), 62.

World Health Organization. (2023). *Regulatory Considerations on Artificial Intelligence for Health.* World Health Organization.

Yates, S., Hill, K., Blackwell, C., Davis, A., Padley, M., Stone, E., Polizzi, G., D'Arcy, J., Harris, R., & Sheppard, P. (2024). *A Minimum Digital Living Standard for Households with Children-Overall Findings Report.*

Zink, A., & Rose, S. (2020). Fair regression for health care spending. *Biometrics, 76*(3), 973–982.

SECTION 3

Maternal health

This theme addresses the systemic failures that result in the stark and preventable differences in survival rates between White women and women from racialised communities in the UK throughout pregnancy and beyond. Chapter 5 draws on recent evidence to chart the egregious inequities in maternal health outcomes for women from minority ethnic groups, while Chapter 6 focuses on one contributing aspect of this inequity through attention to the quality and cultural appropriateness of interpretation services provided in maternity services within the NHS.

In Chapter 5, Felker, Harrison, Carson, Alderdice, Quigley, and Knight draw on literature and data from Mothers and Babies: Reducing Risks through Audits and Confidential Enquiries across the UK (MBRRACE-UK) to evidence the inordinate disparities in mortality and morbidity between women from racialised communities and women of the White ethnic majority in the UK and Ireland. As the risk of maternal death for minority ethnic women remains the same across the social and economic spectrum, Felker et al. refute deprivation models and propose instead a complex of intersecting variables that contribute to maternal health outcomes. They further note that morbidity, with long-term health implications, is higher among minority ethnic women, even after adjusting for deprivation. In addition, many minority ethnic women report feeling unsafe, ignored, disbelieved, and dehumanised in their encounters with maternity services, reducing and delaying engagement. Felker et al. identify several failings, including the lack of individualised care to address specific vulnerabilities in minority ethnic women, poor cultural sensitivity training, a dearth of advocates, and a lack of link workers, which collectively increase their risks of maternal morbidity and mortality.

Chapter 6 centres on one recommendation from the MBRRACE-UK report, maternal interpretation, as a driver of inequity in maternal health outcomes in England. Baz, Sheard, MacFarlane, and MacLellan argue that poor interpretation provision constitutes racism across three domains: as interpersonal racism, through lack of cultural competency and humility; as institutional racism, through poor policy and race-ignorant norms; and as structural racism, through negligent provision for those

DOI: 10.4324/9781003466093-8

in maternity care. They locate this dereliction of duty along intersectional lines, where race, ethnicity, gender, religion, and immigration status intersect to discriminate against women holding more than one of these characteristics. Without appropriate interpretation, informed consent cannot accurately be given for any service or intervention. Baz et al. note that interpreter provision has erroneously focused on the 'language problem', which ignores the power relations embedded in translation and influences how information is interpreted. Finally, Baz et al. highlight the need for a Critical Race Theory-centred approach to redress the privileging of British culture and values in maternal interpretation, so that the heightened vulnerabilities of pregnancy are not compounded by cultural marginalisation for minority ethnic women.

CHAPTER 5

The impact of ethnicity on maternal health outcomes

Allison Felker, Siân Harrison, Claire Carson, Fiona Alderdice, Maria Quigley, and Marian Knight

Definitions (race and ethnicity, women, and mothers)

Both race and ethnicity are social constructs based on individual characteristics that inform the way we think about and relate to others. Ethnicity is a widely used concept in the United Kingdom (UK), describing groups with shared ancestry, traditions, language, national origins, or cultural practices. Race more directly describes the artificial categorisation of individuals based on physical characteristics, such as skin colour, which is rooted in unfounded ideas of a racial hierarchy. When the concepts of race and ethnicity are conflated, the negative framing of race is placed on minority ethnic groups, in a process of racialisation. We use the term 'minority ethnic women' to describe those women who do not identify as White British, but note that minority ethnic women comprise more than one in three women in the UK and are far from a homogenous group.

We use the terms 'women' and 'mother' throughout this chapter to refer to those who are pregnant and give birth. We acknowledge that not all people who are pregnant and give birth identify as women or mothers.

Introduction and aims of the chapter

In this chapter, we draw on the UK literature to highlight key examples of race and health inequity in maternal health outcomes. We show that there is a complex pattern of maternal health outcomes, and that these vary among women of racialised ethnicities. We attempt to dissect the complex multifactorial roots underlying these inequalities, including how they are influenced by economic and social factors, behaviours, and expectations. This complexity is a testament to the broad range of intersecting factors that impact maternal health and that vary for women of different ethnicities, locations, and contexts.

The impact of ethnicity on maternal health outcomes within the UK has long been a topic of discussion for various health initiatives, policy decisions, and advocacy

DOI: 10.4324/9781003466093-9

messages. In recent years, the UK government's Women and Equalities Committee and Health and Social Care Committee have published reports on Black maternal health (House of Commons Health and Social Care Committee, 2025; House of Commons Women and Equalities Committee, 2023), the National Health Service (NHS) Race and Health Observatory critically reviewed existing policy interventions to tackle ethnic health inequalities in maternal and neonatal health (Esan et al., 2022) and the Labour government pledged to reduce inequalities in maternal mortality for Black and Asian women (Labour Party, 2024) including the announcement of a National Maternity and Neonatal Investigation (Department of Health and Social Care et al., 2025) as part of the new 10 Year Health Plan (Department of Health and Social Care, 2025). Yet, despite ongoing and previous efforts to reduce inequalities in maternal health outcomes, slow progress has been made.

Maternal mortality

Annual reports of UK confidential enquiries into maternal deaths, conducted by the MBRRACE-UK collaboration (Mothers and Babies: Reducing Risk through Audits and Confidential Enquiries across the UK), demonstrate persistent inequalities in the rate of maternal death occurring during pregnancy or up to six weeks after the end of pregnancy for women from Black and Asian ethnic backgrounds. When MBRRACE-UK reporting began in 2014, Black women in England had rates of maternal death three times higher than White women. Using these same data, Asian women had an approximate two-fold higher rate of death (Knight et al., 2014). In the ten years since the initial MBRRACE-UK report, these figures have not changed (Felker et al., 2024); in fact, they may have worsened. In 2022–2024, the rate of maternal mortality for Black women was 32.42 per 100,000 maternities, substantially higher than the rate of 24.50 per 100,000 maternities reported for 2009–2012 (Felker & Knight, 2026). Between 2009 and 2024, the relative risk of maternal death for Black and Asian women compared to White women remained largely unchanged (Felker & Knight, 2026), though surveillance conducted during the years of the COVID-19 pandemic (2020–2022) found that the majority of women who died from COVID-19 infection were from minority ethnic groups, around a third of whom were Pakistani and 15% were Black (Felker et al., 2024).

Several research studies have been undertaken using MBRRACE-UK data to further investigate the ethnic inequalities in maternal mortality, including the impact of pre-conception health and health behaviours on maternal outcomes. A national cohort study of surveillance data for 1,894 women who died during or up to a year after the end of pregnancy in the UK from 2009–2018 was used to investigate the characteristics and causes of death by aggregated ethnic groups (Knight et al., 2022). There were no significant differences between the aggregated ethnic groups regarding medical or mental health comorbidities or different causes of death, which shows that pre-existing health conditions alone cannot account for ethnic inequalities in maternal mortality. However, the proportion of Black and Asian women living in the most deprived areas was higher than that of White women, indicating an intersectionality of risk factors for maternal death within these populations (Knight et al., 2022). Exploring this intersection of ethnicity and socioeconomic status was the focus of a similar study utilising a cohort of 801 women who died during or up to six weeks after pregnancy in the UK from 2009 to 2019 (Vousden et al., 2024). Using both routine data comparators from national birth registries and a bespoke control group from UK Obstetric Surveillance System (UKOSS) studies, researchers demonstrated that Black women remained at a significantly increased risk of maternal death independent of social deprivation. Indeed, unlike White women, for whom the risk of maternal death increased with increasing deprivation, the risk of maternal death for Black women was the same across all socioeconomic quintiles. Women from Black and Asian ethnic backgrounds also remained at a higher risk of maternal death after adjusting for smoking, body mass index (BMI), and other comorbidities, again demonstrating that pre-existing conditions or health behaviours alone cannot explain the inequalities in maternal mortality rates (Vousden et al., 2024). While a serious and relatively rare event, maternal mortality is an important barometer for more widespread inequalities in maternal health outcomes and experiences of care.

Maternal physical morbidity

For every woman in the UK who dies during pregnancy or in the period after pregnancy, we know that more than 100 experience 'near miss events' or severe morbidity, which can be life threatening and impact long-term health. Although the UK does not currently have a national surveillance system for severe maternal morbidity, results from UKOSS studies conducted between 2005–2006 (Knight et al., 2009) and 2005–2013 (Nair et al., 2014) demonstrate similar findings to maternal mortality surveillance with regard to ethnic inequalities and severe maternal morbidity. Examples of severe maternal morbidities included in these studies were amniotic fluid embolism, stroke, pulmonary embolism, hypertensive disorders of pregnancy, and peripartum hysterectomy, among others. The risk of any severe maternal morbidity for Black women was more than double that of White Women (Knight et al., 2009; Nair et al., 2014) and for Black Caribbean women in particular, the risk was almost 80% higher (Nair et al., 2014). Asian women, including Bangladeshi, Indian, and Pakistani women, had, on average, a 50% increased risk of severe morbidity compared to White women. The most common cause of morbidity for Black Caribbean and Indian women was sepsis, while women from Bangladeshi, Pakistani, or Black African ethnic groups had a higher incidence of haemorrhagic disorders (Nair et al., 2014).

These findings are supported by more recent nationwide cohort studies using data collected through the English National Hospital Episode Statistics (HES) Admitted Patient Care database between 2016–2021 (Geddes-Barton, Ramakrishnan, et al., 2024) and 2013–2023 (Geddes-Barton et al., 2025), which showed that women from minority ethnic groups had an increased risk of severe maternal morbidity compared to White women (Geddes-Barton et al., 2025; Geddes-Barton, Ramakrishnan, et al., 2024). These studies defined severe maternal morbidity according to the English Maternal Morbidity Outcome Indicator (EMMOI), which includes indicators for both morbid events, such as amniotic fluid embolism or eclampsia, as well as procedures indicating morbidity, such as dialysis or hysterectomy (Nair et al., 2016). Using this indicator, women from Black ethnic groups had an approximately 70–80% increased risk of severe maternal morbidity compared to White women. For Asian women, the risk was around 50% higher, ranging from 30% for Indian women to 80% for Bangladeshi women (Geddes-Barton et al., 2025; Geddes-Barton, Ramakrishnan, et al., 2024). Minoritised ethnic women were also disproportionately represented as living in the most deprived areas (Geddes-Barton et al., 2025; Geddes-Barton, Ramakrishnan, et al., 2024); however, as for maternal mortality, socioeconomic status alone did not explain the observed inequalities in maternal morbidity, as minority ethnic women remained at an increased risk of morbidity after adjusting for deprivation. This was also the case after adjustments were made for age, BMI, smoking status, pre-existing medical conditions, and mental health conditions (Geddes-Barton et al., 2025; Geddes-Barton, Ramakrishnan, et al., 2024; Knight et al., 2009; Nair et al., 2014).

Just as a woman's pre-conception health can impact maternal health and infant outcomes during pregnancy and birth, care during pregnancy and birth, as well as the management of conditions that develop or worsen during pregnancy, can impact health in the immediate and long-term postpartum period. As described previously, women of minoritised ethnicities in the UK face an increased burden of physical morbidity in pregnancy, particularly related to conditions such as pregnancy-induced hypertension, pre-eclampsia, and gestational diabetes. Such pregnancy-related conditions increase the risk of developing chronic health problems, including cardiometabolic conditions such as Type 2 diabetes and cardiovascular disease, with lifelong implications. The physical and emotional impact of pregnancy and birth, and the life upheaval of transition to parenthood, is also a significant period of mental health challenges for women.

Maternal mental health

Mental health problems are among the most common morbidities of the perinatal period, and approximately a third of maternal deaths in the year after pregnancy are due to psychiatric causes (Felker et al., 2025). While death is an extreme outcome of maternal mental health problems, it is estimated that around one in four to one in five women will develop a mental health problem during pregnancy or the first year after childbirth (Howard et al., 2014; Office for Health Improvement and Disparities, 2025). The vast majority of these mental health problems are what are thought to be common disorders, such as depression and anxiety, while more severe disorders, such as psychosis and personality disorders, are rare, with an overall prevalence of around 1.2% (Office for Health Improvement and Disparities, 2025). Nevertheless, it is imperative that all mental health symptoms and conditions are appropriately recognised and managed during pregnancy or in the period following. Pregnancy can exacerbate existing symptoms, trigger new symptoms, or alter how women engage with treatment, and, importantly, maternal mental health conditions have a long-term impact on both women and their children.

Variations in the prevalence of perinatal mental health problems have been reported across different demographic groups; however, variations by ethnicity are not consistently reported. Results from national mortality cohorts showed no difference in the cause of maternal death, including deaths due to psychiatric causes, amongst different ethnic groups; however, small numbers are likely to have limited statistical power in analyses of these specific deaths (Knight et al., 2022). Results from the National Maternity Survey of women who gave birth in England in 2020 found that a higher proportion of White women scored above the cut-off for probable depression on the Edinburgh Postnatal Depression Scale (EPDS), compared to minority ethnic women (25% vs. 21%) (Harrison, Quigley, et al., 2023). However, the difference was not statistically significant after adjustment for other demographic and birth-related factors and, in earlier surveys, prevalence rates for depression have been similar to or even higher in minority ethnic women, compared to White women (Harrison, Quigley, et al., 2023). Measures of anxiety and post-traumatic stress (PTS) were also included in the most recent National Maternity Survey, but the prevalence of anxiety and PTS did not vary significantly by ethnic group (Harrison et al., 2024).

Therefore, the role of ethnicity in self-reported perinatal mental health problems appears to be variable, and it is not possible to draw firm inferences about the overall prevalence in different ethnic groups. Indeed, the results of the recent Office for Health Improvement and Disparities (OHID) analysis of perinatal mental health problems in a primary care sample database were not reported by ethnicity (Office for Health Improvement and Disparities, 2025) as researchers felt there was a risk that perinatal mental health needs amongst minority ethnic women may be under-represented in primary care data. While the prevalence and risk of perinatal mental health problems and maternal mortality or morbidity related to mental health may be difficult to ascertain, there are clear differences in the ways in which women from certain ethnic groups access and engage with care that can greatly affect both their physical and mental health outcomes. This is often compounded by experiences of racism, discrimination or cultural insensitivity, all of which contribute to the complexity underlying inequities in maternal health outcomes.

Why are we seeing differences in maternal health outcomes?

The World Health Organization (WHO) advocates high-quality maternity care for all women, yet access to care, provision of care, and experiences of care for women from different ethnic backgrounds can vary significantly. The findings from a recent inquiry into racial injustice in maternity services in the UK (Birthrights, 2022) showed that minority ethnic women often felt unsafe, ignored, disbelieved and regularly dehumanised. They also reported being subject to racism and coercion by caregivers, not being given the means to make informed decisions or give informed consent and being disproportionately affected by structural barriers to care (Birthrights, 2022).

Access and experiences of care

Antenatal care

Unsurprisingly, inadequate access to and engagement with antenatal services can negatively impact maternal outcomes and increase the risk of severe morbidity or mortality. UK studies have shown that minority ethnic women are more likely to attend their first antenatal appointment later in pregnancy. They also have fewer antenatal appointments and ultrasound scans, and are less likely to attend antenatal classes (Henderson et al., 2013). Differences in minority ethnic women's experiences of care have also been widely reported, including less choice provided for the place of birth, not being involved in decision-making, and not being spoken to in a way that is easily understood (Henderson et al., 2013; Silverio et al., 2023). There is also evidence that Black and Asian women face inequities in the provision of individualised care, including limited recognition and treatment of complex conditions or inadequate clinician knowledge about unfamiliar disorders that are more common among minority ethnic women and that may have impacted their outcomes (Knight et al., 2022). This was also reflected in a greater incidence of biases relating to multidisciplinary care, care by appropriate teams, and senior input or review in Black and Asian women compared to White women (Knight et al., 2022). Issues around continuity of care have also been highlighted as a key barrier to access for certain groups of women, especially those with complexities or experiences of abuse or trauma who will often have to repeat their stories multiple times (Fernandez Turienzo et al., 2021).

Fragmented care pathways were particularly apparent during the COVID-19 pandemic when service pressures disrupted the quality and continuity of maternity care in the UK. In surveys of minority ethnic women's experiences of care during this period, women describe feelings of not being heard and not being fully informed regarding clinical decision-making (John et al., 2021). Social distancing restrictions also prevented some women from receiving in-person consultations, and others delayed seeking medical care due to fear of infection (John et al., 2021). Compounding this was the fact that Black and other minority ethnic women were more hesitant to accept COVID-19 vaccinations during pregnancy (Davies et al., 2022; Galanis et al., 2022), contributing to higher rates of maternal deaths due to COVID-19 amongst Black and Asian women (Knight et al., 2023).

Postpartum care

The physical impact of pregnancy can have long-lasting effects, and the postpartum period is a pivotal period for engagement and intervention. Biases in care relating to medical complexity for Black and Asian women extend into the postpartum period, where continuing care under a specialist physician may be required (Knight et al., 2022). Women from minority ethnic groups have longer lengths of hospital stay after birth (Henderson et al., 2013). Postpartum care in the UK has long been described as a 'Cinderella service', which is often overlooked and under-resourced. As such, it suffers from inadequate funding and patchy provision of services commissioned by different administrative NHS and local authority agencies. Gaps in care often occur as women transition from hospital to midwifery-led care and then to community care by health visitors or general practitioners (GPs). After hospital discharge, minority ethnic women are significantly less likely to see a midwife (Khan, 2021), to have five or more home visits by a midwife, or to have follow-up for their own health in the weeks after birth (Henderson et al., 2013).

While health visitors link into primary care services and aim to provide support in the early weeks postpartum, there is very little research that describes or evaluates these services, or the experiences of women who interact with them. Many women will also not have any contact with their GPs in the first few weeks after giving birth, and minority ethnic women are less likely to register with a GP practice (Bansal et al., 2022). A six-week postpartum check with a GP has long been recommended for new mothers. The National Institute for Health and Care Excellence (NICE) recommends that this covers a variety of topics, including mental health and general well-being, return to physical health and identification of pelvic health issues, family planning and contraception, and pregnancy-related or birth-related conditions requiring ongoing management. However, this only became an essential service under the GP contract in 2020 (National Institute for Health and Care Excellence, 2021). As such, between 2006 and 2021, only 60% of women in England had a record of a six-week check, which varied between 58–68% across minority ethnic groups. Women of Pakistani ethnicity (58%) and any other Black, African, or Caribbean background (60%) had the lowest coverage, while White British women were most likely to receive the check-up (68%) (Zhang et al., 2024). Low rates of postpartum maternal checks were also associated with lower rates of eight-week checks for the infant and immunisations, highlighting the need to provide joined-up care in order to reduce ethnic disparities in care across the life span.

Mental healthcare

As with access to routine maternity care, there is evidence of inequalities in minority ethnic women's access and experience of perinatal mental healthcare. As mentioned, reports on the prevalence of perinatal mental health problems in minority ethnic women are varied. While there is some speculation that the prevalence of perinatal mental health problems is lower in minority ethnic women, potentially due to closer family networks, greater social support, and different cultural expectations regarding motherhood and gender roles (Prady et al., 2013), these theories are speculative due to inconsistent evidence.

What is known is that, for certain ethnic groups, cultural stigma and shame surrounding mental health problems can be more pronounced, leading to reluctance and fear in reporting symptoms or seeking help (Conneely et al., 2023; Pilav et al., 2022). Minority ethnic women are also less likely to trust healthcare professionals, which further reduces the likelihood of disclosure. Black and minority ethnic women and migrant women are less likely to report treatment for anxiety or depression (Moore et al., 2019) and are also less likely to be asked about their mental health antenatally and postnatally compared to White women (Draper et al., 2023b; Harrison, Pilkington, et al., 2023). In a recent survey of Black women's experiences with UK maternity services, nearly half of the women who responded said they were not asked about their emotional well-being or mental health, and many felt that they were not provided with sufficient information about mental health during their pregnancy (Peter & Wheeler, 2022). The measurement of mental health symptoms may also be problematic in certain ethnic groups due to the use of screening tools, which have not been validated on particular groups of women who may present differently (Fellmeth et al., 2022, 2019). Language barriers can also make measurement challenging and unreliable, particularly when interpreters are unavailable and relatives are relied upon to interpret.

Other considerations

Women born outside the UK are four times more likely to have late initiation of care compared to UK-born women (Rowe et al., 2008). This group of women faces additional barriers when accessing care due to unfamiliarity with NHS services, limited social or financial support, and language difficulties that are not always supported by adequate provision of interpreters (Felker et al., 2024; Kenyon et al., 2024). A confidential enquiry investigating ethnic disparities in maternal mortality from 2009 to 2018 found problems identifying and properly managing language needs, particularly amongst Asian women. This included inconsistent use of interpretation services and the use of family members and healthcare professionals as interpreters (Knight et al., 2022). The unique experiences of women with language needs were also identified in a joint MBRRACE-UK maternal morbidity confidential enquiry and perinatal confidential enquiry into the care of women who had recently migrated to the UK and who had language difficulties (Felker et al., 2024; Kenyon et al., 2024). The majority of women included in this confidential enquiry did not receive the interpreting support they needed in order to properly participate in their own care and make informed decisions (Felker et al., 2024; Kenyon et al., 2024).

In addition to barriers put in place by language, limited awareness of and sensitivity to specific cultural beliefs and preferences amongst healthcare professionals may cause migrant women or women of certain ethnic backgrounds to feel isolated and disempowered, leading to a breakdown in trust (Jomeen & Redshaw, 2013). Limitations in the continuity of carers (Obionu et al., 2023) and underrepresentation of minority ethnic groups in the healthcare workforce, particularly in leadership roles, can compound this lack of trust in maternity care services (Fernandez Turienzo et al., 2021; Khan, 2021). The importance of training healthcare professionals in cultural sensitivity and the consistent use of interpreters, advocates, and link workers has long been emphasised in government reports. However, initiatives have tended to be time-limited and geographically scattered, targeted only at numerically significant minority populations. These gaps must be closed in order to provide culturally sensitive, appropriate care at all levels and in all regions of the country.

Racism and discrimination

When considering the impact and extent of ethnic differences on access to and experiences of maternity care, it is important to consider the critical role of racism and discrimination in driving inequality in maternal health outcomes for minority ethnic women. The three-level framework we use to consider the role of racism draws from Nazroo et al., who describe the insidious influence of racism at a structural level, within our institutions, and at an interpersonal level (Nazroo et al., 2020).

Structural racism

Structural racism refers to the ways in which racism is embedded in the systems, policies, and practices that govern healthcare, leading to inequitable outcomes for marginalised ethnic groups. Within maternity care settings, structural racism plays a central role in driving inequalities in maternal health (Fernandez Turienzo et al., 2021). Historical and ongoing discrimination within systems can limit trust amongst minority ethnic women and create the feeling that maternity care is functional and task-focused and therefore unable to recognise individual circumstances and complexities (MacLellan et al., 2022). This includes the recording of complex social circumstances as a 'tick-box' exercise rather than a nuanced discussion, which can allow trust to be built (Draper et al., 2023a, 2023b; Felker et al., 2024; MacLellan et al., 2022).

Institutional racism

Institutional racism refers to how processes and procedures within institutions, such as hospitals and other healthcare settings, are influenced by broader structural biases and discriminatory cultures of practice, including collective acceptance of interpersonal racism amongst staff, all of which can impact the experiences of minoritised groups. A recent confidential enquiry into the care of Asian and Black women who experienced a stillbirth or neonatal death found that, although overall improvements needed for care were graded similarly for Asian, Black, and White women, there was evidence of significant microaggressions in the care of pregnant women belonging to minority ethnic groups (Draper et al., 2023a, 2023b). This includes Asian and Black women's ethnicity and the ethnicity of their partner not being recorded correctly or consistently, and many minority ethnic women's individual circumstances and complexities not being recognised or considered in their care (Draper et al., 2023a, 2023b). Issues with completeness and consistency of ethnicity data collection in health statistics can lead to underreporting or misclassification, which may obscure some inequalities or patterns in maternal outcomes.

Women from minority ethnic groups also express greater concerns about labour and delivery relating to pain management and possible medical interventions than White women (Redshaw & Heikkilä, 2011). This is perhaps not unfounded, as Black African women are significantly more likely to have an emergency caesarean birth than White women (Henderson et al., 2013) and Black women who have an elective or emergency caesarean birth are more likely to receive general anaesthesia over neuraxial analgesia (epidural) compared to White women (Bamber et al., 2023), which can increase the risk of adverse maternal outcomes. Similarly, amongst women giving birth vaginally, Asian women are less likely than White women to receive neuraxial analgesia (epidural) for pain relief during labour (Bamber et al., 2023).

Some institutional factors that influence care can be resolved fairly easily, such as the provision of halal foods in maternity and postnatal wards; however, others represent more challenging, underlying systemic issues. The stretched workforce means that the availability of in-person GP appointments is rare in many parts of the country. For women who require a female practitioner for religious or cultural reasons, this adds another barrier to access.

Interpersonal racism

Interpersonal racism can occur when healthcare providers hold conscious or unconscious biases that influence how they interact with and provide care to women from different ethnic backgrounds. Multiple examples of interpersonal bias have been identified within the antenatal care of women from Black and Asian ethnic backgrounds (Knight et al., 2022). The most frequently observed biases related to a lack of individualised care include an under-appreciation of women's complex and cultural needs, and examples of microaggressions directly related to women's ethnicity. Biases and concerns about the quality of antenatal care received by minority ethnic women were also consistently reported in MBRRACE-UK confidential enquiries, including evidence of various microaggressions and discrimination (Felker et al., 2024; Kenyon et al., 2024).

Lower satisfaction with care during labour and childbirth and poorer childbirth experiences for minority ethnic women have also been reported in several national surveys (Harrison et al., 2025). A recent report on Black maternity experience in the UK found that the most commonly reported attitude of healthcare providers towards Black and Black mixed women was one of dismissiveness and a feeling of being ignored

(Peter & Wheeler, 2025). Women also reported feeling that they are not spoken to in a way they can understand, treated with kindness, or sufficiently involved in decisions (Henderson et al., 2013; Raleigh et al., 2010; Redshaw & Henderson, 2014).

Evidence of dismissiveness and not being listened to was echoed in UK studies reporting instances of minority ethnic women's concerns not being taken seriously or agitations dismissed as mental health problems (Knight et al., 2022; MacLellan et al., 2022). This may result in potential misdiagnosis or delayed or inadequate care. There is also still evidence of Black and Asian women's pain being dismissed due to an unfounded belief that their pain tolerances are higher than those of White women (Knight et al., 2022; Peter & Wheeler, 2025). As such, many women from minority ethnic groups often report limited confidence and trust in staff throughout their maternity care.

Maternal health in a wider context

While racial inequalities in experience and outcomes can be observed and measured, it is an oversimplification to assume that ethnicity alone drives the disparities. Poverty is an independent risk factor for poor maternal health outcomes (Felker et al., 2024; Geddes-Barton, Baldelli, et al., 2024; Vousden et al., 2025), and a higher proportion of women of minoritised ethnicity live in areas of deprivation (Geddes-Barton et al., 2025). Many underlying risks, such as obesity, are influenced by ethnicity and socioeconomic position, and social determinants of health, such as health behaviour, cultural beliefs, social norms, and relationships, are closely entwined with ethnicity and identity.

It is necessary to reflect on the context in which maternity care is delivered, the experiences of those receiving it, and how this sits within the wider structures of our society in order to start to unpick the drivers of inequality in maternal health and to consider how to implement change. While social complexities, domestic abuse, limited social supports, and financial hardship are not unique to women from minority ethnic backgrounds, evidence from the studies outlined earlier, and others, suggests that certain vulnerabilities are overrepresented amongst minority ethnic groups and that minority ethnic women may not have the same access to individualised care as White women.

Efforts to address inequalities in maternity care have been growing, with the promotion of policies to reduce systemic racism and initiatives to improve cultural competence among healthcare professionals and to increase diversity in the healthcare workforce. For example, training programmes that focus on unconscious bias mitigation and enhancing communication skills and cultural sensitivity have been shown to improve the quality of maternity care for minority ethnic women. In addition to these initiatives, greater attention to basic care principles is needed, such as kindness and respect during pregnancy, labour, and childbirth to ensure equitable and compassionate maternity care experiences for women from all backgrounds (Peter & Wheeler, 2025). Numerous grassroots organisations in the UK continue to advocate for the improvement of outcomes for minority ethnic groups, and the political will to address inequality in maternal health is growing with a recent announcement of a national investigation into maternity and neonatal care (Department of Health and Social Care et al., 2025). It is imperative that the findings of this investigation are appropriately actioned to enact change and improve outcomes for all women.

Conclusion

The reasons behind the increased risk of maternal mortality and morbidity for women from certain ethnic groups are multifaceted and interconnected. Minority ethnic women who experience poor outcomes do not always have clear risk factors, such as pre-existing medical conditions. Thus, it is important to consider how all aspects of care, including discrimination, biases, and other barriers to access, may factor into their maternal health outcomes and experiences.

Discussion questions

1. Research across pregnancy, birth, the postpartum, and infancy is unusual because we are often studying an outcome in more than one person including the mother, the baby, the mother-baby dyad, or the family. This can present additional challenges when looking at ethnic inequalities, particularly if the mother and baby are recorded as having different ethnicities. Reflect on how ethnicity is defined, whose ethnicity you would want to consider when studying the following outcomes, and why they may differ: fetal growth, maternal morbidity, birthweight, healthcare utilisation for the mother, and healthcare utilisation for the baby.
2. The factors influencing ethnicity-based inequalities in maternal outcomes are multifaceted and interconnected. In your view, where should efforts and interventions be targeted in order to best reduce inequalities?
3. It is clear that there are many evidence gaps around how ethnicity impacts experiences of and engagement with care, particularly concerning perinatal mental health. What evidence do you think is needed in order to make decisions and target interventions to reduce ethnic inequalities in access to maternity services and maternal outcomes?

Further reading

1. Knight, M., Bunch, K., Vousden, N., Banerjee, A., Cox, P., Cross-Sudworth, F., Dhanjal, M. K., Douglas, J., Girling, J., Kenyon, S., Kotnis, R., Patel, R., Shakespeare, J., Tuffnell, D., Wilkinson, M., & Kurinczuk, J. J. (2022). A national cohort study and confidential enquiry to investigate ethnic disparities in maternal mortality. *EClinicalMedicine*, *43*, 101237. https://doi.org/10.1016/j.eclinm.2021.101237
2. Felker, A., Patel, R., Kotnis, R., Kenyon, S., & Knight, M. (Eds.). (2024). *Saving Lives, Improving Mothers' Care – Lessons Learned to Inform Maternity Care from the UK and Ireland Confidential Enquiries into Maternal Deaths and Morbidity 2020–22*. National Perinatal Epidemiology Unit, University of Oxford. https://doi.org/10.5287/ora-j0yabxa44
3. Harrison, S., Alderdice, F., Fellmeth, G., & Quigley, M. (2025). Inequalities in childbirth experiences: A population-based cross-sectional survey in England during the Covid-19 pandemic [version 1; peer review: 1 approved with reservations]. *NIHR Open Research*, *5*(31). https://doi.org/10.3310/nihropenres.13835.1
4. Peter, M., & Wheeler, R. (2022). *The Black Maternity Experiences Survey: A Nationwide Study of Black Women's Experiences of Maternity Services in the United Kingdom*. Five X More. https://fivexmore.org/blackmereport
5. Birthrights. (2022). *Systemic Racism, Not Broken Bodies: An Inquiry into Racial Injustice and Human Rights in UK Maternity Care*. Birthrights.
6. MacLellan, J., Collins, S., Myatt, M., Pope, C., Knighton, W., & Rai, T. (2022). Black, Asian and Minority Ethnic Women's Experiences of Maternity Services in the UK: A Qualitative Evidence Synthesis. *Journal of Advanced Nursing*, *78*(7), 2175–2190. https://doi.org/10.1111/jan.15233

References

Bamber, J. H., Goldacre, R., Lucas, D. N., Quasim, S., & Knight, M. (2023). A national cohort study to investigate the association between ethnicity and the provision of care in obstetric anaesthesia in England between 2011 and 2021. *Anaesthesia*, *78*(7), 820–829. https://doi.org/10.1111/anae.15987

Bansal, N., Karlsen, S., Sashidharan, S. P., Cohen, R., Chew-Graham, C. A., & Malpass, A. (2022). Understanding ethnic inequalities in mental healthcare in the UK: A meta-ethnography. *PLoS Med*, *19*(12), e1004139. https://doi.org/10.1371/journal.pmed.1004139

Birthrights. (2022). *Systemic Racism, Not Broken Bodies: An Inquiry into Racial Injustice and Human Rights in UK Maternity Care*. Birthrights.

Conneely, M., Packer, K. C., Bicknell, S., Janković, J., Sihre, H. K., McCabe, R., Copello, A., Bains, K., Priebe, S., Spruce, A., & Jovanović, N. (2023). Exploring Black and South Asian women's experiences of help-seeking and engagement in perinatal mental health services in the UK. *Front Psychiatry*, *14*, 1119998. https://doi.org/10.3389/fpsyt.2023.1119998

Davies, D., McDougall, A., Prophete, A., Sivashanmugarajan, V., & Yoong, W. (2022). COVID-19 vaccination: Patient uptake and attitudes in a multi-ethnic North London maternity unit. *Postgraduate Medical Journal*, *98*(1164), 750–755. https://doi.org/10.1136/pmj-2022-141829

Department of Health and Social Care. (2025). *Fit for the Future: 10 Year Health Plan for England*. London: DHSC. https://www.gov.uk/government/publications/10-year-health-plan-for-england-fit-for-the-future

Department of Health and Social Care, NHS England, & The Rt. Hon Wes Streeting MP. (2025). *National Maternity Investigation Launched to Drive Improvements*. https://www.gov.uk/government/news/national-maternity-investigation-launched-to-drive-improvements

Draper, E., Gallimore, I., Kurinczuk, J. J., & Kenyon, S. (Eds.). (2023a). *MBRRACE-UK Perinatal Confidential Enquiry, A Comparison of the Care of Asian and White Women Who Have Experienced a Stillbirth or Neonatal Death: State of the Nation Report*. The Infant Mortality and Morbidity Studies, Department of Population Health Sciences, University of Leicester.

Draper, E., Gallimore, I., Kurinczuk, J. J., & Kenyon, S. (Eds.). (2023b). *MBRRACE-UK Perinatal Confidential Enquiry, A Comparison of the Care of Black and White Women Who Have Experienced a Stillbirth or Neonatal Death: State of the Nation Report*. The Infant Mortality and Morbidity Studies, Department of Population Health Sciences, University of Leicester.

Esan, O. B., Adjei, N. K., Saberian, S., Christianson, L., McHale, P., Pennington, A., Geary, R., & Ayorinde, A. (2022). *Mapping Existing Policy Interventions to Tackle Ethnic Health Inequalities in Maternal and Neonatal Health in England: A Systematic Scoping Review with Stakeholder Engagement*. NHS Race & Health Observatory. https://www.nhsrho.org/wp-content/uploads/2022/12/RHO-Mapping-existing-policy-interventions_December-2022.pdf

Felker, A., & Knight, M. (2026). *MBRRACE-UK Data Brief: Maternal Mortality 2022–2024*. National Perinatal Epidemiology Unit, University of Oxford. https://www.npeu.ox.ac.uk/mbrrace-uk/data-brief/maternal-mortality-2022-2024

Felker, A., Patel, R., Kotnis, R., Kenyon, S., & Knight, M. (Eds.). (2024). *Saving Lives, Improving Mothers' Care – Lessons Learned to Inform Maternity Care from the UK and Ireland Confidential Enquiries into Maternal Deaths and Morbidity 2020–22*. National Perinatal Epidemiology Unit, University of Oxford. https://doi.org/10.5287/ora-j0yabxa44

Felker, A., Patel, R., Kotnis, R., Kenyon, S., & Knight, M. (Eds.). (2025). *Saving Lives, Improving Mothers' Care – Lessons Learned to Inform Maternity Care from the UK and Ireland Confidential Enquiries into Maternal Deaths and Morbidity 2021–23*. National Perinatal Epidemiology Unit, University of Oxford. https://doi.org/10.5287/ora-4javr692x

Fellmeth, G., Harrison, S., McNeill, J., Lynn, F., Redshaw, M., & Alderdice, F. (2022). Identifying postnatal anxiety: Comparison of self-identified and self-reported anxiety using the

Edinburgh Postnatal Depression Scale. *BMC Pregnancy Childbirth*, *22*(1), 180. https://doi.org/10.1186/s12884-022-04437-0

Fellmeth, G., Opondo, C., Henderson, J., Redshaw, M., McNeill, J., Lynn, F., & Alderdice, F. (2019). Identifying postnatal depression: Comparison of a self-reported depression item with Edinburgh Postnatal Depression Scale scores at three months postpartum. *Journal of Affective Disorders*, *251*, 8–14. https://doi.org/10.1016/j.jad.2019.03.002

Fernandez Turienzo, C., Newburn, M., Agyepong, A., Buabeng, R., Dignam, A., Abe, C., Bedward, L., Rayment-Jones, H., Silverio, S. A., Easter, A., Carson, L. E., Howard, L. M., & Sandall, J. (2021). Addressing inequities in maternal health among women living in communities of social disadvantage and ethnic diversity. *BMC Public Health*, *21*(1), 176. https://doi.org/10.1186/s12889-021-10182-4

Galanis, P., Vraka, I., Siskou, O., Konstantakopoulou, O., Katsiroumpa, A., & Kaitelidou, D. (2022). Uptake of COVID-19 vaccines among pregnant women: A systematic review and meta-analysis. *Vaccines (Basel)*, *10*(5). https://doi.org/10.3390/vaccines10050766

Geddes-Barton, D., Baldelli, S., Karthikappallil, R., Bentley, T., Omorodion, B., Thompson, L., Roberts, N. W., Goldacre, R., Knight, M., & Ramakrishnan, R. (2024). Association between socioeconomic disadvantage and severe maternal morbidity and mortality in high-income countries: A systematic review. *Journal of Epidemiology & Community Health*. https://doi.org/10.1136/jech-2024-222407

Geddes-Barton, D., Goldacre, R., Knight, M., Vousden, N., & Ramakrishnan, R. (2025). Ethnic disparities in severe maternal morbidity and the contribution of deprivation: A population-based causal analysis. *BJOG*. https://doi.org/10.1111/1471-0528.18254

Geddes-Barton, D., Ramakrishnan, R., Knight, M., & Goldacre, R. (2024). Associations between neighbourhood deprivation, ethnicity and maternal health outcomes in England: A nationwide cohort study using routinely collected healthcare data. *Journal of Epidemiology & Community Health*, *78*(8), 500–507. https://doi.org/10.1136/jech-2024-222060

Harrison, S., Alderdice, F., Fellmeth, G., & Quigley, M. (2025). Inequalities in childbirth experiences: A population-based cross-sectional survey in England during the Covid-19 pandemic [version 1; peer review: 1 approved with reservations]. *NIHR Open Research*, *5*(31). https://doi.org/10.3310/nihropenres.13835.1

Harrison, S., Pilkington, V., Li, Y., Quigley, M. A., & Alderdice, F. (2023). Disparities in who is asked about their perinatal mental health: An analysis of cross-sectional data from consecutive national maternity surveys. *BMC Pregnancy Childbirth*, *23*(1), 263. https://doi.org/10.1186/s12884-023-05518-4

Harrison, S., Quigley, M. A., Fellmeth, G., Stein, A., & Alderdice, F. (2023). The impact of the Covid-19 pandemic on postnatal depression: Analysis of three population-based national maternity surveys in England (2014–2020). *The Lancet Regional Health–Europe*, *30*, 100654. https://doi.org/10.1016/j.lanepe.2023.100654

Harrison, S., Quigley, M. A., Fellmeth, G., Stein, A., Ayers, S., & Alderdice, F. (2024). The impact of the Covid-19 pandemic on postnatal anxiety and posttraumatic stress: Analysis of two population-based national maternity surveys in England. *Journal of Affective Disorders*, *356*, 122–136. https://doi.org/10.1016/j.jad.2024.04.003

Henderson, J., Gao, H., & Redshaw, M. (2013). Experiencing maternity care: The care received and perceptions of women from different ethnic groups. *BMC Pregnancy Childbirth*, *13*, 196. https://doi.org/10.1186/1471-2393-13-196

House of Commons Health and Social Care Committee. (2025). *Black Maternal Health: Third Report of Session 2024–26*. House of Commons. https://committees.parliament.uk/publications/49523/documents/263985/default/

House of Commons Women and Equalities Committee. (2023). *Black Maternal Health: Third Report of Session 2022–23*. House of Commons. https://committees.parliament.uk/publications/38989/documents/191706/default/

Howard, L. M., Molyneaux, E., Dennis, C. L., Rochat, T., Stein, A., & Milgrom, J. (2014). Non-psychotic mental disorders in the perinatal period. *Lancet*, *384*(9956), 1775–1788. https://doi.org/10.1016/s0140-6736(14)61276-9

John, J. R., Curry, G., & Cunningham-Burley, S. (2021). Exploring ethnic minority women's experiences of maternity care during the SARS-CoV-2 pandemic: A qualitative study. *BMJ Open*, *11*(9), e050666. https://doi.org/10.1136/bmjopen-2021-050666

Jomeen, J., & Redshaw, M. (2013). Ethnic minority women's experience of maternity services in England. *Ethnicity & Health*, *18*(3), 280–296. https://doi.org/10.1080/13557858.2012.730608

Kenyon, S., Gallimore, I., Evans, T., Page, G., Felker, A., & Fenton, A. (2024). *MBRRACE-UK Perinatal Confidential Enquiry, The Care of Recent Migrant Women with Language Barriers Who Have Experienced a Stillbirth or Neonatal Death: State of the Nation Report.* TIMMS, Department of Population Health Sciences, & University of Leicester.

Khan, Z. (2021). Ethnic health inequalities in the UK's maternity services: A systematic literature review. *British Journal of Midwifery*, *29*(2), 100–107. https://doi.org/10.12968/bjom.2021.29.2.100

Knight, M., Bunch, K., Felker, A., Patel, R., Kotnis, R., Kenyon, S., & Kurinczuk, J. J. (Eds.). (2023). *Saving Lives, Improving Mothers' Care – Lessons Learned to Inform Maternity Care from the UK and Ireland Confidential Enquiries into Maternal Deaths and Morbidity 2019–21*. National Perinatal Epidemiology Unit, University of Oxford. https://doi.org/10.5287/ora-kzkpjdbpg

Knight, M., Bunch, K., Vousden, N., Banerjee, A., Cox, P., Cross-Sudworth, F., Dhanjal, M. K., Douglas, J., Girling, J., Kenyon, S., Kotnis, R., Patel, R., Shakespeare, J., Tuffnell, D., Wilkinson, M., & Kurinczuk, J. J. (2022). A national cohort study and confidential enquiry to investigate ethnic disparities in maternal mortality. *EClinicalMedicine*, *43*, 101237. https://doi.org/10.1016/j.eclinm.2021.101237

Knight, M., Kenyon, S., Brocklehurst, P., Neilson, J., Shakespeare, J., & Kurinczuk, J. (Eds.). (2014). *Saving Lives, Improving Mothers' Care – Lessons Learned to Inform Maternity Care from the UK and Ireland Confidential Enquiries into Maternal Deaths and Morbidity 2009–12*. National Perinatal Epidemiology Unit, University of Oxford. https://doi.org/10.5287/ora-nrymp8wxq

Knight, M., Kurinczuk, J. J., Spark, P., & Brocklehurst, P. (2009). Inequalities in maternal health: National cohort study of ethnic variation in severe maternal morbidities. *BMJ*, *338*, b542. https://doi.org/10.1136/bmj.b542

Labour Party. (2024). *Labour Party Manifesto 2024: Our Plan to Change Britain*. https://labour.org.uk/change/

MacLellan, J., Collins, S., Myatt, M., Pope, C., Knighton, W., & Rai, T. (2022). Black, Asian and minority ethnic women's experiences of maternity services in the UK: A qualitative evidence synthesis. *Journal of Advanced Nursing*, *78*(7), 2175–2190. https://doi.org/10.1111/jan.15233

Moore, L., Jayaweera, H., Redshaw, M., & Quigley, M. (2019). Migration, ethnicity and mental health: Evidence from mothers participating in the Millennium Cohort Study. *Public Health*, *171*, 66–75. https://doi.org/10.1016/j.puhe.2019.03.022

Nair, M., Kurinczuk, J. J., & Knight, M. (2014). Ethnic variations in severe maternal morbidity in the UK – a case control study. *PLoS One*, *9*(4), e95086. https://doi.org/10.1371/journal.pone.0095086

Nair, M., Kurinczuk, J. J., & Knight, M. (2016). Establishing a national maternal morbidity outcome indicator in England: A population-based study using routine hospital data. *PLoS One*, *11*(4), e0153370. https://doi.org/10.1371/journal.pone.0153370

National Institute for Health and Care Excellence. (2021). *NG194: Postnatal Care*. Retrieved June 22, 2025, from https://www.nice.org.uk/guidance/ng194

Nazroo, J. Y., Bhui, K. S., & Rhodes, J. (2020). Where next for understanding race/ethnic inequalities in severe mental illness? Structural, interpersonal and institutional racism. *Sociology of Health & Illness*, *42*(2), 262–276. https://doi.org/10.1111/1467-9566.13001

Obionu, I. M., Onyedinma, C. A., Mielewczyk, F., & Boyle, E. (2023). UK maternity care experiences of ethnic minority and migrant women: Systematic review. *Public Health Nursing*, *40*(6), 846–856. https://doi.org/10.1111/phn.13240

Office for Health Improvement and Disparities. (2025). *Estimated Prevalence of Perinatal Mental Health Conditions in England, 2016 and 2019*. OHID. https://www.gov.uk/government/publications/perinatal-mental-health-condition-prevalence/estimated-prevalence-of-perinatal-mental-health-conditions-in-england-2016-to-2019

Peter, M., & Wheeler, R. (2022). *The Black Maternity Experiences Survey: A Nationwide Study of Black Women's Experiences of Maternity Services in the United Kingdom*. Five X More. https://fivexmore.org/blackmereport

Peter, M., & Wheeler, R. (2025). *The Five X More Black Maternity Experiences Report: Continuing the Conversation on Black Maternal Care in the UK*. Five X More. https://fivexmore.org/black-maternity-experiences-report-2025

Pilav, S., De Backer, K., Easter, A., Silverio, S. A., Sundaresh, S., Roberts, S., & Howard, L. M. (2022). A qualitative study of minority ethnic women's experiences of access to and engagement with perinatal mental health care. *BMC Pregnancy Childbirth*, *22*(1), 421. https://doi.org/10.1186/s12884-022-04698-9

Prady, S. L., Pickett, K. E., Croudace, T., Fairley, L., Bloor, K., Gilbody, S., Kiernan, K. E., & Wright, J. (2013). Psychological distress during pregnancy in a multi-ethnic community: Findings from the born in Bradford cohort study. *PLoS One*, *8*(4), e60693. https://doi.org/10.1371/journal.pone.0060693

Raleigh, V. S., Hussey, D., Seccombe, I., & Hallt, K. (2010). Ethnic and social inequalities in women's experience of maternity care in England: Results of a national survey. *Journal of the Royal Society of Medicine*, *103*(5), 188–198. https://doi.org/10.1258/jrsm.2010.090460

Redshaw, M., & Heikkilä, K. (2011). Ethnic differences in women's worries about labour and birth. *Ethnicity & Health*, *16*(3), 213–223. https://doi.org/10.1080/13557858.2011.561302

Redshaw, M., & Henderson, J. (Eds.). (2014). *Safely Delivered: A National Survey of Women's Experience of Maternity Care 2014*. The National Perinatal Epidemiology Unit, University of Oxford.

Rowe, R. E., Magee, H., Quigley, M. A., Heron, P., Askham, J., & Brocklehurst, P. (2008). Social and ethnic differences in attendance for antenatal care in England. *Public Health*, *122*(12), 1363–1372. https://doi.org/10.1016/j.puhe.2008.05.011

Silverio, S. A., Varman, N., Barry, Z., Khazaezadeh, N., Rajasingam, D., Magee, L. A., & Matthew, J. (2023). Inside the 'imperfect mosaic': Minority ethnic women's qualitative experiences of race and ethnicity during pregnancy, childbirth, and maternity care in the United Kingdom. *BMC Public Health*, *23*(1), 2555. https://doi.org/10.1186/s12889-023-17505-7

Vousden, N., Bunch, K., Kenyon, S., Kurinczuk, J. J., & Knight, M. (2024). Impact of maternal risk factors on ethnic disparities in maternal mortality: A national population-based cohort study. *The Lancet Regional Health–Europe*, *40*, 100893. https://doi.org/10.1016/j.lanepe.2024.100893

Vousden, N., Geddes-Barton, D., Hanley, S. J., Roberts, N., & Knight, M. (2025). Interventions to reduce inequalities for pregnant women living with disadvantage in high-income countries: An umbrella review. *BMC Public Health*, *25*(1), 1140. https://doi.org/10.1186/s12889-025-22283-5

Zhang, C. X., Quigley, M. A., Bankhead, C., Kwok, C. H., Parekh, N., & Carson, C. (2024). Ethnic inequities in 6–8 week baby check coverage in England 2006–2021: A cohort study using the Clinical Practice Research Datalink. *British Journal of General Practice*, *74*(746), e595–e603. https://doi.org/10.3399/bjgp.2023.0593

CHAPTER 6

Language interpretation provision in maternity services

A racialised perspective

Sarah Akhtar Baz, Laura Sheard, Anne MacFarlane, and Jennifer MacLellan

Introduction

The routine use of professionally trained interpreters in healthcare settings can raise standards of care to equal that of patients who do not experience communication barriers (Puthoopparambil et al., 2021). However, a lack of adequate and good-quality professional interpreter provision has been consistently highlighted as a key shortcoming in service provision for ethnic minority[1] and migrant[2] people who have cross-cultural communication needs in English healthcare settings. This inadequacy leads to significant health issues and health inequalities (Rayment-Jones et al., 2021; Gill et al., 2011; MacFarlane et al., 2009). This chapter explores interpreting provision and use in healthcare from a racialised perspective, an under-researched issue that warrants urgent attention.

The use of professionally trained interpreters is known to be the safest support for patients who experience communication barriers (Puthoopparambil et al., 2021). However, previous studies have found that professional interpreters are underused in healthcare, with informal interpreters, including bilingual staff, family and friends, undertaking the interpretations (Rayment-Jones et al., 2021; Gill et al., 2011; MacFarlane et al., 2009). The National Health Service (NHS) Race and Health Observatory (RHO) recommends concerted efforts be made to ensure readily accessible high-quality interpreting services (Kapadia et al., 2022). Providing adequate interpreter provision is particularly crucial for pregnant women[3] whose preferred language is not English, enabling them to access safe, ethical, and efficient maternity care (Cramer, 2017). The MBRRACE-UK (2024) report found that many pregnant women who had recently migrated to the UK with English language challenges did not have their language needs assessed. The lack of provision, combined with this clear need, highlights the continuing shortsightedness in anticipating interpretation provision in this context. While interpreter provision in maternity care remains the focus of this chapter, we will also explore interpreter provision across the healthcare system.

Hamed et al. (2022) argue that it is important to focus on racism 'as the object of research' to provide a more in-depth and complex account of the role racism plays in

DOI: 10.4324/9781003466093-10

healthcare and health inequity. Reasserting the importance of recognising racial discrimination, Pattillo et al. (2023) also argue that racism and its impacts on racialised migrants' access to healthcare are 'remarkably under-researched' as compared to other barriers like communication barriers. The role of racism in interpreter provision is, therefore, a niche and important area of interest. To begin to bridge this knowledge gap, this chapter explores language interpretation provision and use in healthcare settings, with a particular interest in maternity services for ethnic minority and migrant women in England and how this is intricately linked to issues of race and health inequity. We also draw on studies from other European countries to reference the wider interpretation literature and incorporate learning from these contexts. This chapter incorporates Critical Race Theory (CRT) (Meghji & Niang, 2022; Solórzano & Yosso, 2001) to help contextualise interpreter provision in a racialised society.

The chapter advances the topics of race and racialisation to the issue of interpreter provision. It aims to address the following questions:

1. What does a racialised approach offer to contextualising interpreter provision in maternity care?
2. How do race, ethnicity, migration status, and gender intersect with interpreting provision?
3. How can health equity, quality care, and improved interpreter provision for all pregnant women in maternity services be achieved?

The chapter first starts with a background of interpreter provision in England with the key barriers and shortcomings outlined. It then moves on to defining what racism is, introducing CRT, and exploring racism in the area of healthcare. It introduces different dimensions of racism in relation to healthcare, namely the structural, institutional, and interpersonal (Pattillo et al., 2023). The chapter then explores the role racism in healthcare and wider society plays in influencing interpreter provision and policy, by moving beyond the 'language problem' (Piacentini et al., 2019), bringing the two areas of focus (interpreter provision and CRT) together. This chapter takes a racialised approach to contextualising poor professional interpreter provision in maternity care, whilst acknowledging that race intersects with other factors, such as ethnicity, gender, religion, class, and migration status (Solórzano & Yosso, 2001), in producing poor outcomes. A lack of adequate, quality interpreter support has previously been discussed in practice from a perspective of quality and safety of care provision (e.g. Kapadia et al., 2022; Loewenthal et al., 2012); however, this deficit has been explored neither from a racialised perspective, nor in the wider context of the racialised language concerning ethnicity, migration, gender, and race. This chapter aims to address this gap.

Background: Challenges encountered in interpreter provision within maternity care

We start the chapter by outlining the 'problem' and key gap in service provision, namely the inadequate provision of high-quality language interpretation despite its utmost importance in the field of maternity care.

National Health Service England (NHSE) has pledged to improve the health outcomes of mothers and babies by focusing on the populations with greatest experience of ill health who reside in the 20% most deprived areas of England (NHSE, 2022). Women with cross-cultural communication needs are overrepresented within these populations experiencing intersecting disadvantage and poor health, and poor maternal and infant outcomes (Knight et al., 2020; ONS, 2015). Language, communication, and understanding of information are central to the provision of safe maternity care; therefore, when provider and patient do not share a linguistic or cultural background, supporting cross-cultural consultations is essential for pregnant women to be equal partners in their care. All women need access to information about their pregnancy and birth in order to give informed consent. They need to be able to ask questions and understand the answers, and they need to know where to seek help if needed (NHSE, 2016). Research shows that cross-cultural communication adds complexity to this endeavour. Cultural differences between providers and patients can lead to misunderstandings and conflicts, affecting the experience and quality of care (Liamputtong & Suwankhong, 2019). Belief systems, values, practices, and social norms shape a person's understanding of health problems and influence their use of healthcare services and help-seeking behaviours (Teti & van Wyk, 2020; Vaughn, 2019). Some healthcare providers' demonstrations of racist and discriminative attitudes and beliefs about ethnic minority women, migrants and their culture can also negatively influence the care that they receive (Pattillo et al., 2023; Hamed et al., 2022; Kapadia et al., 2022).

Those whose preferred language is not English may neither understand signs and symptoms of pregnancy that are cause for concern, nor know how to seek help. Poor cross-cultural communication may further invalidate consent due to patients not understanding enough to make informed decisions. Informed consent is a legal and ethical principle, making permissible a wide range of conduct that would otherwise be wrongful (Miller & Wertheimer, 2009). It is a positive act that goes beyond acquiescence or compliance. For informed consent to be valid, the person providing consent must understand the risks and benefits of the suggested intervention, and it is incumbent on the person seeking consent to ensure that the person understands what they are consenting to (NHS, 2022). Standards of consent in maternity care have been reported as sub-optimal by pregnant women and clinicians (Gutman et al., 2022; Birthrights, 2020). Thus, altogether, pregnant women with cross-cultural communication needs are at risk of inadequate, unconsented care, leaving them feeling isolated, unsupported, and unable to communicate (Cramer, 2017; Karliner et al., 2007) and worse, potentially receiving interventions they did not want. This represents a significant translational gap between policy and practice, which compromises the NHS's commitment to woman-centred, safe, equitable care (NHSE, 2016; van den Muijsenbergh et al., 2014).

Common barriers reported about the use of interpreters in maternity services in England, the UK, and other European countries are multifactorial and include issues and challenges of (1) interpreter availability, (2) interpreter quality, and (3) organisational factors. This section further considers these issues and the multifactorial challenges in relation to providing high-quality interpreter provision.

Interpreter availability

A systematic review of access to maternity services among immigrant pregnant women describes how they often have no other option than to arrange for family or friends to act as interpreters (Higginbottom et al., 2020). Research focusing on unscheduled maternity care encounters among women with cross-cultural communication needs is limited. However, in the meta-ethnography of Sellevold et al. (2022) covering six countries, participants described acute situations that ended in perceived forced consent as they did not understand what was being said to them. This led to anxiety, trauma and unwanted interventions.

Lack of interpreter availability can be observed across the healthcare system (Kapadia et al., 2022). Loewenthal et al. (2012), who examined interpreter availability within general practitioner (GP) services, found that many patients felt interpreter services were unreliable and that interpreters were untrustworthy. Kapadia et al. (2022) found that in the context of GP services, it is very rare for there to be interpreters for traditional languages like those used by the Roma community, who may not speak the main language of their country (Kapadia et al., 2022). This can make it difficult to communicate healthcare issues. There is often a lack of accessibility to interpreting services, particularly in urgent situations, leading to family interpreting (Kapadia et al., 2022). Similar availability issues are likely present in maternity services. For example, in a recent review of maternal deaths, none of the 17 women who required interpreter support had received appropriate provision at all key points of their maternity care (Cosstick et al., 2022).

Interpreter quality

Healthcare service users have expressed concern about the accuracy of interpretation and confidentiality of services (MacLellan et al., 2022; Sellevold et al., 2022; Crowther & Lau, 2019). Family or friends have been described as unable to properly understand and translate complex medical information (Higginbottom et al., 2020). Collusion and inaccuracy have been identified when informal interpreters, particularly family, have been used in public services, resulting in errors and compromised meaning (Lucas, 2015). Oscarsson and Stevenson-Ågren (2020) report that relatives can sometimes take over the conversation and answer questions themselves. A meta-ethnography by Pangas et al. (2019) reports that even professionally trained interpreters are sometimes unable to understand the medical terminology used in consultations. Whitaker et al.'s (2022) primary care study similarly found that formal interpreters have varying levels of medical terminology preparation for their role within different specialities. Agency requirements to work as an interpreter are inconsistent and vary by provider (Chartered institute linguistics, 2006). Brief, in-house training is often provided by agencies. Interpreters themselves have described receiving insufficient preparation for their role from such training, including learning medical terminology and physiology, or guidance on how to balance 'speaking up' about patient safety while remaining impartial when facilitating communication (Wu & Rawal, 2017). These tensions can impact practitioner trust in their skills (MacFarlane et al., 2020; Brisset et al., 2013) and increase women's preference for family to interpret (Rayment-Jones et al., 2021), despite NICE (2021) guidelines being clear that interpreters should be independent. The Kapadia et al. (2022) review concludes that better investment and resources are required to provide adequate interpreter provision along the maternal healthcare pathway, including more professionally trained interpreters. Currently, there is no minimum standard for interpreter qualification in healthcare and no accountability to ensure competence in interpreting skills.

Organisational factors

Midwives often lament a lack of training in how to access and work with interpreters, a lack of continuity in interpreter support, limited access to appropriate technology, and funding constraints (Bridle et al., 2021; Oscarsson & Stevenson-Ågren, 2020). Inaccurate assumptions from healthcare professionals of a woman's English proficiency are compounded by a lack of time in consultations and in planning for patients' language needs (Bridle et al., 2021; Khan, 2021; Oscarsson & Stevenson-Ågren, 2020). Minoritised women are also not always aware of their right to a trained interpreter (MacLellan et al., 2022).

Absent or irregular professional interpreters undermine midwifery care (Cramer, 2017). This is a risk factor for poor outcomes (Chitongo et al., 2022; Karliner et al., 2007) and can lead to suboptimal assessment of serious medical symptoms (Gutman et al., 2022; Knight et al., 2020), unconsented procedures, such as episiotomy, amniotomy, and internal examinations in labour (van der Pijl et al., 2020), as well as birth trauma (Birthrights, 2020). Poor interpreter provision can contribute to disparities in maternal mortality (Cosstick et al., 2022). Midwives report inefficient care and professional dissatisfaction when they cannot access timely, accurate, trusted, and professionally trained interpreters to support women with cross-cultural communication needs (Bridle et al., 2021). The 2022 NHS RHO evidence review described a lack of consistent and high-quality interpreting services to be a common issue for women who require an interpreter when using maternity services (Care Quality Commission, 2024; Kapadia et al., 2022). Both access to and the quality of interpreting services vary. These continue to contribute to patient safety incidents nationally, where having poor or no spoken English is associated with worse experiences of care (Care Quality Commission, 2024). A Freedom of Information request by MacLellan et al. (2024) found that women who needed an interpreter received an average of three interpreted consultations out of every 14 planned consultations. A lack of adequate interpreter provision disadvantages both healthcare providers, who strive to provide equitable healthcare, and those receiving care.

There are significant barriers to access and shortcomings in the provision of adequate and quality interpreter provision, particularly at crucial ethical and legal points on the maternal health journey, such as in providing informed consent to care or in understanding various medical terminologies. This chapter now moves on to introducing the lens of a 'racialised approach' with which to critique the current state of interpreter provision within healthcare services.

A racialised approach to interpreter provision

Defining racism and introducing CRT

Racial disparities in society create inequalities for ethnic minority, migrant, and other racialised groups in areas such as housing, health, and employment (Bhopal, 2023). 'Race' is a social construct (Bhopal, 2023) embedded in a historical process (Hamed et al., 2022; Spivak, 2000). Manzoor-Khan (2022) notes that 'there is no natural set of races that existed prior to people devising them'; in fact, the concept of race was invented to uphold colonial projects and to justify racism (Pattillo et al., 2023). Racism is defined as 'a system of power related to capitalism and colonialism' (Manzoor-Khan, 2022) that excludes, discriminates, exploits, and oppresses.

Contemporary racism generally manifests as systematic exclusion from access to adequate healthcare and housing (Manzoor-Khan, 2022) and also through 'more normalized covert or invisible processes rather than explicit expressions of racism' (Hamed et al., 2022). Racism, however, can also be more overt, as demonstrated in the right-wing riots of Summer 2024 in the UK. These overt expressions are fuelled by institutional racism and 'institutional power' (Marable, 1992).

To understand racism in contemporary society, it is useful to draw on Critical Race Theory (CRT). CRT is an approach which seeks to dissect contemporary racism and analyse national racialised social systems (Meghji & Niang, 2022). CRT attempts to identify oppressive aspects of society (Tierney, 1993 in Solórzano & Yosso, 2001) and to show how racism intersects with other systems of oppression, such as gender and class inequality. This awareness-making aims to engender individual and societal change (Solórzano & Yosso, 2001; Crenshaw, 1989). CRT centres racism as a central aspect of society predicated on White privilege (Bhopal, 2023), which are the 'specific privileges White groups possess due to their Whiteness and White identity' (Bhopal, 2023). CRT aims to achieve social justice (Meghji & Niang, 2022; Solórzano & Yosso, 2001) and to fully theorise 'race' (Ledesma & Calderón, 2015). CRT helps contextualise how contemporary racism and policies are informed by colonial histories and uphold White Privilege and inequality, bringing 'race' back to its imperialist roots grounded in Empire and colonial expansion rather than just focusing on the contemporary nation state (Meghji & Niang, 2022) and backlash against 'migrants' crossing borders. Bhopal (2023) argues that contemporary racism exists due to the existence of White privilege and reinforces institutional and structural processes. In doing so, a racial hierarchy is created that puts White groups in superior positions of power and advantage. Meghji and Niang (2022) and Bhopal (2023) point to the COVID-19 pandemic as both highlighting and exacerbating racial inequalities in real time. Rattansi (2020) argues that contemporary racism must be explored through a structural and systemic lens. Structural and systemic racism focuses on how interrelationships 'reproduce the subordinate and superior positions occupied by racialized populations' (Rattansi, 2020). By taking a CRT approach, disparities in education, housing, and health between White and ethnic minority people can be linked to the underpinning structural and systemic inequities in society (Bhopal, 2023; Rattansi, 2020).

Racism in healthcare

Considering healthcare, Hamed et al. (2022) argue that racism is a persistent barrier to achieving 'equitable and responsive healthcare'. Due to a dearth of research on race and interpreter provision in English healthcare settings, it is important to look closely at racism and racialised encounters in healthcare more generally and in maternal services specifically. Racism shapes people's health and healthcare experiences via three 'interdependent' dimensions (Pattillo et al., 2023). Firstly, the 'interpersonal' dimension is embedded in the everyday experience of violence and discrimination. Secondly, the 'institutional' dimension which is reflected in policies and norms in institutions leading to discriminative outcomes. And, finally the 'structural' dimension, which includes access to resources. Taken together, these three dimensions significantly impinge on the quality of healthcare that ethnic minority and migrant women receive.

Attitudes of healthcare staff and positive interactions between staff and patients are a critical component of high-quality care for pregnant women. It has been found that some healthcare staff can have racist attitudes and stereotypes about ethnic minorities, which can, in turn, influence the quality of care they provide (Henderson et al., 2013). Other studies have found that some healthcare staff homogenise ethnic minority service users and deny the existence of racism. For example, studies have found that some healthcare professionals consider those who follow the Muslim faith as 'problematic' and 'frustrating' and view Asians as holding irrational religious beliefs (Hamed et al., 2022; Morel, 2019; Vydelingum, 2006). In their scoping review, Pattillo et al. (2023) found discrimination and bias towards migrants in the healthcare system, such as when migrants are labelled as 'hysterical' and their pain dismissed as exaggerated. These biases are often experienced by women, highlighting the intersection of racism, ethnicity, and gender. Holding both power and privilege, some healthcare providers consider their judgments as objective and true, rather than subjective, discriminatory, and racist (Pattillo et al., 2023).

Stereotyping and racist attitudes have also been reported in maternity services (Henderson et al., 2013). In a quantitative study by Henderson et al. (2013), some healthcare staff suggested that if ethnic minority women behaved more like White women, the health disadvantages these groups face would be eradicated. The study also revealed that 'Asian women' are stereotypically perceived as not needing support as they are understood to be well supported by family, and when they do request help, this is perceived as being fussy, non-compliant and demanding (Henderson et al., 2013). A lack of consideration of cultural, social, and economic circumstances can lead to a lack of culturally contextual care (Heys et al., 2021). As such, much attention has been given to interpersonal discrimination, prejudice and racism within healthcare. Although discrimination and racism amongst some healthcare staff in maternity services is evident (see Kapadia et al., 2022) and cannot be denied, this 'bad apple' approach alone (Manzoor-Khan, 2022) overlooks discriminatory policies, systemic barriers, and structural racism, and how these are more prevalent in shaping health inequality and healthcare (Puthoopparambil et al., 2021). It is for these reasons that the NHS RHO (Kapadia et al., 2022) has concluded that NHS England must make a 'serious commitment' to tackle 'racist attitudes and behaviours amongst healthcare staff' and 'address structural dimensions of NHS systems that discriminate against ethnic minority women and their babies'.

Heys et al. (2021) found that disadvantaged, vulnerable, or ethnic minority women's experiences of traumatic birth are accompanied by a lack of consent, poor information giving, poor, and degrading care as recurring concerns. Women had no choice but to accept 'poor, inconsistent and deindividualized care' (Heys et al., 2021). Being seen and listened to would have provided better care for these women. As MacLellan et al. (2022) argue, ethnic minority and migrant women are often undermined and silenced in maternity care. Khan's (2021) work has found poor active listening skills among some healthcare providers. This undermines communication, leaving vulnerable women feeling dismissed and unsafe. This can reduce women's abilities to make informed choices, with significant implications for their care and safety (Kapadia et al., 2022). As shown in the previous section, language and a lack of interpreter support can disadvantage vulnerable women even further by creating barriers to essential aspects of their care (Hsieh & Ma, 2024). Structural factors such as inadequate policy, practice, and procedures inhibit the provision of quality interpretation services. This, in turn, adversely impacts healthcare providers' ability to supply adequate and safe care for mothers.

Different dimensions of racism in healthcare can have adverse impacts on the healthcare that ethnic minorities and migrants receive. Moving beyond the language problem and exploring how the issue of 'language' is constructed in wider racialised structural and institutional discourses around ethnic minority and migrant women in England can help further understand poor interpreter service provision.

Moving beyond 'language' and racialising interpreter provision

While this chapter has primarily focused on interpreter provision, we will now broaden our focus to explore cross-cultural consultations more generally, drawing attention to the linguistic *and* cultural backgrounds of patients *and* providers, and utilise a racialised approach to understanding how the issues of language and interpreter provision are constructed.

There is often a narrow focus on the 'language problem', that is, the issue being that many migrant and ethnic minority people have a 'lack of English language skills'. The belief in interpreting provision and language matching as a solution to this is pervasive. Alternatively, an intercultural communication approach (communication between two cultures) not only provides language support but also offers an opportunity for shared understanding of the diverse practices, knowledge, and positionalities of ethnic minorities and migrants and a readiness to understand other cultures without being judgemental (Piacentini et al., 2019). An individual's understanding of their health and the role of healthcare is shaped by their cultural backgrounds and life experiences. Taking an intersectional approach, a core component of CRT (Solórzano & Yosso, 2001; Crenshaw, 1989), ethnicity, migrant status, and culture intersect with structural and societal factors which burden individuals, impacting their health and healthcare trajectories. In their study, Piacentini et al. (2019) found that interpreters in the community often play a 'navigator' role to help immigrants with aspects such as accessing services, benefits, and housing. Beyond interpreting words, interpreting requires much emotional labour (Hsieh & Ma, 2024). These elements of intercultural communication elucidate the complexity of cross-cultural communication and challenge the interpreter's independent role as an impartial support to patient and providers. Paying attention to these elements can be helpful in improving interpreter provision beyond language matching and helping to improve intercultural and cross-cultural understandings, resolve misunderstandings, and transcend diverse belief systems, values, and practices.

Structural and discriminative policies shape perceptions of healthcare provision for ethnic minorities. Political racialised rhetoric often frames migrants as 'health tourists' or as being a 'drain on resources' (Piacentini et al., 2019). Ethnic minority women are also often racialised through political discourses around race, ethnicity, religion, and gender in relation to citizenship and social integration (Bredström & Gruber, 2015). These discussions are shaped by colonial legacies and the positioning of these women as harbingers of cultural difference. On the one hand, they are viewed as unwilling to integrate and on the other, as in need of containment within the boundaries of their community (Alexander, 2013). The English language is often seen as central to citizenship and integration; thus, there is a continued emphasis on assimilation through learning English and showing loyalty to the nation (Bloch et al., 2013; Kalra & Kapoor, 2009). Ethnic minority and migrant women, in particular those who are Muslim, are often labelled as different and the 'ethnic other' (Bredström & Gruber, 2015). These racialised approaches, which neglect their agency, are reflective of colonial narratives that have consistently racialised and problematised ethnic minority women as the 'inferior other' (Pattillo et al., 2023; Manzoor-Khan, 2022; Heys et al., 2021). Wider debates around citizenship and identity directly feed into discussions surrounding interpreter provision, including arguments around whether migrants have a 'duty' to learn English and discourse around the perceived high cost of interpreter provision to the NHS (MacFarlane et al., 2009). The problemisation of ethnic minority and migrant women locates the burden on them to change, without recognising the complicity of the nation's colonial past and its persistent classification of former colonial subjects as inferior, rather than adapting the system to meet their language needs.

It is important to consider the policies that shape the broader health landscapes in which ethnic minorities and migrants live (Castañeda et al., 2015). This assertion can also be extended to established ethnic minority populations in England. While the previous assertions may seem far from interpreter provision in maternity care, they can potentially shape policy around integrating interpreter provision in healthcare teams with fair pay and conditions, and the need for appropriate skills and recognition among interpreters working in healthcare settings. Puthoopparambil et al. (2021) state that 'conscious and unconscious societal racism and ethnocentrism were considered as possible reasons for the lack of political will to establish routine use of trained interpreters'. This leads to questions of whether particular ethnic groups are 'deserving' enough for this provision (Piacentini et al., 2019). 'Deservingness' refers to 'how some groups, but not others, are considered worthy of attention, investment, and care, particularly against the backdrop of the retrenchment of the welfare state and increasing healthcare costs' (Castañeda et al., 2015). Deservingness can influence how social and health resources are allocated. Language difference affects access to power, resources and services. Piacentini et al. (2019) found immigration status, language, and accent all affect perceived deservingness. They report that an individual's immigration status is often a focus in clinical appointments, and even where there are well-intentioned efforts to provide equitable healthcare services, there are complexities in interactions shaped by overlapping factors including ethnicity, language, local and regional identities, and migration experiences (Piacentini et al., 2019). These tensions can lead to medical mistrust and feelings of not being taken seriously and a resultant delay in healthcare seeking (Baz et al., 2023; Pattillo et al., 2023; Shahid & Dogra, 2022). There can also be fear amongst service users of stigma, judgement, and unpleasant and prejudicial attitudes (Heys et al., 2021). When talking about medical mistrust amongst the Muslim community, Shahid and Dogra (2022) argue that this is shaped by historical mistrust and structural factors. They explore mistrust in government policies both in the past, in relation to colonial legacies and austerity, and during the COVID-19 pandemic. Mistrust can lead to alternative healthcare seeking, the spreading of misinformation and delay in medical treatment and accessing healthcare. Feelings of mistrust are shaped by structural and systemic racism. Distrust may lead to women not wanting to speak to an interpreter regardless of the interpreter's identity, which creates serious implications and vulnerabilities, particularly within maternity care.

This section has teased out some of the wider pervasive racist discourses embedded within society's structures, institutions, and policies that influence negative attitudes towards ethnic minority and migrant populations. This includes how these discourses shape healthcare experiences, germinating feelings of distrust on both sides and culminating in poor interpreter provision and uptake. Such discourses need to be acknowledged when exploring professional interpreter provision and the practical improvements required.

Concluding thoughts

This chapter highlights a significant gap in the provision of adequate, high-quality interpreters and interpretation services in maternity services. It advocates for the urgent need to improve and optimise the use of professionally trained interpreters in this setting. We have discussed this in relation to ethnic minority and migrant women in England who are accessing maternity services. Language, communication, and understanding of information are central to safe, ethical and efficient maternity care (Cramer, 2017), particularly in relation to consent (Birthrights, 2020; Gutman et al., 2022). Currently, perinatal women with cross-cultural communication needs are at risk of inadequate, unconsented care, leaving them at risk of receiving care they do not want or unknowingly agree to, as well as feeling isolated and unable to make themselves understood at this critical stage in their life course (Cramer, 2017; Karliner et al., 2007). This can leave women reliant on informal interpretation provision from family or friends, which contravenes NICE (2021) guidelines and the NHSE's commitment to woman-centred, safe, equitable care (NHSE, 2016; van den Muijsenbergh et al., 2014). The chapter illustrates the systematic, structural, and institutional barriers to and shortcomings of interpreter provision in healthcare and maternity settings. These include lack of interpreter availability, poor interpreter quality, insufficient medical terminology training, and organisational barriers.

This chapter illustrates the importance of contextualising interpreter provision in the intersectional matrix of inequality (Crenshaw, 1989) for those ethnic minorities, migrants, and refugees on the receiving end of services. A CRT framework, combined with a colonialism and White privilege lens (Manzoor-Khan, 2022; Bhopal, 2023), helps identify and contextualise how racism operates at societal, structural, institutional, and interpersonal levels (Meghji & Niang, 2022; Solórzano & Yosso, 2001). Furthermore, the racialisation and politicisation of the 'language problem' can feed into narratives and the practice of interpreter provision while ignoring the nuance of and labour involved in cross-cultural communication. The chapter highlights the importance of accounting for structural and institutional racism and recognising how racialised policies and attitudes about migrants and ethnic minority women shape healthcare experiences and 'deservingness' of resource allocation. This is situated in the context of a society where a 'lack of English language skills' is perceived as a problem. Wider debates around citizenship, social integration, and assimilation can, albeit indirectly, shape the lack of attention being paid to providing high-quality interpreter provision. The role of structural, institutional, and interpersonal racism (Pattillo et al., 2023) must be considered when optimising interpreter provision.

This chapter has significant policy and practice implications, as well as theoretical contributions to the study of race in healthcare, maternity services, and cross-cultural communication. A key gap in the field yet to be explored is how these broader racialised narratives of the 'language problem' and 'deservingness' directly shape policy, practice, and provision in the field of interpreter provision. How do stereotypical tropes depicting migrants as undeserving of specific healthcare needs within a crippling healthcare system, or as racialised groups seen as less than and 'other', influence attitudes towards improving language provision? Exploring such questions is just as critical to achieving safe, confidential, and equitable maternity care for those with language needs as are the practical barriers to interpreter provision. Working toward solving the challenges of interpreter provision in maternity services will ensure that pregnant women can confidently communicate their needs at a critical point in their life course.

Discussion questions

1. Why is it important to provide high-quality professionally trained interpreters in the area of maternity care?
2. How does not meeting the language and communication needs of diverse users constitute structural racism?
3. What practical interventions and changes to policy would be needed to ensure those whose first language is not English receive equitable care?

Notes

1 Ethnic minority definition: Modood's work offers a comprehensive definition of ethnic minority. Ethnic minorities are those people of non-European descent who themselves or their families migrated to Britain. These are foremost people from the former British Empire and Commonwealth, including the Caribbean, Africa, Hong Kong, and South Asia (Modood, 2005). Ethnic minority groups' experiences are shaped by racism, 'attitudes, behaviours and structures of dominant groups' as well as their own heritage, including response to exclusion, religion, and collective action, and finally the 'political and economic relations between groups in Britain' (Modood et al., 2002, 1997).

2 Migrant definition: The International Organization for Migration's (IOM, 2024) definition of migrant is 'an umbrella term, not defined under international law, reflecting the common lay understanding of a person who moves away from his or her place of usual residence, whether within a country or across an international border, temporarily or permanently, and for a variety of reasons. The term includes a number of well-defined legal categories of people, such as migrant workers; persons whose particular types of movements are legally defined, such as smuggled migrants; as well as those whose status or means of movement are not specifically defined under international law, such as international students'. An immigrant refers to a person who comes to another country to live there permanently (Cambridge dictionary).

3 The term 'pregnant women' is used in this chapter, although not all pregnant individuals may identify with this term.

Further reading

Bhopal, K. (2023). Critical race theory: Confronting, challenging, and rethinking white privilege. *Annual Review of Sociology*, *49*, 111–128.

Bloch, A., Solomos, J., & Neal, S. (2013). *Race, Multiculturalism and Social Policy*. Palgrave Macmillan.

Meghji, A., & Niang, S. M. (2022). Between post-racial ideology and provincial universalisms. *Sociology*, *56*(1), 131–147.

Puthoopparambil, S. J., Phelan, M., & MacFarlane, A. (2021). Migrant health and language barriers. *Health Policy*, *125*, 1085–1091.

References

Alexander, C. (2013). Marriage, migration, multiculturalism: Gendering the Bengal diaspora. *Journal of Ethnic and Migration Studies*, *39*(3), 333–351.

Baz, S. A., Fang, C., Carpentieri, J., & Sheard, L. (2023). 'I don't know what to do or where to go': Experiences of accessing healthcare support from the perspectives of people living with long COVID and healthcare professionals. *Health Expectations*, *26*(1), 542–554.

Bhopal, K. (2023). Critical race theory: Confronting, challenging, and rethinking white privilege. *Annual Review of Sociology*, *49*, 111–128.

Birthrights. (2020). *Holding It All Together: Understanding How Far the Human Rights of Women Facing Disadvantage Are Respected during Pregnancy, Birth and Postnatal Care.* Birthrights.

Bloch, A., Solomos, J., & Neal, S. (2013). *Race, Multiculturalism and Social Policy.* Palgrave Macmillan.

Bredström, A., & Gruber, S. (2015). Language, culture and maternity care. *Nordic Journal of Migration Research*, *5*(2), 58–66.

Bridle, L., Bassett, S., & Silverio, S. (2021). 'We couldn't talk to her': A qualitative exploration of UK midwives' experiences of navigating women's care without language. *International Journal of Human Rights in Healthcare*, *14*(4), 359–373.

Brisset, C., Leanza, Y., & Laforest, K. (2013). Working with interpreters in health care: A systematic review and meta-ethnography of qualitative studies. *Patient Education and Counseling*, *91*(2), 131–140.

Care Quality Commission. (2024). *National Review of Maternity Services in England 2022–2024.* Care Quality Commission.

Castañeda, H., Holmes, S. M., Madrigal, D. S., Young, M. D., Beyeler, N., & Quesada, J. (2015). Immigration as a social determinant of health. *Annual Review of Public Health*, *36*, 375–392.

Chartered Institute of Linguists. (2006). *IoLET Qualifications.* Chartered Institute of Linguists.

Chitongo, S., Pezaro, S., Fyle, J., Suthers, F., & Allan, H. (2022). Midwives' insights into barriers to providing effective perinatal care for ethnic minority women with high-risk pregnancies. *Women and Birth*, *35*(2), 152–159.

Cosstick, E., Nirmal, R., Cross-Sudworth, F., Knight, M., & Kenyon, S. (2022). The role of social risk factors in ethnic disparities in maternal mortality. *eClinicalMedicine*, *52*, 101612.

Cramer, E. (2017). The impact of professional language interpreting in midwifery care. *International Journal of Childbirth*, *7*(1), 1–14.

Crenshaw, K. (1989). Demarginalizing the intersection of race and sex. *University of Chicago Legal Forum*, *1989*(1), 139–167.

Crowther, S., & Lau, A. (2019). Migrant Polish women overcoming communication challenges in Scottish maternity services. *Midwifery*, *72*, 30–38.

Gill, P. S., Beavan, J., Calvert, M., & Freemantle, N. (2011). The unmet need for interpreting provision in UK primary care. *PLoS One*, *6*(6), e20837.

Gutman, C. K., Lion, K. C., Fisher, C. L., Aronson, P. L., Patterson, M., & Fernandez, R. (2022). Breaking through barriers: Language-concordant communication as a facilitator of equitable emergency care. *JACEP Open*, *3*(1), e12627.

Hamed, S., Bradby, H., Ahlberg, B. M., & Thapar-Björkert, S. (2022). Racism in healthcare: A scoping review. *BMC Public Health*, *22*, 988.

Henderson, J., Gao, H., & Redshaw, M. (2013). Experiencing maternity care among women from different ethnic groups. *BMC Pregnancy and Childbirth*, *13*, 196.

Heys, S., Downe, S., & Thomson, G. (2021). 'I know my place': A meta-ethnographic synthesis of disadvantaged women's negative maternity care experiences. *Midwifery*, *103*, 103112.

Higginbottom, G. M. A., Evans, C., Morgan, M., Bharj, K. K., Eldridge, L., Hussain, B., & Salt, K. (2020). *Access to and Interventions to Improve Maternity Care Services for Immigrant Women*. NIHR Journals Library.

Hsieh, E., & Ma, X. (2024). Healthcare interpreting as a socially contextualized activity. In S. Tyulenev & W. Luo (Eds.), *The Routledge Handbook of Translation and Sociology*. Routledge.

International Organization for Migration (IOM). (2024). *About Migration*. International Organisation for Migration. https://www.iom.int/key-migration-terms#:~:text=Migrant%20%E2%80%93%20An%20umbrella%20term,%20not,for%20a%20variety%20of%20reasons

Kalra, V. S., & Kapoor, N. (2009). Interrogating segregation, integration and community cohesion. *Journal of Ethnic and Migration Studies*, *35*(9), 1397–1415.

Kapadia, D., Zhang, J., Salway, S., Nazroo, J., Booth, A., Villarroel-Williams, N., Bécares, L., & Esmail, A. (2022). Ethnic Inequalities in Healthcare: A Rapid Evidence Review. *NHS Race and Health Observatory*. https://nhsrho.org/wp-content/uploads/2023/05/RHO-Rapid-Review-Final-Report_.pdf

Karliner, L. S., Jacobs, E. A., Chen, A. H., & Mutha, S. (2007). Do professional interpreters improve clinical care for patients with limited English proficiency? *Health Services Research*, *42*(2), 727–754.

Khan, Z. (2021). Ethnic health inequalities in the UK's maternity services. *British Journal of Midwifery*, *29*(2), 100–107.

Knight, M., Bunch, K., Tuffnell, D., Shakespeare, J., Kotnis, R., Kenyon, S., & Kurinczuk, J. (2020). *Saving Lives, Improving Mothers' Care*. University of Oxford.

Ledesma, M. C., & Calderón, D. (2015). Critical race theory in education. *Qualitative Inquiry*, *21*(3), 206–222.

Liamputtong, P., & Suwankhong, D. (2019). Culture as a social determinant of health. In P. Liamputtong (Ed.), *Perspectives on Social Determinants of Health* (pp. 51–82). Oxford University Press.

Loewenthal, D., Mohamed, A., Mukhopadhyay, S., Ganesh, K., & Thomas, R. (2012). Reducing barriers to accessing psychological therapies. *British Journal of Guidance & Counselling*, *40*(1), 43–66.

Lucas, S. E. (2015). Child interpreting in social work. *Transnational Social Review*, *5*(2), 145–160.

MacFarlane, A., Huschke, S., Pottie, K., Hauck, F. R., Griswold, K., & Harris, M. F. (2020). Barriers to trained interpreter use in refugee consultations. *BMC Family Practice*, *21*(1), 1–8.

MacFarlane, A., Singleton, C., & Green, E. (2009). Language barriers in health and social care consultations. *Health Policy*, *92*, 203–210.

MacLellan, A., Collins, S., Myatt, M., Pope, C., Knighton, W., & Rai, T. (2022). Black, Asian and minority ethnic women's experiences of maternity services in the UK. *Journal of Advanced Nursing*, *78*(7), 2175–2190.

MacLellan, J., McIlven, A., & Kenyon, S. (2024). Provision of interpreting support for cross-cultural communication in UK maternity services: A freedom of information request. *International Journal of Nursing Studies Advances*, *6*, 1–9.

Manzoor-Khan, S. (2022). *Tangled in Terror: Uprooting Islamophobia*. Pluto Press.

Marable, M. (1992). *Black America*. Open Media.

MBRRACE-UK. (2024). *Saving Lives, Improving Mothers' Care 2024: Lay Summary*. National Perinatal Epidemiology Unit. MBRRACE-UK_Maternal_Report_2024 _Lay_Summary_V1.0.pdf

Meghji, A., & Niang, S. M. (2022). Between post-racial ideology and provincial universalisms. *Sociology*, *56*(1), 131–147.

Miller, F. G., & Wertheimer, A. (2009). *The Ethics of Consent: Theory and Practice*. Oxford University Press.

Modood, T. (2005). Ethnicity and political mobilisation in Britain. In G. C. Loury et al. (Eds.), *Ethnicity, Social Mobility and Public Policy* (pp. 457–474). Cambridge University Press.

Modood, T., Berthoud, R., Lakey, J., Nazroo, J., Smith, P., Virdee, S., & Beishon, S. (1997). *Ethnic Minorities in Britain*. Policy Studies Institute.

Modood, T., Berthoud, R., & Nazroo, J. (2002). 'Race', racism and ethnicity. *Sociology*, *36*(2), 419–427.
Morel, S. (2019). Inequality and discrimination in access to urgent care in France. *Social Science & Medicine*, *232*, 25–32.
NHS. (2022). *Consent to Treatment*. https://www.nhs.uk/tests-and-treatments/consent-to-treatment/
NHS England. (2016). *Better Births: Improving Outcomes of Maternity Services in England*. https://www.england.nhs.uk/wp-content/uploads/2016/02/national-maternity-review-report.pdf
NHS England. (2022). *Core20PLUS5*. https://www.england.nhs.uk/about/equality/equality-hub/national-healthcare-inequalities-improvement-programme/core20plus5/
NICE. (2021). *Antenatal Care (NG201)*. https://www.nice.org.uk/guidance/ng201/chapter/Recommendations#information-and-support-for-pregnant-women-and-their-partners
ONS. (2015). *People Who Cannot Speak English Well Are More Likely to be in Poor Health*. Office of National Statistics.
Oscarsson, M. G., & Stevenson-Ågren, J. (2020). Midwives' experiences of caring for immigrant women. *Sexual & Reproductive Healthcare*, *24*, 100505.
Pangas, J., et al. (2019). Refugee women's experiences negotiating maternity care. *International Journal of Nursing Studies*, *90*, 31–45.
Pattillo, M., et al. (2023). Racism against racialized migrants in healthcare in Europe. *International Journal for Equity in Health*, *22*, 1–14.
Piacentini, T., et al. (2019). Moving beyond the 'language problem'. *Language and Intercultural Communication*, *19*(3), 256–271.
Puthoopparambil, S. J., Phelan, M., & MacFarlane, A. (2021). Migrant health and language barriers. *Health Policy*, *125*, 1085–1091.
Rattansi, A. (2020). *Racism: A Very Short Introduction* (2nd ed.). Oxford University Press.
Rayment-Jones, H., et al. (2021). Project20. *PLoS One*, *16*(5), e0251020.
Sellevold, V. L., Hamre, L. L., & Bondas, T. E. (2022). Language challenges in midwifery care. *European Journal of Midwifery*, *6*, 1–13.
Shahid, H. J., & Dogra, S. A. (2022). The Muslim gaze and the COVID-19 syndemic. *Religions*, *13*, 788.
Solórzano, D. G., & Yosso, T. J. (2001). Critical race and LatCrit theory. *International Journal of Qualitative Studies in Education*, *14*(4), 471–495.
Spivak, G. C. (2000). Translation as culture. *Parallax*, *6*(1), 13–24.
Teti, M., & van Wyk, B. (2020). Qualitative methods without borders. *International Journal of Qualitative Methods*, *19*, 1–3.
Tierney, W. (1993). *Building Communities of Difference*. Bergin & Garvey.
van den Muijsenbergh, M., et al. (2014). Communication in cross-cultural consultations. *Primary Health Care Research & Development*, *15*(2), 122–133.
van der Pijl, M. S. G., et al. (2020). Left powerless. *PLoS One*, *15*(5), e0233114.
Vaughn, L. (2019). *Psychology and Culture*. Routledge.
Vydelingum, V. (2006). Nurses' experiences of caring for South Asian patients. *Nursing Inquiry*, *13*(1), 23–32.
Whitaker, K. L., et al. (2022). Addressing language as a barrier to healthcare access. *British Journal of General Practice*, *72*(714), 4–5.
Wu, M. S., & Rawal, S. (2017). It's the difference between life and death. *PLoS One*, *12*(10), e0185659.

SECTION 4

Mis/Trust in services

The next theme is one that resides at the core of ethnic and racial inequity: trust. A foundational aspect of all relationships, trust significantly shapes racialised communities' willingness to engage with the healthcare system, the quality of those engagements, and the health outcomes that result. Chapter 7 explores the role of mistrust and its effects among Gypsy, Traveller, and Roma communities in England and Scotland. In Chapter 8, mistrust is elaborated in relation to Black African migrant, refugee, and asylum-seeking groups as they navigate access to mental healthcare.

MacFadden, Atkin, and Jones begin Chapter 7 with clear evidence that among all racialised communities in the UK, those who identify as Gypsy, Traveller, and Roma have the worst health outcomes. These are underpinned by social and economic exclusion, pervasive discrimination, historical mistrust, and barriers to accessing and engaging with the healthcare system. After revealing statistics outlining the significant gaps in life expectancy, maternal and child outcomes, children's health, suicide, and depression, MacFadden et al. turn their attention to qualitative evidence gathered across four sites in England and Scotland, underpinning these numbers. With a focus on maternity, early years, and child dental health, they elaborate on three themes around accessing and receiving healthcare, the role of trust in healthcare encounters, and strategies to enhance experiences and outcomes. Tackling systemic racism and resultant exclusion requires new approaches, including working with Gypsy, Traveller, and Roma communities to co-design services and interventions, a flexible approach for travel and movement, coupled with holistic approaches across families. Changes in healthcare are not enough; the social determinants of health and the attitudes across society also need addressing for long-term improvements.

In Chapter 8, Mafuba, Nyashanu, and Gibson foreground the voices of Black African (African) asylum seekers, refugees, and migrants in their quests to meet their mental health needs. With a focus on the West Midlands in England, the authors draw on Serrant-Green's Screaming Silences conceptual framework to spotlight the marginalised and previously silenced perspectives of their participants. While fear of immigration

DOI: 10.4324/9781003466093-11

and deportation underpins resistance to seeking mental health support, respondents also reflect on their minimal care and neglect by professional services. With this focus, Mafuba et al. dispel the common trope that lack of engagement arises from the service users alone, showing instead that dismissive practices from the healthcare sector actively discourage Black Africans from receiving timely and appropriate mental healthcare. While applauding the agency of their research participants, who draw on spiritual support and other culturally familiar practices in lieu of professional care, Mafuba et al. propose that mental health providers engage with this agency to collaboratively reshape mental health services to restore trust and better serve their needs.

CHAPTER 7

The role of trust in improving health among Gypsy, Roma, and Traveller communities

Alison McFadden, Karl Atkin, and Helen Jones

Introduction

This chapter draws on qualitative case study research with Irish Travellers in London, Romany Gypsies and Irish Travellers in West Yorkshire, Slovak Roma people in Sheffield, and Scottish Gypsy/Travellers in Fife. The case studies, conducted in 2016–2018, explored the different ways mainstream health services engaged with Gypsy, Roma, and Traveller people and the extent to which this engagement focused on negotiating and developing trust.

Throughout this chapter, we use the phrase *Gypsy, Roma, and Traveller people* following the terminology used by policymakers in the UK (House of Commons Women Equalities Committee, 2019). However, we acknowledge the contested nature of these labels and the rich, diverse identities, histories, and cultural and linguistic heritages they subsume. We are aware that these ethnic labels are context dependent. For example, in the UK, the term 'Roma' is used to denote recently arrived migrants, mostly from Eastern and Central Europe. Outside of the UK, Roma is a broader term covering heterogeneous populations. Commonalities across Gypsy, Roma, and Traveller people are a cultural tradition of nomadism even if they no longer travel, and experiences of discrimination, stigma, and social exclusion.

Estimates of the size of the Gypsy, Roma, and Traveller population in the UK vary. Gypsy or Irish Traveller was included as an ethnic grouping for the first time in the 2011 UK Census with Roma first included in 2021. In the England and Wales 2021 Census, about 71,400 individuals identified as Gypsy or Irish Traveller, and 103,100 people as Roma (Office for National Statistics, 2023). In the Scottish 2022 Census, the numbers were 3,300 Gypsy/Travellers and 3,100 Roma (Barton & Zayed, 2024). However, these figures are known to grossly underestimate the true population sizes, as many Gypsy, Roma, and Traveller people prefer not to disclose their identity due to stigma and a 'trust gap' between Gypsy, Roma, and Traveller people and the state (The Traveller Movement, 2022). Organisations working with Gypsy/Travellers in Scotland estimate the population size to be 15,000–20,000 (Scottish Government, 2024). Older

DOI: 10.4324/9781003466093-12

estimates of the Gypsy, Roma, and Traveller population in the UK include the Council of Europe (2012) estimate of 150,000–300,000 people and that of Brown et al of up to 500,000 (Brown et al., 2013). Gypsy, Roma, and Traveller people, therefore, are a significant ethnic minority grouping in the UK and the largest minority ethnic grouping across Europe (Ghimisi, 2021).

The lack of robust data on Europe's largest ethnic grouping is an indication of the degree of systemic and institutional racism faced by Gypsy, Roma, and Traveller people. It is also an issue for analysing health outcomes. Not only do we not know the size of the population, but the NHS ethnicity data categories in England are based on the 2001 Census, which did not include options for Gypsy, Roma, or Irish Traveller (Understanding Patient Data, 2024). Although the NHS in Scotland, Wales, and Northern Ireland include various categories for Gypsy, Roma, and Traveller people, there is reluctance among Gypsy, Roma, and Traveller Communities to use them because of distrust of how such data could be used (Understanding Patient Data, 2024). This distrust is based on historic abuse and erasure during events such as the Holocaust, including a lack of recognition in Holocaust reparation, in addition to more recent events, such as the 'Tinker Experiment', where statutory agencies threatened to take children into care if families continued their nomadic lifestyles (Watson et al., 2025). Consequently, data on health outcomes and inequalities are based on small scale often localised studies and explain why current statistics are lacking for many outcomes. Furthermore, the Roma population is often grouped with Gypsies and Travellers, without considering specific issues that may affect Roma. The Roma population in the UK may have more in common with other socially disadvantaged migrant populations than with Gypsy and Traveller people (Office for Health Improvement and Disparities, 2022).

Despite the lack of robust data, there is consistent evidence that for decades, Gypsy, Roma, and Traveller people have experienced the poorest health outcomes of any minority group in the UK. Life expectancy estimates vary, but all suggest a significant gap compared to the general population. Based on the Republic of Ireland data, the All Ireland Traveller Study reported differences between Irish Travellers and the general population of 15 years less for men and 11 years less for women (HSC Public Health Agency, 2010). A study in Leeds found average life expectancy was 25 years less for Gypsies and Travellers compared to the general population (Baker, 2005). Data on life expectancy for the Roma population in the UK is lacking; however, the European Commission (2014) estimated a life expectancy gap of between 5 and 20 years across Europe.

In the 2021 Census, Gypsies and Irish Travellers were more than twice as likely to rate their health as bad compared with the England and Wales population (Office for National Statistics, 2023). Aspinall (2014) and Parry et al. (2007) reported that Gypsy and Traveller children have the poorest health of any group in the UK, with high rates of accidental injury, infections, and accident and emergency attendance (Beach, 2006; Dar et al., 2013) and low/variable uptake of childhood vaccinations (La Placa & Smith, 2016). Maternal and infant health inequalities include higher rates of pregnancy loss, preterm birth and low birthweight infants, and higher rates of caesarean section (Ekezie et al., 2024; Hollinshead et al., 2023). Friends Families and Travellers (2024) reported that inequalities in mental health are alarming with very high rates of suicide, anxiety, and depression. Smith et al. (2020) argue that, while an established social gradient in diagnosis and cancer survival puts Gypsy, Roma, and Traveller communities at a particular disadvantage, when compared to White majority and other minority groups, high rates of smoking, poor diet, diabetes, significant levels of socioeconomic deprivation, and lower uptake of human papillomavirus (HPV) vaccine significantly increase their risk of common cancers.

The reasons for such poor health are complex and beyond the scope of this chapter to examine. Gypsy, Roma, and Traveller communities experience stark economic and social inequalities, which impact the social determinants of health (Crew, 2024). Chronic under-provision of culturally appropriate site provision for Gypsy and Traveller homes, largely driven by discriminatory public attitudes, leaves Gypsy and Traveller people with little or no choice but to live in unsuitable places that detrimentally impact health. Mapping of all Gypsy and Traveller sites in England, Scotland, and Wales by Bloch and Quarmby (2025) found that many present a risk to residents' health due to their geographical proximity to pollutants, such as industrial sites or busy main roads and infestations with vermin and flies, and are also separated from settled communities resulting in isolation that exacerbates difficulty in accessing public services (see also (Friends Families and Travellers, 2022; Williams, 2021).

A report by the House of Commons Women and Equalities Committee (2019) highlighted that Gypsy, Roma, and Traveller people have poor education, employment, and criminal justice outcomes in the UK. Inequalities faced by Gypsy, Roma, and Traveller people are underpinned by racism in their everyday lives, and a more deep-seated structural discrimination when accessing public services. Although vastly under-reported, high levels of hate crime are experienced by Gypsy, Roma, and Traveller people (Greenfields & Rogers, 2020), and a national survey by Abrams et al. (2018) found that more people expressed negative attitudes toward Gypsies, Roma, and Travellers than any other group. Thus Gypsies, Roma, and Travellers are highly stigmatised groups which profoundly affect their health and well-being, particularly mental health.

Health inequalities are exacerbated for Gypsy, Roma, and Traveller people by the multiple barriers they face when accessing healthcare, including preventative public health interventions such as screening and immunisations. These include bureaucratic barriers such as being asked to provide proof of address to register with a GP or dentist, difficulty in reaching services, inflexible services, low levels of general and health literacy and language barriers, poor communication between healthcare staff and service users, and hostile attitudes and lack of cultural awareness of some healthcare staff (McFadden et al., 2018). Cultural sensitivities preventing open discussion about some health issues, such as mental health, also play a role (Friends Families and Travellers, 2024).

In this context, it is unsurprising that Gypsy, Roma, and Traveller peoples' relationships with health and social care services and healthcare personnel are pervaded by mistrust. In this sense, Spalvieri et al. (2024) describe not trusting health services as a rational and protective response. This lack of trust is frequently highlighted as contributing to health inequalities and lack of engagement with health services, but as far as we are aware, it has not been explored in depth regarding Gypsy, Roma, and Traveller communities. Robust evidence is lacking on effective strategies that health services can use to enhance engagement with Gypsy, Roma, and Traveller communities and to what extent they focus on developing trust.

The research

We chose a case study design to generate an in-depth understanding from multiple perspectives of the complex nature of engagement between Gypsy, Roma and Traveller communities and mainstream health services and their impact on trust in real-life contexts (Crowe et al., 2011). To focus our work, we used maternity, early years, and child dental health services as exemplars of mainstream health services. Four case study sites were chosen to reflect different approaches to engagement. Each case study comprised individual and small-group in-person interviews with mothers of pre-school children, focus group discussions with healthcare practitioners and individual in-person or telephone interviews with key informants from third-sector organisations. We used maximum variation sampling to ensure inclusion of Gypsy, Roma, and Traveller mothers with children of different ages, and diverse living arrangements, such as those living on private or local authority sites or in bricks and mortar housing. We recruited mothers through third-sector organisations in three sites and healthcare practitioners in one site. We conducted the interviews with mothers flexibly, whereby other family members were included if the mother wished. Study participants included 37 mothers, five grandmothers and one father, 54 healthcare practitioners and 13 third-sector organisation staff. Across the case studies, we included English Romany Gypsies, Irish Travellers, Scottish Gypsy/Travellers, and migrant Slovak Roma participants. See Box 1 for details of the case studies.

The study was approved by the East Midlands – Leicester Central NHS Research Ethics Committee (16/EM/0028).

First, we analysed the data separately for each case study and then combined themes across the dataset.

Findings

We developed three key themes.

1. The first theme explores experiences of accessing and receiving healthcare. It sets the context within which the negotiation of trust can be understood.
2. In the second theme, we build on these experiences, focusing on how participants perceived the role of trust (or lack of) when reflecting on the engagement between Gypsy, Roma, and Traveller mothers and mainstream health services.
3. The final theme explores strategies either experienced or proposed that participants believed could enhance trust and thereby improve health experiences and outcomes. Strategies covered those used by mainstream health services, third-sector organisations or a collaborative approach of both.

Accessing appropriate healthcare

Against a backdrop of complex health needs, participants struggled to access appropriate care. A fundamental barrier is the difficulty in registering with dentists and GP practices. All participants were registered with a GP, although for many this was not a straightforward process. Many experienced discrimination, and women's stories highlighted GP practices either directly or indirectly refusing to register them. Women recounted reasons given by practices for not registering them, including 'the practice was full' and 'there were too many families registered with the same name'. Both of which offer a good example of indirect discrimination faced by Gypsy, Roma, and

Traveller communities. Some practices requested proof of address, which is unnecessary and challenging for those living on temporary sites. GP practices have no contractual obligation to seek evidence of identity or proof of address. If necessary, patients can be registered using the GP surgery address. One GP practice had asked for a bank statement before a mother and her children could be registered. Many of these cases were successfully challenged by advocacy workers from third-sector organisations. However, a lack of awareness of individual rights is a significant barrier to accessing healthcare. In one area, women living on an authorised council site told us that they could not register with the nearest GP but had to travel some distance to a practice that would accept them:

> *With the doctors it's very hard to get an appointment. Where we should have a doctor's round this area. We shouldn't go all the way up there for a doctor's.*
> *(mother)*

A worker from a third-sector organisation explained that one reason for this was that previously, an outreach mobile health service visited the site, which may have worsened issues with GP registration:

> *In the past with a health bus that used to go up onto [the site], and was a real substandard service. Sometimes it would have a doctor on it, sometimes it wouldn't, quite often it was just a nurse. It was supposed to go up twice a week and would end up going once a fortnight and things like this. But this health bus was used as a reason by lots of local GPs why they didn't need to register people at their surgery, . . . and the reason a lot of our members are registered at a practice which is at least seven miles from the site.*
> *(third-sector worker)*

This is a further example of discrimination and inequity where Gypsy and Traveller communities are not offered the same range or quality of services as the general population. Their health needs are regarded as problematic and challenging, requiring a specialist service and therefore, not a concern of mainstream provision. This can also contribute to the invisibility of communities, which further reinforces the assumption that a response from mainstream provision is not required.

Accessing child dental services was even more problematic. Poor child dental health is not only associated with general overall health, healthy eating, and pain, but Guarnizo-Herreño and Wehby (2012) suggested links to poor educational outcomes and mental well-being. This is particularly pertinent to marginalised communities where low educational attainment and bullying at school are prevalent. Participants suggested different reasons why they were not registered with a dentist. In some areas, participants had to travel unacceptable distances to access dental care. A health visitor suggested that few Roma families were registered with a dentist:

> *There are enough dentists but they're not in the right areas. So, if you live in some parts of the city, it's easily accessible. But I would say like one in twenty of the families I visit have a dentist, if that.*
> *(healthcare practitioner)*

Our participants recognised that access to NHS dental care was difficult for everyone across the UK. However, the high levels of poor oral health among Gypsy, Roma, and Traveller people and the additional barriers of access due to discrimination mean that the consequences of lack of access to dental care are likely to affect this population disproportionately.

A punitive approach by dentists was also an issue with women reporting being removed from dental practices because of missed appointments. Case study two was notable in that good access to dentists was reported, and a reminder that good practice is possible. Participants in this case study appreciated a health promotion initiative whereby free toothbrushes and toothpaste were provided, and tooth-brushing was reinforced in local primary schools. Despite this, there were high levels of dental problems described in casual terms, suggesting that this was normalised, even for very young children:

> *We've all got our own regular dentist. As a matter of fact, I've got an appointment tomorrow . . . our six month check-up for our teeth. . . . One of the young ones, the three year old, yesterday, he got four teeth out*
>
> *(grandmother)*

Other obstacles to accessing healthcare included a lack of public transport routes near to sites. When using public transport, participants risked hostile attitudes, such as a woman who recounted a bus driver throwing her change on the bus floor. Mothers also told us that taxi services refused to come to sites, thereby creating additional barriers to access.

Alongside difficulties accessing care, we heard many accounts of poor care or care that did not meet the women's expectations. These experiences most frequently revolved around patronising attitudes of some health professionals and women feeling that they were not being heard or their concerns not being taken seriously. This was particularly concerning when it related to their children's health:

> *Even if you tell them that they're poorly, they're really, really poorly and they need to see someone, they say, 'well, we haven't got any more appointments'*
>
> *(mother)*

Women not only felt they were not listened to, but at times, felt they were not believed and their accounts questioned. One mother described a particularly distressing experience when she had taken her young child repeatedly to the GP, who clearly did not take her concerns seriously. Sadly, the child died of an infection:

> *They never checked her properly and she died with pneumonia. They never checked her chest properly. Said it was clear. They never gave me antibiotics or anything. And she was there three times because I wasn't happy with her.*
>
> *(mother)*

Specific challenges for Roma people who had migrated to the UK included a lack of interpreter services. Interpreting services when offered were for Eastern European languages via language line and not for the specific Roma dialect or language spoken by the participants. This not only made care difficult to realise but may have deterred communities from accessing care, in the first instance.

The role of trust

The mothers, healthcare professionals, and third-sector workers in our study agreed that trust was central to accessing good-quality healthcare and improving health. For the women, this was mostly discussed in the context of developing trusting relationships with individual healthcare practitioners. One Romany Gypsy mother spoke about the importance of trusting health professionals with her life and the lives of her children. She exemplified her trust in a GP with whom she had experienced continuity of care over several years:

> *But I do think seeing the one person all the time is better. It's like my doctor, I see the one doctor now all the time and it's better. Because you don't have to go through your whole life story with them, they know you when they see you.*
>
> *(mother).*

Continuity of care, including established relationships, is an important condition of this trust and has assumed a particular significance, given the difficulties women faced in accessing services. Conversely, women talked about losing trust when different practitioners gave different advice:

> *You'll see them once, and that's it, you'll see another person . . . and he could say a different thing altogether.*
>
> *(mother)*

Conflicting or differing advice from healthcare professionals is a common criticism of health services by service users from all backgrounds. Making sense of different opinions and asking pertinent questions may be more challenging for those who have experienced hostile attitudes or when explanations are not tailored to the literacy level of the service user.

An Irish Traveller mother spoke of how she trusted a new dentist who had taken time to overcome her child's fear before starting treatment. This followed a bad experience with a previous dentist:

> *That dentist had to build this (child's) trust up because he was frightened of the other dentist. . . . And he built his trust up every time we were going in until he got things so he could start doing his teeth*
>
> *(mother)*

Taking time was also highlighted as a critical factor in fostering trust with midwives. This made the mothers feel valued and offset previous experiences of discrimination:

> *I found it is good when you can go to see the midwife at the local children's centre. And then you see the one midwife all the time because it's an appointment, . . . she wasn't rushed . . . so I think it was better as more one-to-one support.*
>
> *(mother).*

Women were more likely to trust healthcare practitioners who acknowledged their needs and were caring:

> *She [health visitor] was a lovely woman. She came out to see me not long ago, six months check-up. She come out to see me because I had bad depression. Like some days I'd sit and cry all day. But I told her, and she was there for me when I had depression.*
>
> *(mother)*

Relationships built with individual practitioners, described as kind, respectful, reliable, and non-judgemental, provided examples of good practice. Participants were able to develop trusting relationships with such practitioners:

> *I start using the GP, then the GP gives me a midwife, and the midwife, I have a conversation with her every month or every two weeks. She's always asking me questions and looking [at] my baby, how is she growing, and [checking] the heart. This is okay. I feel happy.*
>
> *(mother)*

That such care is not common made examples of good practice important to families. The mothers were influenced by previous good experiences and gave examples of healthcare practitioners with whom they felt comfortable, could rely on, and who were supportive, along with examples of those with whom they had built up relationships over years who had kept their confidence:

> *You build trust with somebody, when we build that up and we keep that trust.*
>
> *(mother)*

However, women and third-sector workers suggested that Gypsy, Roma, and Traveller people find it difficult to trust others, which is not surprising given the high levels of discrimination and racism experienced in their daily lives. This spilled over into relationships with healthcare practitioners to the extent that women saw it as fortunate rather than an expectation if they encountered a kind, respectful practitioner. When asked if she trusted healthcare practitioners, one woman succinctly put it:

> *It depends because you don't know if they're out to get you or to help you.*
>
> *(mother)*

Initial contact with practitioners, therefore, generates uncertainty and anxiety. Mothers are not sure what to expect. Underpinning this perception of healthcare practitioners being 'out to get you' was a specific fear of referral to social services and child removal:

> *There's always a fear, your biggest fear is someone coming to take the kids off you.*
>
> *(mother)*

This fear is not unfounded. With regard to Gypsy, Roma, and Traveller families, child protection systems in England have been described as systemically and culturally racist

(European Roma Rights Centre, 2018). This is because of the assumptions made by child protection professionals that Gypsy, Roma and Traveller children, due to their lifestyle, are more at risk of harm than other children. The 'Tinker Experiment' provides further evidence of this (see above).

While none of the mothers we spoke to had experienced a child being removed from their care, many related stories of children being taken into care. Sometimes these were vicarious experiences of family members, but more often were cases they had heard of through word-of-mouth or social media. That women believed these stories, despite the lack of direct experience, reflects the deep-seated lack of trust among communities, in which care was regarded as more likely to be controlling than nurturing. The fear of social services intervention was also evident in the Roma community. A health visitor recounted the response of a Roma family who had been referred to social services:

> *I've just visited a family who told me that once social care got involved, they did go back to Slovakia for two weeks but now they've hid for three months until eventually they're registered back at the GP.*
>
> *(healthcare practitioner)*

Women's experiences highlighted tensions in how they perceived the role of health visitors; on one hand as providers of valuable support, but on the other as monitoring families on behalf of the State. This could lead to reluctance to engage with health services or to take children to hospital, as discussed during an interview with a group of Irish Traveller mothers:

M1 *If you need them (health visitors) you've got to call upon them. But if you've been in a hospital with a child then they're on top of you. I know they have to, but that's the way I felt.*

M2: *I think that's a bit much, though. If you go to the hospital with a child, a child's fell over, you've got the health visitor the next day. . . .*

M1: *It's making half the people frightened to go to the hospital.*

These mothers talked about needing to trust healthcare practitioners to address health issues. This may offer services a foundation on which to build:

M3: *Because if you don't have trust in someone you're not going to be at ease, you won't confide in them, you won't ask them questions. And you don't want them there so you're on your tip-toes.*

It seemed that women felt they were on a tightrope, balancing their children's need for healthcare with the risk of unnecessary scrutiny and the possibility of blame. This generated mistrust. The mothers continued the discussion in terms of their concerns about lack of confidentiality and disclosure of information between services:

M1 *Travellers, we're very private anyway. It takes a lot to confide in each other. Where with health professionals, we should be able to relax and confide in them to the point where they won't take it anywhere else.*

M2: It's a bad experience that we had in the past. Sometimes you're there and you're having a one-to-one and you think well that's a one-to-one that's the end of it, and before you know it you've got a lot of problems. They've been going behind your back and they're telling this one, telling that one.
Interviewer: Telling other health professionals?
M2: Yes. And you don't need that.

This shows the significance of healthcare practitioners understanding the importance of confidentiality and ensuring that the need to disclose information to other services is explained and, where possible, permission from the patient sought. Without this, service users will feel unsafe disclosing information, irrespective of the significance of such information to meeting care needs.

Mothers related many instances when they had acted on their own initiative because they did not trust the response from health services:

> *But to be honest with you, all the doctors and midwives and health visitors, sometimes you've got to go on your own intuition. You can't trust them entirely.*
> *(mother)*

This usually related to their children's health and included taking children to accident and emergency departments. Women faced a particular dilemma when negotiating their distrust of services, alongside the need to access the best possible care for their child. In making these decisions, mothers drew on their own or a family member's past experiences or their own intuition about their child's health:

> *You don't want to go to the hospital but sometimes you have to because that's the only way you can get your kid seen to.*
> *(mother)*

One mother gave an example that validated her decision:

> *And one time they [GP practice] go to me 'we'll do call-back.' I said, 'okay then.' Waited, and she [child] was really sick, so I took her into the hospital, and two o'clock that afternoon they gave me a call-back, and she was on the hospital bed dripped-up and everything because she was very sick. And if I had waited for that phone call anything could have happened to her.*
> *(mother)*

These examples of women's agency can be contrasted with the earlier example of a mother's concerns about her child not being taken seriously with a tragic outcome. This suggests that the burden of assessing the seriousness of symptoms and deciding how to access appropriate care rests with the patient and family rather than with healthcare practitioners.

Women told us that sometimes they disagreed with the proposed care plan. This was most often influenced by previous experiences:

> *I went to the doctor's and the doctor said 'I'll bring you to the hospital' to get him checked out and they kept him in overnight. They were going to send him*

home, and I said no, because my mummy's sister's child passed away with that, and that made me scared then.

(mother)

This mother's child was diagnosed with whooping cough and as in other examples, an experience of a family member influenced the mother to distrust the proposed care plan and insisted the child was kept in hospital.

Several Roma mothers also felt that their own instincts were important, particularly as previous experiences suggest any trust is contingent. Trust, therefore, cannot be taken for granted by healthcare professionals and requires continual (re)negotiation. One mother said, 'you can trust, but not 100%'. Another Roma mother recounted asking for a second opinion when she did not trust her child's diagnosis. A father described getting conflicting information about his child's health; his trust was negatively affected by short appointment times and a language barrier.

This was the only father who participated in the study; he accompanied his wife during the interview. We were told by our participants (mothers, healthcare practitioners, and third-sector organisation workers) that in Gypsy and Traveller communities, men are rarely involved in care of young children and were reluctant to engage with health services. The exception to this was when they were needed to provide transport to appointments. One healthcare practitioner told us that the men often attended pregnancy scan appointments. We don't have any evidence for the role of men with regard to the Roma participants other than the one father who attended an interview. More broadly, however, Havlin (2015) suggests migration may impact gender roles due to the absence of female relatives, meaning that men become more involved in childcare and domestic work than they would have been in their country of origin.

Strategies to increase trust and engagement

We asked participants how they thought health services could build trust with Gypsy, Roma, and Traveller people and ensure timely access to appropriate care. For the mothers, developing trusting relationships with individual practitioners was key. An example was given of a midwife visiting a site regularly and facilitating the transition to other services. The community had confidence in this practitioner. However, typical of many accounts we heard, this role had ended. The short-term nature of such initiatives could, therefore, undermine trust, irrespective of positive intent.

The mothers and third-sector workers also spoke about the importance of advocacy by third-sector organisations. The mothers more commonly mentioned activities such as accompanying them to appointments to ensure appropriate healthcare was offered, explaining medical terminology, translating for the Roma community, and supporting registration with GPs. This type of advocacy helped women feel safe, navigate complex health systems, and challenge discrimination on their behalf. Farrer et al. (2015) argue that advocacy is particularly important for disadvantaged and marginalised communities in challenging inequities and giving voice to those who feel disempowered.

She's happy of [the third sector organisation staff]. They're sorting out herself when she's been poorly. They take her to midwife'.

(mother through an interpreter)

Third-sector workers additionally focused on the importance of collective advocacy activities such as ensuring the voice of communities was heard in policy fora and working for Gypsy, Roma, and Traveller rights. Some mothers also recognised the importance of these activities:

> *Having a healthcare provider worker like her, when there's meetings about healthcare for certain communities she could go to them, put Travellers on the list, push forward the issues.*
>
> *(mother)*

Flexibility was a common theme in the responses of healthcare practitioners. This could mean flexible appointment times, being adaptable in terms of geographical boundaries and preparing for community members' seasonal travelling. This was of particular concern for pregnant women with one practitioner discussing the importance of giving women the confidence to access services when travelling:

> *If they are going to move on during the pregnancy, that they know how to access services wherever they move on to, or they know who to ask . . . putting them in touch with services in that area is really important in getting that confidence to reach out and ask for care.*
>
> *(healthcare practitioner)*

A mother highlighted an additional challenge when families are moved on by police before they can access healthcare and went further to suggest a solution:

> *I think . . . for Travelling people that travels, little caravans or something that they can walk in and be seen to by a midwife. . . . Because I do think there's a lot of women when they're having children, Travelling women do get neglected. . . . I know in one way it's their own fault, but in another way it's not because if they have nowhere to go. And then they pull into camp and get shifted the first thing in the morning, they don't get the time.*
>
> *(mother)*

There were mixed views about outreach services. Where such activities were embedded in mainstream services, such as midwifery and health visiting, these were valued by women, practitioners and third-sector organisations. However, some third-sector workers were concerned about outreach services potentially providing a substandard service (as highlighted earlier regarding a mobile health bus), while absolving mainstream services of responsibility to provide care. Such services were also thought to further stigmatise communities by seeing them as 'special'. Conversely, some practitioners felt that dedicated outreach services for one community could result in an inequitable service for the majority population. Perceptions of 'special' services may create resentment in practitioners. One practitioner recognised this tension saying:

> *To make sure that the most marginalised don't get more marginalised, but also to make sure that the mainstream of society is getting good care in services as well.*
>
> *(healthcare practitioner)*

Outreach services, however, were not appreciated by all participants with some suggesting they did not welcome healthcare practitioners arriving without an appointment and would prefer to attend a clinic. Asking about preferences, without assuming what they are is, therefore, an important part of negotiating trusting relationships.

A further element of building trust was recognising the impact of the social determinants of health on Gypsy, Roma and Traveller communities and the role of trusted healthcare practitioners to link to other services. In one area, a midwife provided this:

> *I think someone like that is very key. Because she didn't just touch on health things, it opened up doors for other areas as well, so she was involved in housing. . . . But because she was the first point of contact in [the area] as a healthcare provider everyone came through her.*
>
> *(mother)*

This was recognised by third-sector organisations who spoke about how concerns with issues such as education or finance could lead to discussions about health. Gypsy, Roma, and Traveller people experience discrimination in all aspects of their lives, and unless this is addressed more widely, it is a challenge to developing trust with health services. Many healthcare practitioners told us they used more holistic approaches, such as dentists who asked about nutrition and a GP practice that provided a 'whole family' session that had increased uptake of immunisations. A social prescribing outreach service by nurses was appreciated by mothers. Unfortunately, this service was discontinued after one year due to lack of funding.

Of all the suggested strategies, the one with the strongest support from mothers and third-sector organisations was training community members to focus on improving health and engaging with health services. Various terms were used, such as 'health advocates', 'health navigators', or 'peer health workers'. The advantages of these roles included being trusted by and understanding the culture and priorities of their communities as well as being a link to health services. For non-English speaking Roma communities, these roles included interpreting during appointments and translating letters.

All participants talked about the importance of healthcare practitioners developing an understanding of Gypsy, Roma, and Traveller people and their cultures. For example, one Irish Traveller mother told us that a health visitor asked her why she lived in a house and not a caravan. This suggests the health visitor held stereotypical views and was unaware that most Gypsies and Travellers live in brick and mortar housing. Other examples included preferences for female practitioners, although the participants in London were keen to emphasise that they were not the only minority ethnic group with this preference. It appeared these women felt validated that their preferences were not exceptional. The strong emphasis on cleanliness was also an area where participants felt their culture was not understood, for example, by practitioners making home visits and not asking where they should sit, place their equipment, or wash their hands.

Many third-sector organisations had been involved in, or offered, training on equalities, cultural competence or Gypsy, Roma, and Traveller health needs. This approach generally seemed to be favoured, though some healthcare practitioners felt that learning by experience was equally valuable. One third-sector worker expressed frustration at not knowing whether the training was effective:

> *We helped put that [training] together and gave a lot of information for that, but then I don't know how that's been received and whether people feel any differently towards the Gypsy Traveller community from doing it.*
>
> *(third-sector worker)*

While valued by the mothers, and effective in building trust at an individual level, strategies that relied on dedicated healthcare practitioners providing services specifically for Gypsy, Roma, or Traveller communities were vulnerable to changes in personnel or relied on short-term funding. Such approaches were therefore unsustainable, and the trust built with an individual practitioner could be lost. Some practitioners in such roles told us that they themselves experienced mistrust from colleagues in mainstream services. One service had overcome the challenge of precarious dedicated roles because the midwife providing maternity care specifically for Gypsy, Roma, and Traveller communities had progressed to a strategic role where she was able to embed the service in policy. This suggests such roles could be part of longer-term strategic plans to meet the needs of marginalised disadvantaged groups.

Conclusion

Our findings focused on how trust between marginalised and disadvantaged communities and health services is essential to meet healthcare needs and reduce health inequities. Trust between care provider and recipient was suggested by Tofan et al. (2013) to improve quality of care and clinical outcomes. Gypsy, Roma, and Traveller people have many reasons to mistrust health services both historical and continuing to the present day. As stated by Spalvieri et al. (2024), and as our findings illustrate, not trusting health services is a rational and protective response. This is because placing trust in health services involves the service user relinquishing control and thereby making themselves vulnerable (Anderson & Griffith, 2022). Others argue that equity is a prerequisite to building trust with marginalised communities (National Academies of Sciences, Engineering, and Medicine, 2023). This explains the value of locating the experience of Gypsy, Roma, and Traveller communities within broader strategies to challenge racism (Bloch & Quarmby, 2025).

Lack of trust is an expression of systemic racism, in which the needs of Gypsy, Roma, and Traveller communities are rendered invisible, due to a supposed lack of demand. This enables statutory agencies to ignore need, by according them little if any priority (Karlsen et al., 2019; Keating, 2019). A lack of data and bureaucratic processes, which assume a normalised lifestyle, exacerbate this invisibility. However, it is also important to recognise that assumptions about similarities between people routinely ascribed as Gypsy, Roma, and Traveller within healthcare settings may cause offence and mistrust and underpin poor care.

When need is acknowledged, however, a further aspect of systemic racism becomes apparent. The experiences of Gypsy, Roma, and Traveller communities become misrepresented and interpreted within the context of essentialised myths and stereotypes, which further reinforce communities' lack of trust in statutory agencies. Problems become located within the community, who are blamed for their own healthcare needs, rather than being seen as a failure of care agencies to facilitate inclusion and diversity (Chattoo & Atkin, 2012). Nonetheless, our findings suggest possible strategies to break this cycle of racism.

Policy implications

There are positive steps health services can take to build trust with Gypsy, Roma, and Traveller communities. Individual trusting relationships are contingent on a service user's belief that a healthcare practitioner is trustworthy. By this, we mean that the individual practitioner listens, is caring, reliable, honest and respects confidentiality as argued by Mullarkey et al. (2011). These are skills and attributes that service users should expect from all healthcare practitioners. However, ingrained historical and ongoing societal and structural discrimination may have heightened practitioners' expectations of aggression from Gypsy and Traveller communities. A starting point to earning trust would be for practitioners to acknowledge these responses and understand as suggested by Tyler and Campbell (2024) that apparent aggression may be a consequence of stigma and shame. This should be central to practitioner training. We also show that trust takes time to develop and is fragile for example, when confidentiality is broken or when a valued service is no longer available. If this occurs, trust may be hard to regain. Even when individual practitioners develop trusting relationships with Gypsy, Roma, and Traveller service users, this does not necessarily extend to mainstream health services. Policy-led, strategic (and integrated) approaches are needed.

One effective way to build trust and address health inequities is through involving Gypsy, Roma, and Traveller communities in co-designing services and interventions that focus on community priorities. This is likely to be best achieved in collaboration with third-sector organisations who are trusted by the community. Listening to community needs and priorities is an important foundation for developing effective policy but must be followed by action. There are multiple examples of local health needs assessments for Gypsy, Roma, and Traveller populations, but without follow through, these engender cynicism which is counter-productive to building trust. Using an asset-based approach will lead to more effective engagement by recognising and enhancing community strengths.

While an unprecedented event, the pandemic highlighted both community strengths (Renedo et al., 2023) and the need for more inclusive health policy that places those with the poorest outcomes and highest need at its centre. This avoids developing specific services that see communities as 'problems to be solved', thereby risking further stigmatisation. The principles of proportionate universalism as proposed by Marmot et al. (Department of Health, 2010) are as relevant now as they were over a decade ago. The proposition is that reducing inequalities in health requires universal actions at a 'scale and intensity that is proportionate to the level of disadvantage' (p. 9). This approach avoids the development of specialist services that can be further stigmatising and resented by mainstream service users. More accessible and flexible services are required because delays in seeking healthcare may mean needs are more urgent. This is particularly relevant for dental health services.

We found examples of well-intentioned and valued interventions that were discontinued when short term funding ended. This was not only disappointing to Gypsy,

Roma, and Traveller service users and providers but also led to further mistrust. Service initiatives need to acknowledge that building trust takes time, and until that trust is gained, new interventions or services will not be able to demonstrate 'effectiveness' in terms of improved health outcomes. Typically, funding was provided for 12 months. Sustainable funding for say, five years or more, with explicit aims of developing trust and increased engagement with services, is needed. Health service collaboration with third-sector organisations that are trusted by communities is likely to be the most effective approach. Alongside this, funding for third-sector organisations may well achieve more return on investment than funding health services.

Addressing data gaps is also imperative as without robust data, we cannot know the level of health inequality experienced by Gypsy, Roma, and Traveller communities. Alongside improving data must be a commitment to using the data to facilitate change. However, as we suggested in the introduction to this chapter, data is unlikely to improve without first building trust.

Finally, building trust with Gypsy, Roma, and Traveller people cannot be achieved by health services alone. We have provided evidence of the systemic neglect and racism towards Gypsy, Roma, and Traveller that pervades policy, service provision and the attitudes and behaviours of frontline professionals. Action is needed at government and societal levels to address the wider determinants of, and the structural barriers to health. This includes addressing the ingrained prejudice and discrimination towards Gypsy, Roma, and Traveller people in all aspects of their lives.

Discussion questions

1. What factors contribute to lack of trust between Gypsy, Roma, and Traveller people and health services?
2. How are Gypsy, Roma, and Traveller people's experiences of structural racism different from those of other population groups and in what ways are they similar?
3. What policies are likely to be most effective in improving health and reducing health inequalities for Gypsy, Roma, and Traveller people?

Further reading

Crew, T. (2024). Disadvantaged, discriminated against and ignored: The experiences of Romani and Gypsy Travellers. In L. Gregory & S. Iafrati (Eds.), *Diversity and Welfare Provision* (pp. 117–135). Policy Press.

Greenfields, M., & Rogers, C. (2020). *Hate: "As Regular as Rain" A Pilot Research Project into the Psychological Effects of Hate Crime on Gypsy, Traveller and Roma (GTR) Communities*. GateHerts.

McFadden, A., Siebelt, L., Gavine, A., Atkin, K., Bell, K., Innes, N., . . . MacGillivray, S. (2018). Gypsy, Roma and Traveller access to and engagement with health services: A systematic review. *The European Journal of Public Health*, *28*(1), 74–81.

Spalvieri, S., Morgan, L., & Wait, S. (2024). *Earning Trust: A Foundation for Health Equity*. The Health Policy Partnership.

Watson, A., Collins, B., Bodine-McCoy, A., Eastwood, O., Jernigan, M., Rasmussen, L., & Wood, M. (2025). *Archival Research Conducted to Explore 20th Century Policies Affecting Gypsy/Traveller Communities in Scotland*. Scottish Government.

Case study 1

Approach to engagement

This case study was based around a third-sector organisation in West Yorkshire. The organisation aimed to improve the lives of Gypsies and Travellers through health-related activities, including telephone, drop-in, and outreach advocacy; community health educators training sessions; developing partnerships with other organisations to increase accessibility of services such as the Health Protection Agency and local GP practices; supporting health practitioners to develop cultural competence and engagement skills; and working with partners to conduct health-related research and consultation, both locally and nationally.

Of interest to our research was an innovative collaboration with local maternity services to provide an integrated pathway for Gypsy, Roma, and Traveller women. The local maternity care provision included a service which provided essential support for pregnant women and their families from minority ethnic communities including Gypsy, Roma, and Travellers families.

Population

The population of Romany Gypsies and Irish Travellers was estimated to be around 3000. The City Council provided one overcrowded site of 41 pitches on the outskirts of the city, although two thirds of the Gypsy and Traveller community lived in bricks and mortar housing, and an estimated 25 families lived in unauthorised sites.

Research participants

- 10 mothers (lived in brick-and-mortar housing or on the council site; some had previously lived roadside)
- 8 healthcare practitioners
- 4 third-sector organisation staff.

Case study 2

Approach to engagement

Case study two was conducted in Fife, Scotland, focusing on Scottish Gypsy/Travellers. This case study was selected because, unlike the other three case studies, it reflected an approach to community engagement that was led by the NHS, and the locality was mainly rural. We were also aware of an oral health promotion initiative involving Gypsy/Travellers in the area. A local health needs assessment (LNA) highlighted dental health and registration with GPs as areas of concern. The LNA recognised an NHS delivered social prescribing service 'Keep Well' as a good vehicle for improving health outcomes. The LNA recommendations included co-ordinated working for roadside encampments, more flexible health services, creation of a multi-agency group to progress partnership working, and appointment of health inclusion workers specifically for Gypsy/Traveller communities.

Population

The 2011 Census reported 316 Gypsy/Travellers living in the county, the fourth largest population of Gypsy/Travellers in Scotland. Of these, 43% lived in a house or bungalow, 42% lived in a flat or tenement, and 12% lived in a caravan or other mobile structure. The Council provides accommodation on three sites with a total of 50 pitches. There are also variable numbers and size of unauthorised sites, especially during the Travelling season of March to October.

Participants

- 6 mothers and 2 grandmothers (all lived on one council site)
- 10 healthcare practitioners
- 2 third-sector organisation staff.

Case study 3

Approach to engagement

Case study three focused on the migrant Roma community in a large city in South Yorkshire. We chose this case study based on a third-sector organisation, the Darnall Well-being Project, which provided advocacy and support for the Slovak Roma population in the city. The case study focused on maternity, early years and dental health services.

Population

In 2012, there were an estimated 2100 Slovak Roma living in three socioeconomically deprived areas of the city. Community tensions between the Roma and other communities had attracted national media attention.

Participants

- 7 mothers (1 mother spoke English, and an interpreter was present for 6 interviews) and 1 father
- 25 healthcare practitioners
- 4 third-sector organisation staff.

Case study 4

Approach to engagement

The fourth case study focused on Irish Travellers living in two London boroughs, where there were relatively large numbers of Gypsy and Traveller people. We selected this case study because of the relatively large population of Irish Travellers living in the context of a very diverse general population, and the pressures on accommodation and health services within the city. We were aware of two third-sector organisations working in the area. The case study focused on maternity and early years' health services.

Population

The estimated size of the Gypsy and Irish Traveller population in London was 13,500.

Participants

- 14 mothers and 3 grandmothers (living on council sites or in brick and mortar houses
- 11 healthcare practitioners
- 3 third-sector organisation staff.

References

Abrams, D., Swift, H., & Houston, D. (2018). *Developing a National Barometer of Prejudice and Discrimination in Britain*. Equality and Human Rights Commission.

Anderson, A., & Griffith, D. M. (2022). Measuring the trustworthiness of health care organizations and systems. *The Milbank Quarterly*, *100*(2), 345.

Aspinall, P. (2014). *Hidden Needs: Identifying Key Vulnerable Groups in Data Collections: Vulnerable Migrants, Gypsies and Travellers, Homeless People, and Sex Workers*. University of Kent.

Baker, M. (2005). *Gypsies and Travellers: The Leeds Baseline Census 2004–2005*. Leeds Racial Equality Council.

Barton, C., & Zayed, Y. (2024). *Gypsies, Roma and Travellers: Statistics*. House of Commons Library.

Beach, H. (2006). Comparing the use of an accident and emergency department by children from two local authority Gypsy sites with that of their neighbours. *Public Health*, *120*(9), 882–884.

Bloch, A., & Quarmby, K. (2025). Environmental racism, segregation and discrimination: Gypsy and Traveller sites in Great Britain. *Critical Social Policy*, *45*(1), 94–114.

Brown, P., Scullion, L., & Martin, P. (2013). *Migrant Roma in the United Kingdom: Population Size and Experiences of Local Authorities and Partners*. University of Salford.

Chattoo, S., & Atkin, K. M. (2012). Race, ethnicity and social policy: Theoretical concepts and the limitations of current approaches to welfare. In *Understanding Race and Ethnicity: Theory, History, Policy and Practice* (pp. 19–40). Policy Press.

Council of Europe. (2012). *Estimates on Roma Population in European Countries: Document Prepared by the Support Team of the Special Representative of the Secretary General of the Council of Europe for Roma Issues*. https://www.coe.int/en/web/roma-and-travellers/publications

Crew, T. (2024). Disadvantaged, discriminated against and ignored: The experiences of Romani and Gypsy Travellers. In L. Gregory & S. Iafrati (Eds.), *Diversity and Welfare Provision* (pp. 117–135). Policy Press.

Crowe, S., Cresswell, K., Robertson, A., Huby, G., Avery, A., & Sheikh, A. (2011). The case study approach. *BMC Medical Research Methodology*, *11*(1), 100–108.

Dar, O., Gobin, M., Hogarth, S., Lane, C., & Ramsay, M. (2013). Mapping the Gypsy Traveller community in England: What we know about their health service provision and childhood immunization uptake. *Journal of Public Health*, *35*(3), 404–412.

Department of Health. (2010). *Healthy Lives, Healthy People (the Marmot Review): Our Strategy for Public Health in England* (Vol. 7985). The Stationery Office.

Ekezie, W., Hopwood, E., Czyznikowska, B., Weidman, S., Mackintosh, N., & Curtis, F. (2024). Perinatal health outcomes of women from Gypsy, Roma and Traveller communities: A systematic review. *Midwifery*, *129*, 103910.

European Commission. (2014). *Tackling Health Inequalities: EU Support to Improve Health across All Sectors of Society*. European Union.

European Roma Rights Centre. (2018). *The Fragility of Professional Competence. A Preliminary Account of Child Protection Practice with Romani and Traveller Children in England*. European Roma Rights Centre.

Farrer, L., Marinetti, C., Cavaco, Y. K., & Costongs, C. (2015). Advocacy for health equity: A synthesis review. *The Milbank Quarterly*, *93*(2), 392–437.

Friends Families and Travellers. (2022). *Briefing: Health Inequalities Experienced by Gypsy, Roma and Traveller Communities*. Friends, Families & Travellers.

Friends Families and Travellers. (2024). *Tackling Mental Health Inequalities for Gypsy, Roma and Traveller People*. Friends, Families & Travellers.

Ghimisi, A. (2021). The new European Union Strategic Framework for Roma Integration 2020–2030: Insights and recommendations for the national strategic frameworks. *Journal of Research and Innovation for Sustainable Society*, *3*(1), 64–68.

Greenfields, M., & Rogers, C. (2020). *Hate: "As Regular as Rain" A Pilot Research Project into the Psychological Effects of Hate Crime on Gypsy, Traveller and Roma (GTR) Communities*. GateHerts.

Guarnizo-Herreño, C. C., & Wehby, G. L. (2012). Children's dental health, school performance, and psychosocial well-being. *The Journal of Pediatrics*, *161*(6), 1153–1159.

Havlin, T. (2015). Shift in social order–shift in gender roles? Migration experience and gender roles. *Current Issues in Personality Psychology*, *3*(3), 185–191.

Hollinshead, R., Gavin, M., & Byram, A. (2023). *Guidance: Tackling Maternal Health Inequalities in Gypsy, Roma and Traveller Communities*. Friends, Family and Travellers.

House of Commons Women and Equalities Committee. (2019). Tackling inequalities faced by Gypsy, Roma and Traveller communities. *Seventh Report of Session 2017–2019*.

HSC Public Health Agency. (2010). *Health Intelligence Briefing: The All Ireland Traveller Health Study*. Northern Ireland: Public Health Agency.

Karlsen, S., Roth, M., & Bécares, L. (2019). Understanding the influence of ethnicity on health. In *Understanding 'Race' and Ethnicity* (pp. 159–180). Policy Press.

Keating, F. (2019). Understanding 'race', ethnicity and mental health. In *Understanding 'Race' and Ethnicity* (pp. 201–226). Policy Press.

La Placa, V., & Smith, D. (2016). The health and wellbeing of gypsies and travellers in settled housing: A narrative review of the evidence and policy. *International Journal of Social Science Studies*, *4*, 87.

McFadden, A., Siebelt, L., Gavine, A., Atkin, K., Bell, K., Innes, N., . . . MacGillivray, S. (2018). Gypsy, Roma and Traveller access to and engagement with health services: A systematic review. *The European Journal of Public Health*, *28*(1), 74–81.

Mullarkey, M., Duffy, A., & Timmins, F. (2011). Trust between nursing management and staff in critical care: A literature review. *Nursing in Critical Care*, *16*(2), 85–91.

National Academies of Sciences, Engineering, and Medicine. (2023). *The Roles of Trust and Health Literacy in Achieving Health Equity: Clinical Settings*. National Academic Press.

Office for Health Improvement and Disparities. (2022). *Improving Roma Health: A Guide for Health and Care Professionals*. Gov.UK. https://www.gov.uk/guidance/improving-roma-health-a-guide-for-health-and-care-professionals

Office for National Statistics. (2023). *Gypsy or Irish Traveller Populations, England and Wales: Census 2021*. Office for National Statistics.

Parry, G., Van Cleemput, P., Peters, J., Walters, S., Thomas, K., & Cooper, C. (2007). Health status of Gypsies and Travellers in England. *Journal of Epidemiology & Community Health*, *61*(3), 198–204.

Renedo, A., Stuart, R., Kühlbrandt, C., Grenfell, P., McGowan, C. R., Miles, S., Marston, C. (2023). Community-led responses to COVID-19 within Gypsy and Traveller communities in England: A participatory qualitative research study. *SSM-Qualitative Research in Health*, *3*, 100280.

Scottish Government. (2024). *Improving the Lives of Scotland's Gypsy/Travellers 2: Action Plan 2024–2026*. Scottish Government.

Smith, D., Newton, P., Berlin, J., & Barrett, S. (2020). A community approach to engaging Gypsy and Travellers' in cancer services. *Health Promotion International*, *35*(5), 1094–1105.

Spalvieri, S., Morgan, L., & Wait, S. (2024). *Earning Trust: A Foundation for Health Equity*. The Health Policy Partnership.

Tofan, G., Bodolica, V., & Spraggon, M. (2013). Governance mechanisms in the physician–patient relationship: A literature review and conceptual framework. *Health Expectations*, *16*(1), 14–31.

The Traveller Movement. (2022, November 29). *Number of Gypsy, Roma, and Traveller People Disclosing Ethnicity in Census Increases by 110,000*. https://travellermovement.org.uk/news/5719#_ftn1

Tyler, I., & Campbell, S. (2024). *Poverty Stigma: A Glue That Holds Poverty in Place*. Joseph Rowntree Foundation.

Understanding Patient Data. (2024). *Work with Us: Equitable Data Collection for Gypsy, Roma & Traveller Communities*. https://understandingpatientdata.org.uk/work-us-equitable-data-collection-gypsy-roma-traveller-communities

Watson, A., Collins, B., Bodine-McCoy, A., Eastwood, O., Jernigan, M., Rasmussen, L., Wood, M. (2025). *Archival Research Conducted to Explore 20th Century Policies Affecting Gypsy/Traveller Communities in Scotland*. Scottish Government.

Williams, J. (2021). *Climate Change Is Racist: Race, Privilege and the Struggle for Climate Justice*. Icon Books.

CHAPTER 8

Uptake of mental health services

A case of Black sub-Saharan Afrikan migrant communities in the West Midlands of England, UK

Last Mafuba, Mathew Nyashanu, and Linda Gibson

Introduction

Globally, mental health disorders represent a growing public health challenge. According to the World Health Organization (WHO, 2025), approximately one in eight individuals worldwide live with a mental health condition. The percentage of individuals experiencing mental illness is higher in low- or middle-income countries compared with high-income countries; yet within high-income settings, people from global majority communities continue to experience elevated mental health needs (Henry, 2020). In England, people of Black heritage, especially those of sub-Saharan Afrikan[1] descent, encounter some of the worst mental health outcomes and the lowest engagement with mental health services (Bignall et al., 2019). When they do access services, it is frequently during acute crises, through law enforcement and not primary care services (Payne-Gill et al., 2021). Recent data collected between April 2024 and March 2025 indicate that Black individuals were detained under the Mental Health Act at a rate of 262.4 per 100,000, compared to just 65.8 per 100,000 for white individuals (NHS England Digital, 2024). This is despite Black communities constituting only 4.2% of the United Kingdom's (UK's) population (ONS, 2022). Once detained, they are faced with ethnically based prejudice and discrimination by health professionals (Adams et al., 2014; Ayinde & Gillum, 2014). There is evidence to suggest that they experience variation and inequality during assessments and are likely to be offered drug treatments over psychological therapies (Payne-Gill et al., 2021). They also face disproportionate levels of coercion, including restraint, seclusion, prolonged hospital stays, and readmissions (Rugkasa & Canvin, 2011; Care Quality Commission, 2025). After discharge, they are more often placed on Community Treatment Orders (CTOs), allowing their continued monitoring and potential readmission, a practice less frequently applied to white patients (NHS England Digital, 2024).

These disparities have prompted ongoing academic and policy debates. While some researchers attribute them to socioeconomic inequalities, including persistent poverty and exclusion (Jones & Patel, 2021), others point to the deep-rooted influence

DOI: 10.4324/9781003466093-13

of structural racism in healthcare systems (Nazroo et al., 2018). At the same time, under-resourced mental health services across the board have contributed to a climate of limited access for all, particularly for marginalised communities (Cummins, 2015).

Efforts to address inequalities in access often falter because of a persistent tendency to view Black communities as a homogeneous group. These erase distinctions between Afrikan and Caribbean heritage groups, and worse, obscure individual lived experiences by categorising all non-white populations under the 'BAME' label. Such homogenisation disregards cultural nuance, lived histories, and community-specific understandings of mental health (Earl et al., 2015). Additionally, many studies focus heavily on administrative records and service usage data, with little engagement with the voices of those most affected (Lawrence et al., 2021).

In contrast, this chapter prioritises first-person narratives to explore what prevents Black sub-Saharan Afrikan individuals in the West Midlands of England, UK, from seeking mental health support. Through this approach, the research aims to capture the experiential knowledge of participants and foreground the social and structural barriers they encounter. The study is theoretically anchored in the concept of 'screaming silences', as outlined later.

Conceptual framework

The research was informed by a conceptual framework grounded in the notion of 'screaming silences', a construct rooted in anti-essentialist theory that challenges the idea of a single, fixed reality. Instead, it emphasises multiple realities shaped by context, history, and lived experience (Serrant-Green, 2011). From this foundation, The Silences Framework (TSF) emerged, providing a methodology for surfacing marginalised or unspoken perspectives, particularly in research with underrepresented populations (Serrant-Green, 2011). Figure 8.1 gives a visual representation of the TSF's four main stages.

TSF is particularly well-suited to studies exploring sensitive or stigmatised subjects, as it seeks to uncover the narratives that are frequently absent from mainstream

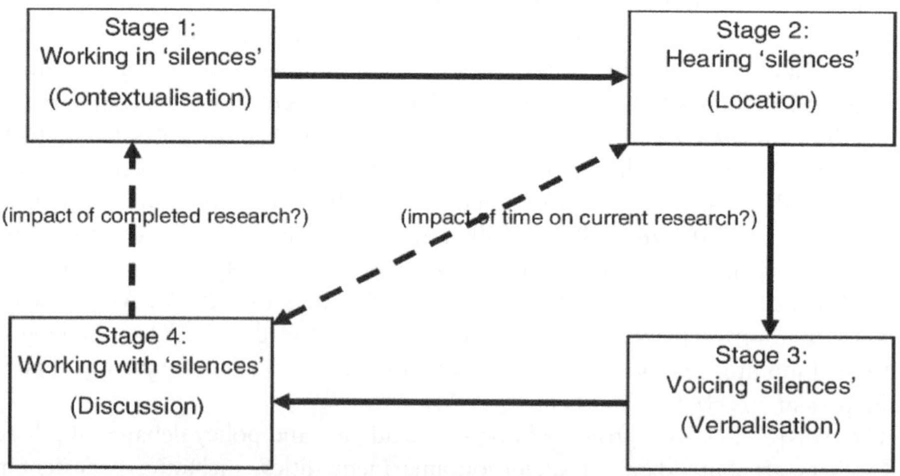

Figure 8.1 The Silences Framework (Serrant-Green 2011).

discourse. For this research, TSF facilitated the examination of overlooked dimensions of Black sub-Saharan Afrikan communities' engagement with mental health services in the UK. Although TSF contains five stages, this study adopted only four. Stage 5 of the framework is dedicated for action planning and is only applicable to studies that use their findings to change service delivery or community action (Serrant-Green, 2011). The data collection and analysis at Stage 3 employed Interpretative Phenomenological Analysis (IPA), which enabled a close exploration of participants' subjective experiences, drawing meaning from their social, cultural, and political contexts. This is a qualitative methodology designed to explore and interpret the lived experiences of participants (Smith et al., 2022). IPA views human beings as 'experiential experts' who, through language and cognition, can describe and make sense of their lived experiences.

To deepen the analysis, Critical Race Theory (CRT) was applied during Stage 4. CRT interrogates the ways in which race and systemic racism influence lived experiences and institutional practices. It operates on the premise that racism is not an anomaly but a structural and enduring feature of society (Delgado & Stefancic, 2017). In healthcare, CRT exposes how systems often deny or devalue the experiences of racialised individuals, particularly when those experiences contradict dominant assumptions of neutrality or universality (Yosso, 2005).

The integration of TSF, IPA, and CRT creates a multifaceted lens through which to understand the barriers facing Black sub-Saharan Afrikan communities in accessing and utilising a white-privileged healthcare system in a structurally racist and unjust society. By combining an emphasis on silenced voices, deep experiential insight, and a critical interrogation of structural power, this framework enables a rigorous, grounded analysis of the low uptake of mental health services in these communities.

While racism is a broad and global phenomenon, this chapter specifically focuses on racial inequality between Black and white populations in the UK, framed through the historical relationship between England and sub-Saharan Afrika. This context is essential for understanding how colonial legacies and racial hierarchies continue to influence access to care and experiences within the mental health system. As such, to provide context to this study, the next section will give an overview of the social environment inhabited by Black sub-Saharan Afrikans in England.

The social environment resided by Black sub-Saharan Afrikans in England

Both TSF and CRT emphasise the importance of acknowledging the broader social contexts in which marginalised communities exist. These environments significantly influence the health outcomes of such populations, often acting as underlying contributors to poor mental health and limited recovery opportunities (Serrant-Green, 2011).

Black sub-Saharan Afrikan communities in England frequently find themselves navigating hostile and unequal social terrains shaped by colonial legacies, entrenched structural racism, and socioeconomic disadvantage. In the West Midlands where this study took place, these challenges are particularly acute. The region has some of the highest deprivation levels in England, with 25% of its population living in poverty (Joseph Rowntree Foundation, 2022). According to the 2021 UK census, individuals of Black sub-Saharan Afrikan origin make up 2.5% of England's 14.4% global majority population (Office for National Statistics, 2022). Despite this relatively small proportion, they experience pronounced inequalities in access to healthcare, employment, housing, and education (Joseph Rowntree Foundation, 2022). Between 2017 and 2020, more than 45% of Black individuals were living in poverty, a rate nearly twice that of white individuals and significantly above the national average by 23% (Joseph Rowntree Foundation, 2022). Many arrive to find an unwelcoming environment, often exacerbated by immigration restrictions and xenophobic local attitudes (Nyashanu et al., 2024).

A major structural barrier is the UK's 'hostile environment' policy, introduced in 2012 to deter irregular migration. These policies restrict access to public services, including healthcare, by linking service eligibility to immigration status (Kirkup & Winnett, 2012). As a result, many sub-Saharan Afrikan migrants live under conditions of chronic insecurity, avoiding contact with services out of fear of deportation or legal consequences (Webber, 2019). Even among those with legal status, lingering fears and a deep mistrust of state institutions persist.

This climate of exclusion, coupled with economic hardship and cultural dislocation, significantly affects mental well-being. It also creates cumulative stressors that are not always visible to mental health practitioners, further complicating efforts to access timely and appropriate care. These social realities serve as a backdrop to the participant experiences explored in the next section.

Methodology

This study adopted a qualitative approach to explore the lived experiences of Black sub-Saharan Afrikan individuals navigating mental health services in the West Midlands. A total of 21 participants were recruited from ten sub-Saharan Afrikan countries: Cameroon, Ethiopia, Gambia, Ghana, Ivory Coast, Kenya, Malawi, Nigeria, Uganda, and Zimbabwe. These countries (bar Ethiopia) are former British colonies and members of the Commonwealth, except for Ethiopia, which was occupied by Italy, and the Ivory Coast, which was colonised by France. While Zimbabwe is a former British colony, it is currently under suspension from the Commonwealth and is undergoing an application to rejoin. It is also important to note that while Cameroon was colonised by France, its southern region became partly colonised by Britain after the Second World War and is a member of the Commonwealth.

Participants were identified using purposive and snowball sampling techniques through trusted community networks. These included Black-majority churches, local businesses, barbershops, and the Inini peer support group. The Inini peer support group, operated by Inini Initiative, a social enterprise founded by Mafuba to support migrant integration, played a central role in recruitment. As the majority of Inini members are of Black sub-Saharan Afrikan heritage, engagement with potential participants was both accessible and culturally appropriate. Mafuba's established relationships with various faith and community groups, and the trust she holds within these communities, further supported outreach.

Initial contact with participants was facilitated through community leaders, with only those expressing interest invited for an interview. Eligibility was based on availability and willingness to participate. Of the 21 participants, 18 were recruited from Inini; 17 had been active members for at least six months, while one had only attended twice. Additionally, two participants were mental health professionals working with migrant populations, and one was a reverend at a local Black church.

The sample comprised 13 men and 8 women, ranging in age from 23 to 60 years (mean age 42 years). All but one participant had migrated from sub-Saharan Afrika; the exception was born and raised in the UK to Afrikan-born parents. Eighteen individuals had migrated directly from Afrika, while two had resided briefly in other European countries before arriving in the UK. Participants held a range of immigration statuses: six were naturalised British citizens, seven were asylum seekers awaiting decisions from the Home Office, two held indefinite leave to remain, five were undocumented, and one was British born. On average, participants had lived in the UK for 17 years. Participant demographics are set out in Table 8.1.

Data collection was conducted using semi-structured interviews designed to encourage open, exploratory dialogue and to ensure cultural sensitivity. Interviews were audio-recorded with consent and transcribed verbatim by the authors. The data was analysed using IPA, which allowed for a detailed, context-sensitive exploration of personal experiences.

Findings were organised into two overarching themes: (1) barriers influencing participants' decisions to seek help for poor mental health and (2) obstacles encountered when accessing and navigating mental health services. These themes are interwoven, with many participants highlighting overlapping issues such as systemic marginalisation, economic precarity, immigration-related barriers, and complex mental health needs. While each story is unique, the shared patterns suggest these challenges are structural and intergenerational, rather than isolated or individual.

Table 8.1 Participants' Demographic Information

Pseudonym	*Gender*	*Age*	*Country of Origin*	*Period in the UK*	*Immigration Status*
Afolabi	F	49	Gambia	28 years	Naturalised
Agbo	M	31	Cameroon	2 years	Undocumented
Akosua	F	59	Zimbabwe	7 years	Asylum seeker
Akua	F	49	Malawi	14 Years	Asylum seeker
Almaz	M	38	Ghana	20 years	Indefinite leave to remain
Ashura	F	51	Ghana	18 years	Undocumented
Chiyedza	F	54	Kenya	23 years	Undocumented
Samora	M	45	Zimbabwe	21 years	Undocumented
Jabu	M	35	Ivory Coast	24 years	Asylum seeker
Kamal	M	35	Zimbabwe	10 years	Asylum seeker
Kodjo	M	35	Cameroon	12 years	Undocumented
Kudzayi	F	27	Zimbabwe	17 years	Naturalised
Kwame	M	54	Ethiopia	11 years	Asylum seeker
Lobengula	M	34	Gambia	3 years	Asylum seeker
Mumbi	M	49	Uganda	23 years	Naturalised
Mupezeni	M	27	Zimbabwe	17 years	Indefinite leave to remain
Punha	F	23	Nigeria	23 years	British born
Sankara	M	60	Zimbabwe	22 years	Naturalised
Setorwu	F	43	Kenya	26 years	Naturalised
Shabalala	M	45	Ghana	17 years	Naturalised
Tafadzwa	M	42	Malawi	18 years	Asylum seeker

Theme 1: Barriers to seeking help for mental health concerns

Participants shared deeply personal accounts of how their social environment shaped their attitudes toward mental health and their decisions about seeking support. Their narratives revealed a landscape of fear, exclusion, cultural misunderstanding, and systemic hardship. These findings are presented through three interconnected sub-themes.

Regularisation of immigration status and fear of deportation

Uncertainty surrounding immigration status emerged as a significant barrier to mental health support. Participants described prolonged waiting periods for Home Office decisions and the financial strain of legal fees, which compounded their psychological distress. Many were reluctant to approach public services, including health providers, for fear that their immigration status might be exposed, triggering detention or deportation.

> *Everything is a fight – to get food, to get housing, to get everything, to get anything. And then it's, you know, your mental health as well, especially battling with things and trying to get status, trying to get a job, and trying to sustain a livelihood.*
>
> *– Kudzayi, 27 years*

> *[I]mmigration is like a, a disability almost . . . I feel stuck and disabled socially to do many things that people would normally do to survive.*
>
> *– Jabu, 35 years*

> *[W]hen you have to pay for your applications. . . . With my indefinite [leave to remain] I was rejected the first time and had to appeal . . . . It's not easy. It's very hard. I've seen people where there's you, there's your wife, or you have just two kids and you have to renew for the four of you*
>
> *– Almaz, 38 years*

The three participants above reflect on the daily challenges of living, where the added pressures of Home Office applications add layers of complexity, challenge, and financial burden, whilst also trying to exist in the day to day. The participant below reflects on how these pressures become even more pronounced when faced with urgent need for medical care.

> *At one point I was really scared of going to the hospital. . . . I just had that, um, perception that the hospital is like a no, no, due to your immigration status. . . . I can say maybe for a couple of years, I was just staying away from hospitals . . . within that time, I had some symptoms which had to develop in my body . . . . I got operated at that time, you know, and it was something which maybe I could have avoided. . . . I was almost dying, you know*
>
> *– Kodjo, 35 years*

The pervasive fear and bureaucracy involved in immigration processes created a hostile context that made prioritising mental health nearly impossible for many.

Racism, isolation, and the loss of identity

Several participants recalled experiencing racial hostility shortly after arriving in the UK. Whether through overt abuse, subtle microaggressions, or systemic discrimination, their sense of safety and belonging was compromised.

> *You never sometimes knew how far you could go; you know. Somebody will abuse you on the streets [and] you can't say anything back. You've got to hold your tongue. You got to. When you go to work, you've got to really behave yourself. You've got to make sure [everything is] right, the papers are right, the right NI, the right everything.*
>
> *– Setorwu, 43 years*

> *In the UK, there is a lot of racism. I find that a lot of the racism that I encounter isn't outright people shouting the N-word at me; it's people subtly doing stuff. It's work; I mean previous jobs being racist, being systematically racist. It's, you know, people excluding me from things because of my colour, you know, and it's uncomfortable because it's so subtle. . . . it kind of feels like I am constantly kind of being gas lit by people. It also feels uncomfortable.*
>
> *– Punha, 23 years*

> *I had a police officer stop me repeatedly just for driving through certain areas. It's like every Black guy in a car is a drug dealer.*
>
> *– Almaz, 38 years*

> *One of our neighbours was so, so challenging. He didn't understand us. He didn't welcome us . . . as soon as we moved into that house, he cut branches and threw them over the fence into our yard just to say, 'you're not welcome'.*
>
> *– Sankara, 60 years*

Both overt and subtle racism are being described in the above statements. In parallel, some described a loss of cultural and professional identity. Previous achievements were often invalidated or dismissed, contributing to low self-esteem and alienation.

> *Well, first is the cultural shock. You come here, you lose everything; your identity, professional, personal identity is gone. So, uh, I was comfortable according to the xxxx standard. Yes. Uh, social status, extremely well respected. . . . That was the hardest part for me, and uh, at some point I wanted to go back because I've never worked in a factory ever in my life. . . . And the people there are not nice at all. They are very nasty people. Yeah. It's ruthless.*
>
> *– Kamuzu, 45 years*

This intersection of racism and cultural erasure led to profound psychological stress and, for some, feelings of regret about migrating. Added to this is loneliness, of no longer being part of a community of support.

> *You know how it is out here in the UK. . . . It's not about your neighbours, about anyone. It's just you and your own family, . . . I've realised it's who the British*

> *are; each one minds their own business. . . . Somebody is mourning next door, you cannot even go and, you know, show your, uh, support in terms of, uh, emotional support. . . . . For me, it's so awkward because I come from a society where people are people, because you know about your neighbour, you care about your surroundings.*
>
> – *Akosua, 59 years*

Low mental health awareness and stigma

Many participants lacked prior exposure to the concept of mental health or did not recognise their symptoms as warranting professional support. Some learned about mental health issues only through community groups like Inini. Cultural norms, often shaped by religious beliefs or traditions discouraged vulnerability and promoted silence over help-seeking.

> *The first time I heard about mental health was at Inini. Before that, no one talked about it.*
>
> – *Kodjo, 35 years*

> *I can only speak from a person who is Afrikan who grew up in an Afrikan family, raised by Afrikans. Like mental health is not an issue. It's something that's overlooked. Particularly, in my family we have this attitude of you've just gotta keep it moving, whatever it is, . . . my mother just said, well why would you get counselling, what is it going to do. . .? What I have seen is people just sweeping things under the carpet. It's like, this has happened, let's move on because we can't stay in the tragedy, there's no transitional period of like, okay hold on, still trying to figure out what is going on. You appear soft in that way. Yeah, so um, pretty much just, sweeping it under the rug.*
>
> – *Kudzayi, 27 years*

> *I'll go to God. I'll open the Bible . . . He'll take care of me.*
>
> – *Tafadzwa, 42 years*

These cultural expectations, combined with limited-service awareness, led many to internalise distress or seek support only when in severe crisis.

The narratives reveal that Black sub-Saharan Afrikan communities in the West Midlands face multiple, interconnected barriers to accessing mental health services. Immigration status emerges as a central issue, with financial strain, fear of deportation, and legal insecurity discouraging engagement with mainstream services to many who historically came from British colonies. These challenges are compounded by racial discrimination, social exclusion, and loss of identity resulting from underemployment and diminished social status. Limited mental health awareness, stigma, and lack of familial or community support further isolate individuals and prevent help-seeking. Together, these factors create a cycle of fear, isolation, and unmet mental health needs. However, a few of these individuals managed to navigate these obstacles and accessed support but were further presented with more challenges as shown in the next section.

Theme 2: Challenges in navigating mental health services

While some participants eventually sought help, doing so often led to new challenges within the system. Their accounts exposed a mental health infrastructure that was unresponsive, culturally detached, and often reactive rather than preventative. The subthemes below highlight the most common barriers encountered during their attempts to engage with mental healthcare.

Disbelief, delays, and diagnostic gaps

Many participants described being dismissed or not taken seriously by mental health professionals until their condition deteriorated significantly. Initial requests for help were often deflected or delayed, and some were denied access to care based on rigid referral systems or narrow criteria.

> *There used to be a mental health unit just less than three minutes from where I lived. I went, and I knocked on the door. . . . You can't come in. The referral process is this; call this number. I called the number, and they referred me to say, oh, can you get to this place? I went to that place. And they said, um okay, we recognise you've used mental health services before. . . . Like how can you tell? So, I explained to them, then they said, but you're not a professional?. . . . They sent me back home. They said, we will send a team to come out. And this team didn't come for four days. . . . When they finally came, the day they came, the state of my room; the moment they get in the house they called the police. The state of my room, I was unwell. I'd been aware and I went to seek for help. By the time I get the help it's almost a week. . . . The next thing within the half hour, I was in the same unit that I'd knocked to say I need some help. . . . I was detained.*
>
> *– Samora, 45 years*

Some reported being overlooked because they appeared 'high functioning', masking internal struggles. Others were misdiagnosed due to language barriers or cultural misunderstandings, undermining trust in the system.

> *What happened is, I had to wait a year to get into therapy and in that year I got worse. So, it would have been better if I had support from when I was like, look I'm struggling. . . and it would have been better if they actually have engaged with me as if I was a person as opposed to kind of a robot. . . because I pass as high functioning I am not taken seriously.*
>
> *– Punha, 23 years*

> *It starts with language. If you don't understand the person you're communicating with, how do you come up with a diagnosis? It's very difficult*
>
> *– Sankara, 60 years*

In the following case, the participant was advocating on behalf of others, trying to prevent a tick box exercise from institutionalising someone in a mental health crisis.

> *Had I not been there, objecting to what the system was trying to do, I think they might have actually taken these people to xxxx (name of psychiatric hospital) and given them a bed and put them on medicine. But I challenged the diagnosis and asked how certain they were that that was the most appropriate action, and whether the other methods couldn't be tried. . . . What I object to is a one-size-fits-all type of system, which is like a tick-box exercise. I've ticked eight out of 10 boxes; I think you should be put into the xxxx (name of mental health institution)*
>
> *– Kamal, 35 years*

These experiences reflect a reactive, overburdened system that fails to offer early intervention or culturally tailored assessment. They also point to support from within the community and family to advocate and question.

Treatment approaches: Medication as a default

A common frustration among participants was the tendency for services to offer medication without addressing underlying causes or exploring alternatives. Medication was often perceived as inappropriate or actually harmful.

> *They are quite the whole medical model of giving people medication. . . . There are tangible reasons why I was feeling the way that I was and giving me anti-depressants as opposed to therapy wasn't actually useful.*
>
> *– Punha, 23 years*

> *I was given some medication, . . . I was in a slumber for two or three days. I didn't know which was which until I had an aunt who came and. . . saw me, and she said they had to stop. . . She's a mental health nurse. . . I believe it was one of the things that actually managed to take me out of this situation; otherwise >pause< I would have just gone into the system and probably never have managed to recover to be able to talk to you today.*
>
> *– Samora, 45 years*

> *I personally do not really believe in taking medicine. . . it becomes fatal. . . when you prescribe something, that medication then gives you a side effect, so you end up with a prescription for something else.*
>
> *– Kudzayi, Female, 27 years*

An overreliance on pharmaceutical interventions, without proper context or communication, was questioned by participants as not the right solution for the specific challenges faced. This contributed to feelings of distrust and fear of consequences from the medication.

Disconnection in talking therapies

While some participants had tried counselling, most found the format ineffective. Therapies often failed to connect with the realities of participants' lives, instead offering generic approaches seen as more suited to white, middle-class clients.

> *I have been through counselling for long . . . but now no. . . . The best way to treat me is to give me freedom because this situation is the one causing this mental problem.*
>
> *– Chiyedza, 54 years*

> *. . . leaving me in my dark room for entire week and giving me once a week appointment to have this kind of conversation that, uh, forces me, uh, to relive my terrible past experience. . . I think that is not helpful.*
>
> *– Kwame, 54 years*

> *. . . They use compassion-focused group therapy, and it is very idealistic. . . . They were like to think about what makes you feel good and peaceful. . . . Do I have the luxury to sit and do nothing? And it's something they didn't get because most of the people they treated are middle-class white women, so of course they could.*
>
> *– Punha, 23 years*

This mismatch between participants' lived realities and therapy models resulted in disengagement and reinforced perceptions that services weren't designed for them.

Lack of empathy and cultural competency

Several participants criticised the impersonal and rigid nature of mental health services. The absence of cultural understanding, and at times basic empathy, led to feelings of being misunderstood or dehumanised.

> *It's just now, a well-managed system that doesn't actually focus on the human being but just on supplying them with whatever they require. There has to be somebody who's dedicated. . . reassure that person and give them the confidence to want to get better.*
>
> *– Samora, 45 years*

> *When I came, when my daughter was sick, she was sick because of, uh, the cancer, but she was also mentally sick in terms of, she had gone through a very, uh, stressful relationship. . . . She was emotionally affected, and they kept treating the cancer, but she was not getting better because I think they were not looking at her psychological problems, but they kept looking at the medical problem and she was like, almost losing it.*
>
> *– Akosua, 59*

The above participants highlight the lack of holistic concern for the human being in their care. People can have complex challenges and each aspect needs attention. This also includes that healthcare professionals need to be aware how trauma from the past continues to inform the present and future.

> *After I spoke about my past experience, uh, I, I remember, uh, once my therapist was telling me, you know, that was in the past. Now you need to remind yourself,*

> *you are here in a safe country, that's not going to happen to you. How can I tell myself, still while, um, worrying about being sent back, uh, to my country.*
>
> *– Kwame, 54 years*

These statements reveal a system where cultural ignorance and bureaucratic procedures undermine effective care, reinforce marginalisation, and dismiss psychological suffering.

In summary, this overarching theme reveals the layered and reinforcing obstacles that Black sub-Saharan Afrikan individuals encounter within the mental health system, even after taking steps to seek support. Participants revealed how they were treated with scepticism by professionals, facing prolonged wait times, and receiving insufficient care, factors that collectively undermined their trust in the system and impeded their healing. Many reported that their concerns were disregarded unless they were in an acute crisis, treatments were delayed, and diagnoses were often unclear, fostering uncertainty and distress. While medication was frequently offered, it often failed to address the broader social issues contributing to their mental health struggles. Additionally, talking therapies were seen as detached from their everyday experiences and ineffective. The generic, one-size-fits-all nature of services, combined with limited cultural awareness and empathy, left many feeling alienated and unsupported. These overlapping issues illustrate how systemic shortcomings in mental health provision disproportionately impact Black sub-Saharan Afrikan communities, leading to disengagement and prolonged suffering.

Discussion

This chapter interprets the meanings constructed by 21 Black sub-Saharan Afrikan participants in relation to their lived experiences within the social environment of the West Midlands of England. The data revealed a complex web of obstacles to accessing and navigating mental health services, shaped by intersecting historical, social, cultural, and political forces. Two overarching themes emerged: the first captures the barriers participants faced when deciding whether to seek mental health support, while the second focuses on the difficulties they encountered once within the system.

These findings are situated within the wider historical relationship between sub-Saharan Afrika and England; a relationship shaped by colonialism, migration, and enduring racial hierarchies. To analyse the persistence of these systemic inequalities, CRT was applied as an analytical framework. CRT allows for a deeper interrogation of how historical injustices and institutional racism have evolved into structural barriers that continue to affect access to mental healthcare for Black sub-Saharan Afrikan communities.

To further structure the discussion, the themes were categorised into four broader conceptual areas. These categories are not mutually exclusive; instead, they reflect the layered and interconnected nature of systemic oppression. This structure helps illuminate how racism operates across multiple institutional and cultural domains, reinforcing inequality at every stage of mental health service engagement.

Institutional power and racialised structures

A core insight from this study is how institutional structures continue to reinforce racial hierarchies that affect Black sub-Saharan Afrikan communities. From a CRT perspective, racism is not limited to individual actions but is embedded in the frameworks and practices of societal institutions. The accounts of participants highlight how structural factors, particularly those linked to immigration systems, create barriers to mental healthcare. For many, the process of securing legal status in the UK involved prolonged uncertainty, significant financial demands, and systemic obstacles. These challenges were especially pronounced for asylum seekers and individuals on temporary visas (seven of the participants were asylum seekers, while five were undocumented); participants reported high upfront costs for visa renewals, frequent rejections, and the necessity of legal representation, all of which deepened financial stress. CRT frames these immigration practices as forms of systemic exclusion, rooted in racialised policy design. A striking example is the contrasting treatment of asylum seekers from Ukraine and Sudan: while Ukrainians were swiftly granted protection under the Temporary Protection Directive, Sudanese applicants were denied comparable assistance (Heschl, 2022). Critics have argued that such differences in treatment reflect underlying racial bias (ENAR, 2022). These insights align with broader research findings that say legal systems in host countries often impede migrants' access to mental health and other essential services (Lindert et al., 2008; Bissonette, 2020).

Participants also described a heightened sense of vulnerability due to racial profiling, surveillance, and fear of wrongful deportation. These anxieties persisted even among those with documented status. Furthermore, the UK's data-sharing agreement between the NHS and the Home Office has intensified mistrust within Black migrant communities (Hiam et al., 2018). For many, the fear of immigration enforcement created a significant deterrent to seeking mental health support. This highlights how the risk of deportation fosters a persistent feeling of vulnerability and anxiety among individuals. These results are consistent with existing literature, which identifies fear around accessing services as a recurring theme (Held et al., 2020). In particular, concerns about being detained by authorities have been linked to hesitancy in disclosing health-related needs and to the limited availability of healthcare services for undocumented migrants (Mona et al., 2021).

Even when mental health services were accessed, participants often faced long waiting times, particularly in under-resourced urban areas. From a CRT lens, this reflects the racialised geography of service provision, commonly referred to as racial tracking, where marginalised populations are clustered in regions with overstretched healthcare infrastructure.

Another key concern was the absence of cultural sensitivity in mental health assessments. Participants frequently felt misdiagnosed or misunderstood due to the use of Eurocentric diagnostic frameworks. These frameworks often overlook how psychological distress may manifest differently across cultures. The result was either overmedication or inappropriate treatment. CRT attributes such outcomes to the colonial roots of Western psychiatry, where non-Western knowledge systems are marginalised. The interest convergence theory, a component of CRT, posits that policies are unlikely to prioritise minority concerns unless they benefit dominant groups; in this case, predominantly white policymakers (Carter, 2020). Despite recent reform efforts (DHSC, 2018), structural gaps persist. This is supported by claims in the literature which identified racism in the delivery of mental health services in England (The MacPherson Report, 1999; Norfolk, Suffolk & Cambridgeshire Strategic Health Authority, 2003; Blofeld, 2004). Similarly, the continuing legacy of colonial history was also identified as one of the factors influencing the uptake of mental health services among individuals of Black Afrikan descent (Lankelly Chase Foundation, 2013).

These challenges collectively underscore the need to centre Black voices in the design and delivery of mental health services. Institutional transformation is necessary to ensure that services are culturally competent, inclusive, and free from structural discrimination.

Racialised narratives and representation

In addition to legal and bureaucratic challenges, participants described the broader cultural narratives that shape their experiences. Many expressed feelings of exclusion within their local communities and reported chronic stress due to being perceived as outsiders. CRT situates these experiences within a broader framework of structural and historical racism. The assumption of white cultural norms as universal often results in implicit biases within mental health services, leading to cultural misunderstandings and alienation.

Participants also noted inconsistencies in how different refugee populations are treated. The positive reception of Ukrainian refugees contrasted sharply with the rejection and suspicion faced by Afrikan asylum seekers. CRT identifies this as an example of differential racialisation and interest convergence, where support is offered based on political or racial convenience rather than equal human concern. These findings align with previous research indicating that British individuals showed greater willingness to assist, employ, and financially support refugees from Ukraine compared to those from Yemen (Sinclair et al., 2023). This disparity has been attributed to perceptions of greater similarity and lower threat associated with Ukrainians relative to Yemenis (Sinclair et al., 2023). Consequently, these patterns may also extend to Black sub-Saharan Afrikan individuals, who often face marginalisation due to their visible differences from the predominantly white British population. Over time, they have also been subject to negative stereotypes portraying them as dangerous, unmotivated, criminal, or violent (Cooke, 2018).

These systemic biases extend into clinical settings. Participants often reported being ignored, misdiagnosed, or treated only when their conditions had reached a critical point. Such patterns suggest that 'Black distress' is frequently dismissed or pathologised, reinforcing historical power imbalances within health systems. However, these findings contradict the currently held view that Black sub-Saharan Afrikan communities mostly present to mental health services when in crisis (Bignall et al., 2019; Care Quality Commission, 2025).

Representation in media and education was another important theme. Participants highlighted how dominant narratives often portray Black individuals through stereotypes of violence or deviance, which affects how they are perceived within healthcare environments. These portrayals, they argued, contribute to self-censorship, fear of judgement, and reluctance to seek help. Mental health services that view Black individuals as inherently strong or aggressive contribute to coercive interventions, including involuntary hospitalisation. The lack of cultural understanding and practitioner diversity further exacerbates this dynamic, making many feel invisible or criminalised.

Resistance and agency

Despite the barriers mentioned earlier, some participants actively resisted marginalisation through various forms of agency. One of the most impactful forms of resistance expressed by participants was the use of counter-narratives; personal and collective stories that challenge dominant stereotypes and expose systemic inequalities in healthcare. Participants described advocating for family members within medical settings and leaning on extended family and religious networks for both emotional and practical support. These culturally grounded strategies often filled the void left by formal services. Scepticism toward Western medical models also led some individuals to turn to alternative forms of healing, such as spiritual practices and traditional remedies. Others engaged in community education efforts to open up dialogue around mental health and reduce associated stigma. These grassroots actions reflect the ability of Black sub-Saharan Afrikan communities to construct culturally relevant spaces for care, healing, and resilience. Indeed, various scholars have recognised prayer as a key coping mechanism within these communities (Harris, 2020; Codjoe et al., 2019). It can therefore be argued that Black sub-Saharan Afrikan communities do not lack mental health awareness; instead, lived experiences of racism and exclusion from mainstream mental health services shape their reliance on spiritual support and culturally familiar practices.

Overall, participants were not passive recipients of inadequate services but active agents working to reshape them. Their resistance took many forms: narrative, relational, and political and underscored the urgency of redesigning systems from the ground up, guided by those most affected. While community resilience and activism were evident, they are not substitutes for institutional accountability. Systemic change is required to address the roots of exclusion. This includes investing in culturally competent services, removing immigration-related barriers to access, and confronting the institutional racism that persists across healthcare. Meaningful reform must be guided by the lived realities of Black sub-Saharan Afrikan individuals. Their voices, experiences, and strategies for survival offer critical insights for building a mental health system that is both equitable and inclusive.

Conclusion

This chapter highlights the systemic inequities that Black sub-Saharan Afrikan communities face when attempting to access and navigate mental health services in the West Midlands. Using TSF, this methodology enabled participants fearful of being seen or heard in the general society of England, or specifically in the West Midlands, to share in settings that were safe and receptive to hearing their voices and their experiences.

While CRT provided a vital lens for understanding how structural racism shapes Black sub-Saharan Afrikan communities' engagement with mental health services, it is the use of TSF that enabled a deeper understanding of how silence itself operates as both a product of oppression and a mode of survival. At Stage 1, participants' silences were shaped by living under conditions of racialised surveillance, precarious or uncertain migration status, and the persistent threat of immigration enforcement in the West Midlands of England (Stage 2). These conditions rendered silence a reasonable and protective response and not an absence of need. At Stage 3, through this research, participants articulated experiences that are routinely marginalised within mental health discourse, reframing distress as a response to systemic injustice rather than individual pathology. At the discussion level (Stage 4), it becomes evident that these narratives function as catalysts for both healing and action, challenging dominant assumptions that Black sub-Saharan Afrikan communities are disengaged from mental healthcare.

Instead, the findings demonstrate that silences are actively produced by hostile systems and that enabling them to be spoken exposes the urgent need for institutional accountability and reform. Importantly, TSF recognises that speech acts do not merely describe experience but enact change; voiced silences reverberate as forms of validation, resistance, and collective meaning-making. Therefore, attending to what has been silenced and to what speaking these silences does is important for building an equitable and inclusive mental health system.

Discussion questions

1. How do structural racism and immigration policies intersect to shape access to mental health services for Black sub-Saharan Afrikan communities in the UK?
2. In what ways can culturally responsive and community-led approaches challenge the limitations of the current mental health system?
3. What does the concept of 'screaming silences' reveal about whose voices are heard or ignored in mental health discourse and policy?

Note

1 The spelling 'Afrika' instead of 'Africa' is used in this chapter as a deliberate act of decolonial resistance.

Further reading

Aas, K. F., & Bosworth, M. (Eds.). (2013). *The Borders of Punishment: Migration, Citizenship, and Social Exclusion*. Oxford University Press.

Bignall, T., Jeraj, S., Helsby, E., & Butt, J. (2019). *Racial Disparities in Mental Health*. Race Equality Foundation.

Delgado, R., & Stefancic, J. (2017). *Critical Race Theory: An Introduction* (2nd ed.). New York: New York University Press.

Nazroo, J. Y., Bhui, K. S., & Rhodes, J. (2018). Where next for understanding race/ethnic inequalities in severe mental illness? *Sociology of Health & Illness*, *40*(4), 735–750.

Serrant-Green, L. (2011). The sound of 'silence': A framework for researching sensitive issues or marginalised perspectives in health. *Journal of Research in Nursing*, *16*(4), 347–360.

References

Adams, A., Vail, L., Buckingham, C. D., Kidd, J., Weich, S., & Roter, D. (2014). Investigating the influence of African American and African Caribbean race on primary care doctors' decision making about depression. *Social Science & Medicine*, *116*, 161–168.

Ayinde, H., & Gillum, R. F. (2014). Cardiovascular disease mortality in sub-Saharan Africa and the Caribbean. *Ethnicity & Disease*, *24*(4), 495–501.

Bignall, T., Jeraj, S., Helsby, E., & Butt, J. (2019). *Racial Disparities in Mental Health*. Race Equality Foundation.

Bissonette, A. (2020). Legal barriers and their impact on migrants' access to psychosocial support in host countries. *Journal of Migration and Health*, *7*, 45–58.

Blofeld, J. (2004). *Report of the Independent Inquiry into the Death of David "Rocky" Bennett*. Commissioned by the Norfolk, Suffolk and Cambridgeshire Strategic Health Authority and the Department of Health.

Care Quality Commission. (2025). *Monitoring of the Mental Health Act in 2023/24*. Retrieved October 15, 2025, from https://www.cqc.org.uk/publications/monitoring-mental-health-act/2023-2024?utm_source=chatgpt.com

Carter, C. (2020). Mental health social work "must do better" as study finds less staff diversity than in rest of profession. *Community Care*. Retrieved October 19, 2025, from https://www.communitycare.co.uk/2020/09/18/mental-health-social-work-must-better-race-study-finds-lower-average-staff-representation/

Codjoe, L., Barber, S., & Thornicroft, G. (2019). Tackling inequalities: A partnership between mental health services and Black faith communities. *Journal of Mental Health*, *28*(3), 225–228.

Cooke, B. G. (2018). Creating a stereotype of a race as dangerous, unintelligent, and lazy: Examining consequences of cultural and psychological conditioning in America. In *Socio-Economic and Education Factors Impacting American Political Systems: Emerging Research and Opportunities* (pp. 1–28). IGI Global.

Cummins, I. (2015). Discussing race, racism and mental health: Two mental health inquiries reconsidered. *International Journal of Human Rights in Healthcare*, *8*(3), 160–172.

Delgado, R., & Stefancic, J. (2017). *Critical Race Theory: An Introduction* (2nd ed.). New York: New York University Press.

Department of Health and Social Care. (2018). *Modernising the Mental Health Act: Final Report of the Independent Review of the Mental Health Act 1983*. Chair: Sir Simon Wessely. GOV.UK.

Earl, T. R., Fortuna, L. R., Gao, S., Williams, D. R., Nieghbors, H., Takeuchi, D., & Algeria, M. (2015). An exploration of how psychotic-like symptoms are experienced, endorsed, and understood from the National Latino and Asian American Study and National Survey of American Life. *Ethnicity & Health*, *20*(3), 273–292.

European Network Against Racism. (2022). *Racist Double-Standards Persist at EU Ukraine Borders and Beyond*. [Online]. Retrieved October 19, 2025, from https://www.socialplatform.org/news/european-network-against-racism-racist-double-standards-persist-at-eu-ukraine-borders-and-beyond/?utm_source=chatgpt.com

Harris, J. (2020). Prayer as a coping mechanism for mental health problems: An exploration. *Journal of Mental Health and Spirituality*, *22*(3), 210–225.

Held, R., Phillips, J., Clarke, S., & Johnson, M. (2020). Fear as a barrier to service utilisation: Understanding the impact on access to health services. *Journal of Health Services Research*, *15*(2), 123–136.

Henry, B. F. (2020). Typologies of adversity in childhood & adulthood as determinants of mental health & substance use disorders of adults incarcerated in US prisons. *Child Abuse & Neglect*, *99*, 104251.

Heschl, L. (2022). A Refugee is a Refugee is . . . a Refugee? Differential treatment of persons in need of protection and non-discrimination law. *Peace Human Rights Governance*, 7(1), 107–141.

Hiam, L., Steele, S., & McKee, M. (2018). The NHS and home office memorandum of understanding: Data sharing and its implications. *The Lancet Public Health*, *3*(7), 341–342.

Jones, R., & Patel, S. (2021). Social deprivation and mental health service uptake: A global perspective. *International Journal of Social Psychiatry*, *67*(5), 437–448. Sage Publications.

Joseph Rowntree Foundation. (2022). *The Essential Guide to Understanding Poverty in the UK*. London. JRF Analysis Unit. Retrieved October 19, 2025, from https://www.jrf.org.uk/uk-poverty-2022-the-essential-guide-to-understanding-poverty-in-the-uk

Kirkup, J., & Winnett, R. (2012, May 25). Theresa May interview: "We're going to give illegal migrants a really hostile reception. *The Telegraph*.

Lankelly Chase Foundation. (2013). *Review of a Short Consultation Exercise on Ethnic Inequalities in Mental Health by Lankelly Chase Foundation, Mind, the Afiya Trust and the Centre for Mental Health*. London: Lankelly Chase Foundation.

Lawrence, E., Fearon, P., Morgan, C., & Dazzan, P. (2021). Follow-up of the AESOP (Aetiology and Ethnicity in Schizophrenia and Other Psychoses) study: Ten-year outcomes and ethnic disparities. *British Journal of Psychiatry*, *219*(6), 487–495.

Lindert, J., Schouler-Ocak, M., & Priebe, S. (2008). Legal frameworks and their impact on access to psychosocial interventions for migrants in host countries. *International Journal of Migration, Health and Social Care*, *4*(2), 10–19.

Macpherson, W. (1999). *The Stephen Lawrence Inquiry: Report of an Inquiry*. https://assets.publishing.service.gov.uk/government/uploads/system/uploads/attachment_data/file/277111/4262.pdf

Mona, J., Patel, R., Sanchez, L., & Williams, A. (2021). Fear of police detainment as a barrier to accessing mental health services: An analysis. *Journal of Mental Health and Wellbeing*, *22*(4), 405–418.

Nazroo, J. Y., Bhui, K. S., & Rhodes, J. (2018). Where next for understanding race/ethnic inequalities in severe mental illness? Structural, interpersonal and institutional racism. *Sociology of Health & Illness*, *40*(4), 735–750. Check citation in-text.

NHS England Digital. (2024). *Mental Health Act Statistics, Annual Figures 2023–24*. [online]. Retrieved October 19, 2025, from https://digital.nhs.uk/data-and-information/publications/statistical/mental-health-act-statistics-annual-figures/2023-24-annual-figures

Norfolk, Suffolk & Cambridgeshire Strategic Health Authority. (2003). *Independent Inquiry into the Death of David "Rocky" Bennett* (HSG (94)27). Norwich: Author.

Nyashanu, M., Mbalinda, S. N., Madziva, R., & Ekpenyong, M. S. (2024). Perceptions and attitudes of Black Sub-Sahara African migrants from war torn zones towards accessing health services in the English West Midlands region, UK. *International Journal of Migration, Health and Social Care*, *20*(1), 19–31.

Office for National Statistics. (2022). *Ethnic Group England and Wales: Census 2021*. Retrieved August 12, 2025, from https://www.ons.gov.uk/peoplepopulationandcommunity/culturalidentity/ethnicity/bulletins/ethnicgroupenglandandwales/census2021

Payne-Gill, J., Whitfield, C., & Beck, A. (2021). The relationship between ethnic background and the use of restrictive practices to manage incidents of violence or aggression in psychiatric inpatient settings. *International Journal of Mental Health Nursing*, *30*(5), 1221–1233.

Rugkasa, J., & Canvin, K. (2011). Researching mental health in minority ethnic communities: Reflections on recruitment. *Qualitative Health Research*, *21*(1), 132–143.

Serrant-Green, L. (2011). The sound of 'silence': A framework for researching sensitive issues or marginalised perspectives in health. *Journal of Research in Nursing*, *16*(4), 347–360.

Sinclair, S., Granberg, E., & Nilsson, P. (2023). The British public's preferences: Greater support for Ukrainian Refugees compared to Yemeni Refugees. *Journal of Refugee Studies*, *36*(1), 65–82.

Smith, J. A., Flowers, P., & Larkin, M. (2022). *Interpretative Phenomenological Analysis: Theory, Method and Research* (2nd ed.). London: SAGE.

Webber, F. (2019). On the creation of the UK's 'hostile environment'. *Race & Class*, *60*(4), 76–87.

World Health Organization. (2025). *WHO Special Initiative for Mental Health* [online]. Retrieved August 11, 2025, from https://www.who.int/initiatives/who-special-initiative-for-mental-health

Yosso, T. J. (2005). Whose culture has capital? A critical race theory discussion of community cultural wealth. *Race Ethnicity and Education*, *8*(1), 69–91.

SECTION 5

Chronic conditions and the social determinants of health

In this theme, the two chapters demonstrate that the preconditions for health and wellbeing are inextricably linked to social justice. In Chapter 9, Daquila and Hood discuss how sickle cell disease and the social determinants of health merge with racism and societal disinterest to produce harm. In Chapter 10, Armstrong, Nimmons, and Woodward add deprivation as a further burden to interpersonal and systemic racism that minority ethnic populations face when managing their multiple long-term conditions.

Daquila and Hood's chapter uncovers how many of the challenges faced by those living with sickle cell disease (SCD) in the UK are due to the structural factors inhibiting effective disease management, rather than the biological disease process itself. In Chapter 9, they discuss how the stigma associated with SCD reduces opportunities for routine accommodations that would enable sustained engagement in education and employment. They also reveal how a poor understanding of the disease and its clinical manifestations can lead to accusations of malingering and factitious behaviour when healthcare is sought, further worsening outcomes among people living with this condition. These firmly held biases generate adverse effects for people living with SCD who are accessing care across diverse geographical settings, wherein racism intersects with the social gradient to generate deleterious outcomes. With the implementation of pre-planned and advanced care pathways, some strides to redress suboptimal care are taking place. A collective commitment to listening and the urgent need to eliminate all forms of stereotyping and cultural bias in healthcare remain. Daquila and Hood end by calling for renewed policies that dismantle systemic barriers and encourage multi-sectoral collaboration so that people living with SCD can receive equitable, high-quality care and live longer, healthier lives.

In Chapter 10, Armstrong, Nimmons, and Woodward press for a holistic approach to the management of multiple long-term conditions (MLTCs), one which accounts for the intersectional identities and varying social circumstances of individuals within racialised communities living in the UK. Their chapter demonstrates how impersonalised care can disenfranchise individuals navigating their MLTCs, leading to psychological

DOI: 10.4324/9781003466093-14

distress and poor adherence to suggested treatment plans. These challenges are further compounded by the interpersonal and systemic racism, from within the healthcare system and wider society, that people from these communities face. The downstream consequences of socioeconomic inequality, including insecure housing, poor access to healthy food and digital illiteracy, further compound the day-to-day challenges of managing their conditions. Armstrong et al. emphasise the crucial role that local support groups and collaborative community partnerships play in supporting these individuals and call for increased cultural sensitivity and awareness among healthcare professionals to enable ethnic minority individuals living with MLTCs to feel empowered in the management of their own health.

CHAPTER 9

Invisible in the system

Sickle cell and the struggle for equity

Savanna M. Daquila and Anna M. Hood

Introduction

Sickle cell disease (SCD) is the most common inherited blood condition worldwide (Modell & Darlison, 2008; Piel et al., 2013), affecting ~17,000 people in the United Kingdom (UK) (Foster, 2021). Due to immigration and increased life expectancy, SCD has the fastest-growing prevalence of any genetic condition in the UK. SCD changes the functionality of haemoglobin in red blood cells, hindering its ability to deliver oxygen to tissues and organs throughout the body effectively (Rees et al., 2010). SCD is progressive and unpredictable with acute and chronic medical complications, including acute and chronic pain, fatigue, acute chest syndrome (severe lung-related complication with pneumonia-like symptoms), infections, organ and bone damage, priapism in males (prolonged erections without stimulation), and delayed growth and sexual maturation (Redding-Lallinger & Knoll, 2006; Rees et al., 2010).

The complexity and debilitating nature of SCD lead to high healthcare utilisation (e.g. emergency visits, hospital admissions) (AlJuburi et al., 2012) and continued outpatient care. Given the significant challenges of living with SCD, it is perhaps unsurprising that people living with SCD have a higher risk for psychological (e.g. depression, anxiety) (Jonassaint et al., 2016; Levenson et al., 2008; Reed-Knight et al., 2015) and social challenges (Poku et al., 2018). Due to reduced oxygen delivery (Ohene-Frempong et al., 1998), they also experience significant neurological complications (e.g. infarction, stroke) (DeBaun et al., 2012).

SCD occurs when a child inherits one gene that encodes the abnormal haemoglobin from each parent. People from any ethnic minority group can be born with this lifelong, life-threatening condition; however, the highest prevalence is in people who have African or Caribbean ancestry (Thomson et al., 2023). Importantly, SCD is protective against severe forms of malaria, which provides a survival advantage to individuals carrying one copy of the HbS gene living in those regions (Luzzatto, 2012). Until recently, SCD was a disease of childhood, but with advances in care (e.g. blood transfusion), people now survive into adulthood, albeit with much-shortened life expectancies

DOI: 10.4324/9781003466093-15

compared to the general population (Thomson et al., 2023). Reflecting the benefits of modern therapies and prophylactic treatments to mitigate the complications of disease, high-income countries such as the UK and the United States (US) have reduced morbidity and mortality rates for people living with SCD.

Nonetheless, the post-paediatric to adult healthcare transition period remains particularly vulnerable. A US mortality study from 1999 to 2009 found a sharp increase in deaths for 20–24-year-olds (1.4 per 100,000) compared to 15–19-year-olds (0.6 per 100,000) (Hamideh & Alvarez, 2013). A US study assessing data from 2003 to 2017 had similar findings despite evaluating a more recent period. They found a threefold and twofold higher mortality risk and increased hospitalisation prevalence for 22–24 and 19–21-year-olds, respectively, compared to 16–18-year-olds (Fasipe et al., 2021). There are no published UK data regarding SCD-related mortality rates pre- and post-healthcare transition. However, hospitalisations in England are higher for those aged 20–29 years than for 10–19 and 30–39-year-olds (AlJuburi et al., 2012).

Although SCD was first described over 100 years ago, disease-modifying and curative therapy development stagnated for many years because of inadequate research funding, attributable at least in part to structural inequities, including racism (Hood, 2025; Power-Hays & McGann, 2020). This slow progression is highlighted by the fact that in 2021, the National Institute for Health and Care Excellence (NICE) recommended the first new SCD treatment (Crizanlizumab) in 20 years (Buka et al., 2023). In contrast, NICE has recommended three treatments in the past ten years for cystic fibrosis, a long-term condition commonly impacting white individuals, which is less prevalent in the UK than SCD, showing a racialised bias within funding treatment development. Further compounding existing inequities, the Medicines and Healthcare products Regulatory Agency (MHRA) withdrew the marketing authorisation for Crizanlizumab with immediate effect in January 2024 due to questions around its clinical benefit, representing a significant setback for patients relying on the drug (Jacobs et al., 2024).

Currently, there is a lack of awareness regarding how biological factors are compounded by the social, cultural, institutional, and systemic barriers faced by people living with SCD, including challenges within the educational system, medical systems, and the impact of stigma related to SCD. This chapter will first highlight the health inequities for the broader Black and ethnic minoritised communities living in the UK to provide crucial context. We will then discuss the role of racism and stigma in perpetuating justified mistrust of healthcare institutions and between people living with SCD and their healthcare providers, which may result in individuals avoiding seeking care. Finally, we will identify potential pathways toward restoration and solutions to eliminate inequities for the historically neglected and underfunded SCD population.

Health inequity in the UK

Throughout this chapter, we will use the term 'health inequities' when discussing the systematic challenges faced by ethnic minority populations, particularly those living with SCD in the UK. Critically, we distinguish between inequalities and inequities and do not consider them interchangeable. Inequalities are measurable differences in health between two or more groups in a population; however, inequities are unfair or unjust inequalities due to social environments or status, for example, economic deprivation or racialised status (Williams et al., 2022).

As an example, ethnic minority populations in Britain experience systemic inequities and discrimination in nearly all areas of community engagement, including housing (Shankley & Finney, 2020). Our research systems, however, measure inequalities, such as English ethnic minority populations having less accumulated wealth than their white counterparts, less ability to own their homes, and earning less than 60% of the average income (Harris, 2020). The observation of difference does not provide the complete picture, as we have strong evidence that this inequality is being driven by inequity mechanisms (e.g. exclusion from higher-paid positions, less inherited generational wealth) due to systemic racism's influence on accessing resources necessary for purchasing a home, such as mortgages and credit (Robinson, 2024). Further, these inequities are then additive and multiplicative. People from ethnic minority groups are at higher risk of residing in areas with higher community deprivation, thus limiting their access to healthcare resources. Additionally, as shown during the COVID-19 pandemic, community deprivation – lacking access to essential resources and opportunities – is associated with an increased risk of early mortality (Bosworth et al., 2023).

The deleterious effects of these inequities on health are well-documented. Racialised inequities are found prenatally, with ethnic minority babies having a 48% to 138% greater risk of adverse birth outcomes compared with white British babies (Opondo et al., 2019). Although racism is an undeniable health issue, socioeconomic deprivation, another driver of morbidity and mortality, receives much more attention (Lee et al., 2023). As seen later, research demonstrates racialised inequities in the presence of deprivation. Specifically, one study found that, after adjustment for deprivation, South Asian and Black children with kidney failure were less likely to receive pre-emptive kidney transplantation (Plumb et al., 2021). In 2020, a study found that Black UK patients have experienced prejudice from healthcare professionals because of their ethnicity and the colour of their skin, with 65% of younger people feeling especially discriminated against (Iacobucci, 2022). In 2023, the 10,000 Black British Voices Project showed the significant adverse effects of racism, with less than 1 in 60 respondents feeling they were fairly treated within the 'hostile environment' of the UK healthcare systems (NHS England, NHS Scotland, NHS Wales, and Health and Social Care (HSC) in Northern Ireland), and 87% of respondents reported that they 'expected to receive a substandard level of healthcare because of their racialised identity' (Monrose et al., 2023). Finally, people of African-Caribbean backgrounds are at greater risk of experiencing health inequities, discrimination, coercive treatments, and delayed access to holistic care (Kapadia et al., 2022).

Health inequity for people living with SCD in the UK

The predominantly Black SCD population in the UK faces systemic racism and unequal treatment in healthcare. However, their negative experiences are perpetuated due to damaging inequities in pain management and treatment, where suffering is downplayed and dismissed often because of false beliefs about Black people's ability to tolerate pain (Hoffman et al., 2016). After years of stagnation, the landmark 2021 No One's Listening Sickle Cell and Thalassaemia All-Party Parliamentary Group Report was triggered by a coroner's inquiry into the avoidable death of 21-year-old Evan Nathan Smith at the North Middlesex Hospital in April 2019. Evan experienced a sickle cell pain crisis but had to ring 999 from his hospital bed after being denied oxygen (Mahase, 2020). The coroner's inquiry found that Evan would not have died if the medical staff had recognised his symptoms and treated him sooner. The No One's Listening Report highlighted the growing burden of SCD in the UK, a pattern of several years of substandard care, stigmatisation, and lack of prioritisation, and severe health inequities associated with the long-standing lack of investment in sickle cell research. Notably, the report revealed 'serious care failings and insufficient investment', that there is a 'lack of robust processes needed to ensure a safe transfer of care to adult services', and called for 'major changes in the care of patients living with SCD'.

The report inquiry process found worrying evidence of deeply racialised inequities in the healthcare system for people living with SCD. Specifically, the report demonstrates a pattern of substandard care in general wards and emergency departments. There was a lack of adherence to national standards, low awareness of SCD among staff, and inadequate SCD training. Although specialist haemoglobinopathy services provide better care than general wards, stakeholders repeatedly emphasised the transition from paediatric to adult healthcare as a significant concern. In early 2023, a National Health Service (NHS) Race and Health Observatory report mirrored the inquiry findings and underlined the same need to address and improve healthcare transition for children and young people (CYP) living with SCD (Kmietowicz, 2023). A recent study has also shown that adults living with SCD relate the invisibility of their pain with the racism they encountered in services and describe 'second-class treatment' and being labelled as 'aggressive' (Berghs et al., 2022).

People living with SCD from the most socioeconomically deprived areas and with comorbidities are at the highest risk of SCD readmissions. Using data collected from hospital readmissions for individuals living with SCD between 2005 and 2006, monitored over a five-year period, researchers found that in 2005–2006, approximately 8,000 people were admitted to the hospital for SCD in England. Follow-up over five years revealed that most individuals requiring readmission resided in England's most socioeconomically disadvantaged areas. Notably, individuals in this group also experienced the highest mortality rates. These findings suggest that disparities in healthcare utilisation are closely linked to structural factors, including socioeconomic status, rather than being attributed solely to biological factors related to the SCD

disease process. Critically, these inequities for people living with SCD connect to the broader context of socioeconomic status and racialisation in the UK, where individuals who are in the global majority, the vast majority of the world's population who are not white or of European descent, are often excluded from receiving adequate healthcare.

It is also important to note that the majority of SCD research takes place in England, particularly in London. This geographic concentration introduces a significant inequality in the evidence base. This regional bias means that the experiences of people living with SCD in other parts of the UK, for example, rural areas and regions with fewer minoritised populations, are less likely to be captured in the research literature. Although the concentration of expertise in London delivers essential advances, it also presents a blind spot. Findings and interventions may be tailored to London-centric patient populations and health systems, potentially limiting their relevance or applicability elsewhere. It thus constitutes an important inequality and likely inequity. SCD affects individuals across the UK; however, research often does not reflect the full diversity of lived experience, care settings, or service access.

Stigma and SCD

To understand some of the various barriers individuals living with SCD face in trying to acquire equitable healthcare treatment, it is necessary to understand the multiple forms of discrimination encountered when trying to access care. Two primary forms of discrimination significantly impact the well-being, treatment, and outcomes of individuals living with SCD. Firstly, since a large population of individuals living with SCD belongs to the global majority, it is crucial to recognise the consequences of racialised discrimination within healthcare contexts and beyond (see Figure 9.1). Prejudice can manifest in various ways, such as being given lower doses of medication, experiencing extended waiting times, or being dismissed entirely (Huq & Devakumar, 2024).

Racialised discrimination is compounded by the additional discrimination associated with having SCD, often referred to as health-related discrimination or diagnosis-related discrimination. Previous research has noted that racialised discrimination and health-related discrimination can coalesce to create even more barriers than either discrimination alone for people living with SCD (Hood et al., 2022). Stigmatising experiences, such as being denied care or labelled as 'drug-seeking' when seeking treatment to alleviate their pain, foster mistrust and reluctance to seek support from medical professionals (are Made & List). A systematic review was conducted on health-related discrimination and its influence on the health of individuals living with SCD. Whereas most participants in the included studies resided in the USA, a prevalent theme identified was the impact of discrimination on physiological well-being, with many experiencing discrimination (Bulgin et al., 2018). As a result of these experiences, people seeking care were compelled to find ways to manage their pain without formal support, often in harmful ways, such as isolation or delays in seeking care (Bulgin et al., 2018).

There has been less research conducted in the UK, but studies have also contributed valuable insight into the profound stigma experienced by individuals living with SCD, rooted in both societal misunderstanding and healthcare inequity. A mixed-methods survey of 93 young people (aged 10–19) in England found that 15% reported self-perceived stigma, which was significantly associated with more frequent hospital admissions and visible symptoms; this stigma predicted heightened psychological distress and depressive symptoms (Ani, 2010). A mixed-methods study in English schools surveyed 569 young people living with SCD and conducted 40 in-depth interviews, revealing the dilemma young people faced, for example, whether to disclose their condition and risk being misunderstood, or conceal it and struggle alone, marking them as 'discreditable' and reinforcing stigma in educational settings (Dyson, Atkin, et al., 2010). A qualitative focus-group study revealed that young adults living with SCD frequently perceive themselves as misunderstood and marginalised across key life domains, including education, employment, relationships, and hospital care, highlighting stigma embedded within psychosocial, familial, and institutional landscapes (Thomas & Taylor, 2002).

SCD across the life course

Children and educational settings

Children and young people (CYP) living with SCD in the UK face significant educational issues stemming from both health-related challenges and institutional barriers. Dyson et al., in the UK, sought to understand the extent to which information about SCD is communicated, considering the lower prevalence of SCD in the UK than in other regions such as India or Europe. They focused on the early life experiences of children living with SCD in academic settings, examining whether their diagnosis was represented correctly and considered during various aspects of the educational process, such as ear and eye screenings, absence policies, and academic achievement. Dyson et al. (2007) importantly state that although a child is not defined solely by their disability, they can be limited by systemically discriminatory practices, barriers, and beliefs, some of which exist in an educational setting (see Figure 9.1) that is arbitrarily designed to promote positive development and well-being (Dyson et al., 2007). A follow-up study in 2010 found that nearly one in eight children living with SCD experienced persistent school absences, often due to pain crises or hospital visits. A small number of students can reach or exceed the government's threshold for persistent absence, so it is crucial that there is clear documentation so children are not mislabelled as truants. Unfortunately, schools rarely provide catch-up support. Students were also sometimes denied access to basic needs such as water, toilet breaks, or rest, despite these functions being essential to managing their condition. Over a third of children in the study reported being forced to participate in physical activities inappropriate for their health (Dyson, Abuateya, et al., 2010). These failures reflect structural inequities within the education system, where standardised routines and a lack of chronic illness awareness compromise access and participation for pupils living with SCD.

In the UK, many schools check students' vision and hearing. Thus, greater integration between school and healthcare services could facilitate targeted intervention for symptoms associated with SCD that can directly affect educational attainment. Similarly, SCD-related complications can result in cognitive difficulties (Prussien et al., 2019), particularly in executive function (i.e. goal-directed behaviour, self-control, focus, and following multiple-step directions), becoming more pronounced in late adolescence (Hood et al., 2019). Furthermore, pain crises and access to treatment significantly affect school attendance (Ameringer et al., 2014), risking students living with SCD falling behind, lacking motivation, or forcing themselves through a pain crisis just to attend class. School settings are crucial for children's development, screening for general well-being, and serving as a space for socialisation and identity formation. As such, educators' increased understanding of the complexities of SCD on school performance would assist children and families, as a lack of awareness can reinforce negative racialised stereotypes. For example, a young Black man who lives with SCD, reflecting on his time as a student in England, said,

> In games lessons at school, I'd have real problems completing the cross-country course, because sickle cell leaves you very breathless and short of energy. My teacher didn't understand why I couldn't run, despite being good at indoor sports such as volleyball, badminton, and basketball. He labelled me 'lazy' and 'difficult'. He covered my school reports with adjectives such as these!
>
> *(Dyson et al., 2007)*

Adults and caregivers of adults living with SCD

Many adults living with SCD rely on a carer or caregiver support beyond childhood to assist with navigating healthcare conversations, taking them to and from appointments, and administering medication. The burden placed on caregivers of a family member, partner, or friend can negatively affect the caregiver's quality of life and cause psychological challenges and financial problems, partly due to lost work hours within traditional employment (Besser et al., 2024). A global survey also reported that fatigue and acute pain crises have the most significant effect on caregivers' lives and routines (Jastaniah et al., 2023). This finding suggests that there needs to be increased support and infrastructure not only for the person living with SCD but also for their support system. Charity and non-profit organisations, such as the Sickle Cell Society, can provide some support for caregivers, but a dedicated social care infrastructure is needed to meet the everyday challenges faced.

The COVID-19 pandemic and SCD

In the initial stages of the COVID-19 pandemic, individuals living with SCD in the UK were classified as a highly vulnerable population and were encouraged to shield and practice masking and social distancing. Despite following healthcare protocols, the mortality rate for individuals who identified as Black or another racialised identity was higher compared to the rest of the population (Bosworth et al., 2023; Chaturvedi, 2020). While this was occurring, the world also saw a rise in awareness of the Black Lives Matter movement following the murder of George Floyd in the USA (Sullivan et al., 2021). Given the amalgamation of awareness regarding the physical and social impacts of systemic discrimination and racialisation, Berghs et al. examined the lived experiences of Black individuals living with SCD and their caregivers in England during the COVID-19 pandemic.

Approximately 50 individuals living with SCD (or their parents if the individual was a child) participated and indicated a need for healthcare workers to have a more comprehensive understanding of SCD, as well as enhanced pandemic readiness, psychological services, and pain management. Qualitatively, three themes emerged: the first being that participants experienced psychological challenges in response to learning that they fell within the 'critically vulnerable' population, yet did not receive treatment that met the needs of being so susceptible to this virus, with many participants indicating they had to break shielding protocols to obtain services (Berghs et al., 2022).

Secondly, when individuals broke protocols to receive services, many reported that they encountered clinicians lacking adequate knowledge about SCD and its complications, with many practitioners being unaware of how physical symptoms might present differently on Black skin. Thirdly, being Black and living with SCD also presented an intersectional challenge, where both racism and diagnosis-based discrimination simultaneously occurred, with participants stating they felt compelled to change their mannerisms to appear more 'small' or 'agreeable' to obtain appropriate treatment (Berghs et al., 2022). This research illuminates the intersectional barriers faced by Black individuals living with SCD during the COVID-19 pandemic.

Figure 9.1 highlights the institutional barriers and illustrates the multifaceted social, medical, and structural challenges experienced by individuals living with SCD. Challenges are represented as six interconnected thematic areas. At the top of Figure 9.1,

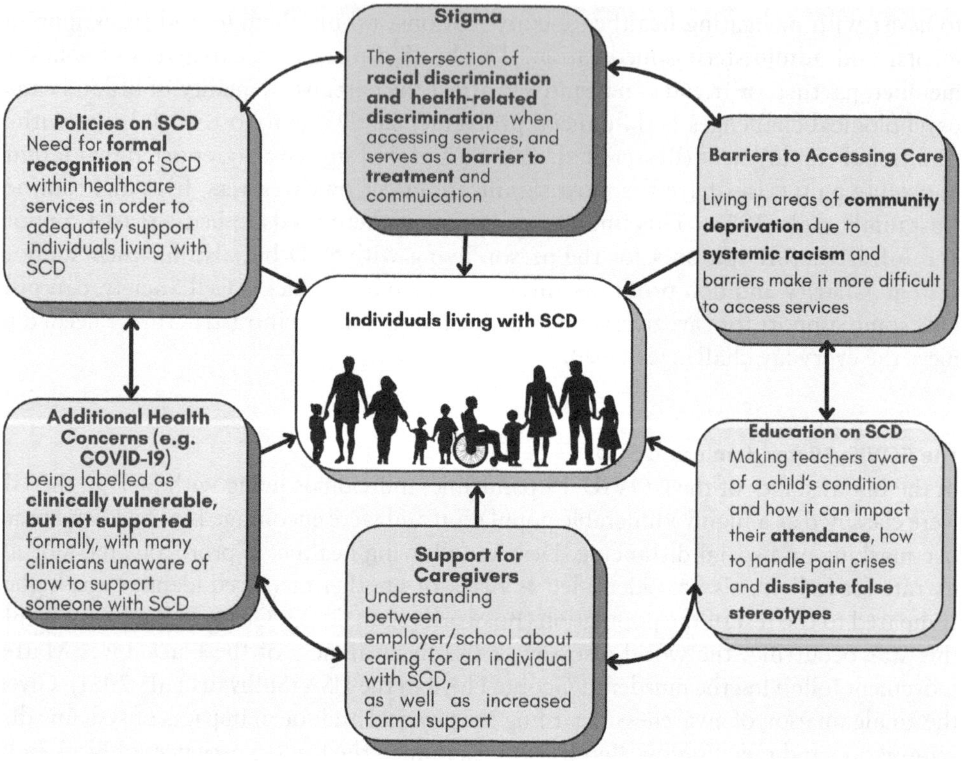

Figure 9.1 Interconnected Systems of Health, Life, and Support for Individuals Living with Sickle Cell Disease.

'Stigma' highlights the intersection of racialised and health-related stigma, which acts as a significant barrier to treatment and communication. Closely linked is 'Barriers to Accessing Care', which points to systemic racism and community deprivation as factors that make healthcare access more difficult. 'Education on SCD' stresses the importance of awareness within schools. Teachers should understand how SCD affects a child's attendance, recognise pain crises, and challenge false stereotypes. Below, 'Support for Caregivers' emphasises the need for understanding from employers and schools, along with better formal support systems for those caring for people living with SCD. 'Additional Health Concerns (e.g. COVID-19)' notes that people living with SCD are often labelled clinically vulnerable but lack proper clinical support, partly because many healthcare providers are unaware of how to meet their needs. This connects to 'Policies on SCD', which calls for formal recognition of the SCD within healthcare systems to ensure consistent and equitable care. Overall, Figure 9.1 portrays the cyclical and interconnected relationship between stigma, systemic inequities, lack of education, insufficient policy recognition, and inadequate caregiver support. Together, these factors create a complex landscape in which individuals living with SCD navigate daily challenges that extend far beyond their immediate health condition. Figure 9.1 emphasises the necessity of a holistic, socially informed approach to healthcare and policy reform that addresses not only clinical needs but also the broader societal determinants of health.

These findings elucidate the systemic barriers and challenges faced by Black individuals living with SCD and how these barriers are often exacerbated within the larger macro context, increasing the risks faced by individuals living with SCD beyond those associated with their diagnosis.

Future implications and policy change

This chapter highlights the systemic barriers faced in nearly every aspect of an individual living with SCD in the UK across various settings and throughout the life course. From educational obstacles to accessing healthcare services, navigating stigma, and enduring a global pandemic, individuals living with SCD consistently encounter health inequities, often in interconnected ways. None of these barriers exists in isolation; for example, children navigating the education system who may fall behind can later be perceived as 'drug-seeking' adults, just by existing. An individual may experience challenges in accessing healthcare services and may be stigmatised or denied care once those services are obtained (see Figure 9.1). Importantly, these barriers are encountered at both the interpersonal and systemic levels, meaning that change cannot be achieved solely through individual shifts but must also be reinforced by policy change.

Policy shifts and collective acknowledgement of harm are critical to creating change and eliminating inequities for individuals living with SCD. Some recent examples include the NHS introducing the 2025 Sickle Cell Disorder National Education Programme. This programme addresses discrimination among healthcare providers by offering education on SCD, its symptoms, and acute pain crises. This educational tool includes two courses: one co-developed with individuals who have lived experience of the disease, covering the fundamentals of SCD and how it clinically manifests, as well as a general overview of what it is like to live with SCD. The second course focuses more on the clinical profile of symptomatology and how to treat symptoms commonly associated with SCD. These types of changes provide a potential pathway to decrease the life-threatening SCD outcomes.

The London Ambulance Service has also begun to address inequities in care. People living with SCD residing in London, England, have long reported inequities in their care when interacting with the system – from delayed response times and paramedics unaware of the disease's severity, to acute pain crises being downplayed or misinterpreted as 'drug-seeking behavior'. A recent co-developed project aims to address these issues through targeted reforms, such as rapid analgesia, chair carry options, and a choice of destination for sickle crises (Sickle Cell Society, 2025). In addition, the introduction of electronically accessible Patient-Specific Protocols and Universal Care Plans, shared digitally with paramedics via the Cleric system, means pre-hospital teams now have instant access to individualised treatment directives, reducing the burden on patients to self-advocate to paramedics while in extreme pain (Sickle Cell Society, 2025). These steps mark a significant shift toward equity in emergency care, illustrating how frontline recognition of bias and structural barriers can lead to meaningful service redesign.

Related to curative therapies, the NICE independent appraisal committee's initial decision was to reject the Clustered Regularly Interspaced Short Palindromic Repeats (CRISPR) gene therapy, exagamglogene autotemcel, also known as exa-cel, as a treatment for SCD in the UK, citing 'several issues with the economic modelling'. Despite the documented inequities and limited medication options, NICE stated that the cost-effectiveness estimate for exa-cel was higher than what NICE usually considers to be an acceptable use of NHS resources (Lipanovic, 2024). Only after people with lived experience and healthcare professionals contributed to the consultation was the use of gene editing therapy made available under a managed access scheme for some people 12 years and over with certain types of severe SCD (Mahase, 2024).

Importantly, the NHS Race and Health Observatory (RHO) has agreed to collaborate with the NICE to tackle persistent and systemic ethnic health inequities, including work to de-bias clinical guidance in SCD. This collaboration aims to improve recommendations and advice to support better patient treatment, safety, and outcomes (Kmietowicz, 2025). Ongoing research, policy advocacy, and growing awareness within educational and healthcare sectors are driving change for people living with SCD, but continued funding, effort, and lasting support are required for long-term systemic change. With continued collaboration between families, schools, healthcare professionals, and policymakers, there is a real opportunity to dismantle these long-standing barriers and ensure that people living with SCD receive the equitable treatment and support they deserve. Yet, the persistence of inequities and the limited visibility of lived experiences reveal how often SCD remains invisible – or worse, ignored – within broader health and social policy conversations. To move forward, we must not only recognise this invisibility but actively challenge it, ensuring that every voice within the SCD community is seen, heard, and valued in shaping a more just and inclusive future.

Summary

This chapter explores how systemic inequities in the United Kingdom (UK) health system continue to shape the experiences of people living with sickle cell disease (SCD), situating these challenges within the broader context of racialised disparities affecting Black communities in the UK. The chapter outlines the historical and structural roots of health inequity, showing how institutional racism and underfunding have contributed to the marginalisation of SCD within healthcare policy and practice. The chapter then examines SCD across the life course, highlighting how individuals face persistent barriers from childhood to adulthood, including stigma, inadequate clinical understanding, and limited access to specialist care.

The discussion of stigma underscores how racialised bias and misconceptions about pain and behaviour compound the everyday struggles of those with SCD. The chapter also reflects on the COVID-19 pandemic, which exposed the fragility of existing support systems and deepened inequities in healthcare access and protection for those deemed 'clinically vulnerable'.

In conclusion, the chapter calls for systemic reform and sustained policy change – grounded in equity, representation, and education – to ensure that people living with SCD are no longer rendered invisible in research, policy, and practice but recognised as a priority within the UK's health and social care landscape.

Discussion questions

1. How are health inequities different from health inequalities, and what are the consequences of each?

2. If a medical clinician were to read this chapter, what changes might they seek to make in their practice or approach to treating someone living with SCD?
3. What are some policies within your community (school, work, etc.) to support individuals living with medically complex conditions, such as SCD? What could they seek to expand on?

Further reading

Bulgin, D., Tanabe, P., & Jenerette, C. (2018). Stigma of sickle cell disease: A systematic review. *Issues in Mental Health Nursing*, *39*(8), 675–686.

Dyson, S. M., Atkin, K., Culley, L. A., Dyson, S. E., Evans, H., & Rowley, D. T. (2010). Disclosure and sickle cell disorder: A mixed methods study of the young person with sickle cell at school. *Social Science & Medicine*, *70*(12), 2036–2044.

Hood, A. M. (2025). Racism in pain management causes needless suffering. *BMJ, 389*, r848. https://doi.org/10.1136/bmj.r848

Jacobs, J. W., Stephens, L. D., Chooljian, D. M., Sharma, D., Adkins, B. D., & Booth, G. S. (2024). Crizanlizumab and sickle cell disease: When should medications have their approval status revoked. *American Journal of Hematology*, *99*, 1016–1018.

Sickle Cell Society. (2025, February). *Sickle Cell Patients' Experiences of the London Ambulance Service* [Report]. https://www.sicklecellsociety.org/wp-content/uploads/2025/02/Sickle-cell-London-Ambulance-Service-report-final.pdf

References

AlJuburi, G., Laverty, A. A., Green, S. A., Phekoo, K. J., Banarsee, R., Okoye, N. V. O., . . . Majeed, A. (2012). Trends in hospital admissions for sickle cell disease in England, 2001/02–2009/10. *Journal of Public Health*, *34*(4), 570–576.

Ameringer, S., Elswick, J. K., & Smith, W. (2014). Fatigue in adolescents and young adults with sickle cell disease: Biological and behavioral correlates and health-related quality of life. *Journal of Pediatric Oncology Nursing*, *31*(1), 6–17. https://doi.org/10.1177/1043454213514632

Ani, C. (2010). *Self-Perceived Stigma in Young People with Sickle Cell Disease: Associations with Psychosocial Distress*. Imperial College London.

Berghs, M. J., Horne, F., Yates, S., Graham, S., Kemp, R., Webster, A., & Howson, C. (2022). Black sickle cell patients' lives matter: Healthcare, long-term shielding and psychological distress during a racialised pandemic in England – A mixed-methods study. *BMJ Open*, *12*(9), e057141–e057141.

Besser, M., O'Sullivan, S. B., Bourke, S., Longworth, L., Barcelos, G. T., & Oluboyede, Y. (2024). Economic burden and quality of life of caregivers of patients with sickle cell disease in the United Kingdom and France: A cross-sectional study. *Journal of Patient-Reported Outcomes*, *8*(1), 110.

Bosworth, M. L., Ahmed, T., Larsen, T., Lorenzi, L., Morgan, J., Ali, R., . . . Raleigh, V. (2023). Ethnic differences in COVID-19 mortality in the second and third waves of the pandemic in England during the vaccine rollout: A retrospective, population-based cohort study. *BMC Medicine*, *21*(1), 13.

Buka, R. J., Roy, N., & Nicolson, P. L. R. (2023). UK media reporting of NICE recommendation of crizanlizumab for patients with sickle cell disease. *EJHaem*, *4*(1), 13–17.

Bulgin, D., Tanabe, P., & Jenerette, C. (2018). Stigma of sickle cell disease: A systematic review. *Issues in Mental Health Nursing*, *39*(8), 675–686.

Chaturvedi, N. (2020, April). Why are people from BAME groups dying disproportionately of Covid-19? *The Guardian*. https://www.theguardian.com/world/2020/apr/22/why-are-people-from-bame-groups-dyi ng-disproportionately-of-covid-19

DeBaun, M. R., Armstrong, F. D., McKinstry, R. C., Ware, R. E., Vichinsky, E., & Kirkham, F. J. (2012). Silent cerebral infarcts: A review of a prevalent and progressive cause of neurologic injury in sickle cell anemia. *Blood, 119*(20), 4587–4596. https://doi.org/10.1182/blood-2011-02-272682

Dyson, S. M., Abuateya, H., Atkin, K., Culley, L., Dyson, S. E., Rowley, D., & Group, M. O. T. S. C. A. E. (2010). Reported school experiences of young people living with sickle cell disorder in England. *British Educational Research Journal, 36*(1), 125–142.

Dyson, S. M., Atkin, K., Culley, L. A., & Dyson, S. E. (2007). The educational experiences of young people with sickle cell disorder: A commentary on the existing literature. *Disability & Society, 22*(6), 581–594.

Dyson, S. M., Atkin, K., Culley, L. A., Dyson, S. E., Evans, H., & Rowley, D. T. (2010). Disclosure and sickle cell disorder: A mixed methods study of the young person with sickle cell at school. *Social Science & Medicine, 70*(12), 2036–2044.

Fasipe, T., Dongarwar, D., Lopez, E., Brown, R., Abadom, M., Mahoney, D. H., & Salihu, H. M. (2021). Hospital use and mortality in transition-aged patients with sickle cell disease. *Hospital Pediatrics, 11*(12), 1303–1310.

Foster, M. (2021). *National Haemoglobinopathy Registry Annual Data Report 2019/20.* National Haemoglobinopathy Registry (NHR), MD/SAS.

Hamideh, D., & Alvarez, O. (2013). Sickle cell disease related mortality in the United States (1999–2009). *Pediatric Blood & Cancer, 60*(9), 1482–1486.

Hoffman, K. M., Trawalter, S., Axt, J. R., & Oliver, M. N. (2016). Racial bias in pain assessment and treatment recommendations, and false beliefs about biological differences between Blacks and whites. *Proceedings of the National Academy of Sciences, 113*(16), 4296–4301.

Hood, A. M. (2025). Racism in pain management causes needless suffering. *BMJ, 389*, r848. https://doi.org/10.1136/bmj.r848

Hood, A. M., Crosby, L. E., Hanson, E., Shook, L. M., Lebensburger, J. D., Madan-Swain, A., . . . Trost, Z. (2022). The influence of perceived racial bias and health-related stigma on quality of life among children with sickle cell disease. *Ethnicity & Health, 27*(4), 833–846.

Hood, A. M., King, A. A., Fields, M. E., Ford, A. L., Guilliams, K. P., Hulbert, M. L., . . . White, D. A. (2019). Higher executive abilities following a blood transfusion in children and young adults with sickle cell disease. *Pediatric Blood & Cancer, 66*(10), e27899–e27899. https://doi.org/10.1002/pbc.27899

Huq, M., & Devakumar, D. (2024). Racism and the health system. *The Lancet, 404*(10454), 741–742.

Iacobucci, G. (2022). Most Black people in the UK face discrimination from healthcare staff, a survey finds. *BMJ, 376*, o273. https://doi.org/10.1136/bmj.o273

Jacobs, J. W., Stephens, L. D., Chooljian, D. M., Sharma, D., Adkins, B. D., & Booth, G. S. (2024). Crizanlizumab and sickle cell disease: When should medications have their approval status revoked. *American Journal of Hematology, 99*, 1016–1018.

Jastaniah, W., Hartfield, R., James, J., Tinga, B., Ingoli, E., de Montalembert, M., . . . Odame, I. (2023). Sickle cell health awareness, perspectives, and experiences (SHAPE) survey: Findings on the burden of sickle cell disease and impact on the quality of life of patients and caregivers in Gulf Cooperation Council countries. *Blood, 142*, 2516.

Jonassaint, C. R., Jones, V. L., Leong, S., & Frierson, G. M. (2016). A systematic review of the association between depression and health care utilization in children and adults with sickle cell disease. *British Journal of Haematology, 174*(1), 136–147.

Kapadia, D., Zhang, J., Salway, S., Nazroo, J., Booth, A., Villarroel-Williams, N., . . . Esmail, A. (2022). *Ethnic Inequalities in Healthcare: A Rapid Evidence Review.* NHS Race and Health Observatory. https://www.nhsrho.org/publications/ethnic-inequalities-in-healthcare-a-rapid-evidence-review/

Kmietowicz, Z. (2023). Patients with sickle cell disease are let down by lack of coordinated NHS care, report finds. *BMJ, 380*, 257. https://doi.org/10.1136/bmj.p257. PMID: 36720482.

Kmietowicz, Z. (2025). Race and health observatory to work with NICE to tackle ethnic health inequalities. *BMJ*, *389*, r913. https://doi.org/10.1136/bmj.r913

Lee, A. R., Kingdon, C. C., Davie, M., Hawcutt, D., & Sinha, I. P. (2023). Child poverty and health inequalities in the UK: A guide for paediatricians. *Archives of Disease in Childhood*, *108*(2), 94–101.

Levenson, J. L., McClish, D. K., Dahman, B. A., Bovbjerg, V. E., Citero, V. D. A., Penberthy, L. T., . . . Smith, W. R. (2008). Depression and anxiety in adults with sickle cell disease: The PiSCES project. *Psychosomatic Medicine*, *70*(2), 192–196.

Lipanovic, D. (2024). Gene-editing sickle cell drug not approved for NHS use in draft NICE guidance. *The Pharmaceutical Journal*. https://pharmaceutical-journal.com/article/news/gene-editing-sickle-cell-drug-not-approved-for-nhs-use-in-draft-nice-guidance

Luzzatto, L. (2012). Sickle cell anaemia and malaria. *Mediterranean Journal of Hematology and Infectious Diseases*, *4*(1), e2012065. https://doi.org/10.4084/MJHID.2012.065. Epub 2012 October 3. PMID: 23170194; PMCID: PMC3499995.

Mahase, E. (2020). Vaccinating the UK: How the covid vaccine was approved, and other questions answered. *BMJ*, *371*, m4759. https://doi.org/10.1136/bmj.m4759

Mahase, E. (2024). Thalassaemia: NICE recommends "life-changing" gene editing therapy. *BMJ*, *386*, q1771. https://doi.org/10.1136/bmj.q1771

Modell, B., & Darlison, M. (2008). Global epidemiology of haemoglobin disorders and derived service indicators. *Bulletin of the World Health Organization*, *86*(6), 480–487.

Monrose, K., Dyke, P., & Semple, M. (2023). *Black British Voices Project*. https://www.bbvp.org

NHS England. (2025). *Sickle Cell Disorder National Education Programme: About*. Learning Hub. https://learninghub.nhs.uk/catalogue/SCD-national-education-programme/about

Ohene-Frempong, K., Weiner, S. J., Sleeper, L. A., Miller, S. T., Embury, S., Moohr, J. W., . . . Gill, F. M. (1998). Cerebrovascular accidents in sickle cell disease: Rates and risk factors. *Blood*, *91*(1), 288–294.

Opondo, C., Gray, R., Hollowell, J., Li, Y., Kurinczuk, J. J., & Quigley, M. A. (2019). Joint contribution of socioeconomic circumstances and ethnic group to variations in preterm birth, neonatal mortality and infant mortality in England and Wales: A population-based retrospective cohort study using routine data from 2006 to 2012. *BMJ Open*, *9*(7), e028227–e028227.

Piel, F. B., Hay, S. I., Gupta, S., Weatherall, D. J., & Williams, T. N. (2013). Global burden of sickle cell anaemia in children under five, 2010–2050: Modelling based on demographics, excess mortality, and interventions. *PLoS Medicine*, *10*(7), e1001484–e1001484.

Plumb, L. A., Sinha, M. D., Casula, A., Inward, C. D., Marks, S. D., Caskey, F. J., & Ben-Shlomo, Y. (2021). Associations between deprivation, geographic location, and access to pediatric kidney care in the United Kingdom. *Clinical Journal of the American Society of Nephrology*, *16*(2), 194–203.

Poku, B. A., Caress, A.-L., & Kirk, S. (2018). Adolescents' experiences of living with sickle cell disease: An integrative narrative review of the literature. *International Journal of Nursing Studies*, *80*, 20–28.

Power-Hays, A., & McGann, P. T. (2020). When actions speak louder than words – Racism and sickle cell disease. *New England Journal of Medicine*, *383*(20), 1902–1903.

Prussien, K. V., Jordan, L. C., DeBaun, M. R., & Compas, B. E. (2019). Cognitive function in sickle cell disease across domains, cerebral infarct status, and the lifespan: A meta-analysis. *Journal of Pediatric Psychology*, *44*(8), 948–958.

Redding-Lallinger, R., & Knoll, C. (2006). Sickle cell disease – Pathophysiology and treatment. *Current Problems in Pediatric and Adolescent Health Care*, *36*(10), 346–376.

Reed-Knight, B., Thompson, B., Bigham, L., Sil, S., Griffin, A., & Johnson, A. (2015). Identification of pica behaviors in youth with sickle cell disease: A quality improvement (QI) project. *Clinical Practice in Pediatric Psychology*, *3*(2), 167–167.

Rees, D. C., Williams, T. N., & Gladwin, M. T. (2010). Sickle-cell disease. *The Lancet*, *376*(9757), 2018–2031. https://doi.org/10.1016/S0140-6736(10)61029-X

Robinson, D. (2024). Race equality in housing: Tracing the postracial turn in English housing policy. *Housing Studies*, 1–22.

Shankley, W., & Finney, N. (2020). 7: Ethnic minorities and housing in Britain. In *Ethnicity, Race and Inequality in the UK*. Bristol, UK: Policy Press. Retrieved July 16, 2025, from https://doi.org/10.51952/9781447351269.ch007

Sickle Cell Society. (2025, February). *Sickle Cell Patients' Experiences of the London Ambulance Service* [Report]. https://www.sicklecellsociety.org/wp-content/uploads/2025/02/Sickle-cell-London-Ambulance-Service-report-final.pdf

Social Metrics Commission. (2020). *Measuring Poverty 2020*. Legatum Institute.

Sullivan, J. N., Eberhardt, J. L., & Roberts, S. O. (2021). Conversations about race in Black and White US families: Before and after George Floyd's death. *Proceedings of the National Academy of Sciences*, *118*(38), e2106366118.

Thomas, V. J., & Taylor, L. (2002). The psychosocial experience of people with sickle cell disease and its impact on quality of life: Qualitative findings from focus groups. *British Journal of Health Psychology*, *7*(3), 345–363.

Thomson, A. M., McHugh, T. A., Oron, A. P., Teply, C., Lonberg, N., Tella, V. V., . . . Murray, C. J. L., & Kassebaum, N. J. (2023). Global, regional, and national prevalence and mortality burden of sickle cell disease, 2000–2021: A systematic analysis from the global burden of disease study 2021. *The Lancet Haematology*, *10*(8), e585–e599. https://doi.org/10.1016/S2352-3026(23)00118-7

Williams, E., Buck, D., Babalola, G., & Maguire, D. (2022). *What are health inequalities? The King's Fund*. https://www.kingsfund.org.uk/insight-and-analysis/long-reads/what-are-health-inequalities

CHAPTER 10

Managing multiple long-term conditions in socioeconomically deprived and ethnically diverse populations

Megan Armstrong, Danielle Nimmons, and Abi Woodward

Introduction

Long-term health conditions are defined as health problems that require ongoing management over at least a year (e.g. depression, chronic kidney disease, and diabetes) that cannot currently be cured. Long-term conditions affect 43% of the adult population in England, and around 70% of all health and social care funding goes to supporting people with these conditions (Ara, 2024). Multiple Long-Term Conditions (MLTC), that is, two or more long-term conditions in an individual, are predicted to rise in those aged over 565 years in the United Kingdom (UK) from 54% in 2015 to 68% in 2035 (Brilleman et al., 2013). The management of MLTC can be challenging due to the heterogeneous nature of the conditions. MLTC lead to an increase in primary care contacts, hospital admissions, and social care costs (Salisbury et al., 2010). People with MLTC have highlighted the need for more holistic and integrated care approaches that prioritise psychosocial concerns, including the promotion of independence (National Institute for Health and Care Research Evidence, 2023).

People living in areas of deprivation are almost twice as likely to have MLTC, which occur on average 10–15 years earlier than those from more affluent groups (Barnett et al., 2012). Additionally, most minoritised ethnic groups are at a higher risk of having MLTC compared to their White British counterparts (Hayanga et al., 2023). This health inequality is likely to be driven by upstream determinants of health where minoritised ethnic groups are disproportionately represented in those with insecure and overcrowded housing, and low-paid employment (Samuel et al., 2021). The more health conditions people have, the higher their chance of death; however, this is significantly increased in Pakistani and Black ethnic groups (Stafford, Knight, et al., 2022). These inequalities on mortality reflect broader economic and social inequalities driven by classism and racism (Mitchell et al., 2023).

People from minoritised ethnic groups have suboptimal disease management, less continuity of care, and higher rates of emergency healthcare admissions (Hayanga et al., 2021; Stafford, Bécares, et al., 2022). These populations have reported feeling

DOI: 10.4324/9781003466093-16

less able to ask their doctor questions, and some perceived their socioeconomic background to influence the care they received and the relationship they had with their healthcare provider (Arpey et al., 2017). These experiences, including that of systemic racism, have led to low levels of trust towards healthcare professionals, as well as the government (Armstrong et al., 2022; Dixon-Woods et al., 2006). Interventions to support people manage their MLTC have been developed, but most research participants are middle-class, White British populations meaning that the interventions are typically less effective for minoritised ethnic groups and people experiencing socioeconomic deprivation (Pan et al., 2020). Furthermore, in general, people with MLTC are often excluded from research, particularly trials in which the aim may be to focus on one long-term condition (Du Vaure et al., 2016).

Experiencing deprivation and being from a minoritised ethnic group are typically explored separately in health research. However, these factors intersect with minoritised ethnic groups disproportionately exposed to deprivation. Asian people overall (15.7%) are among the most likely to live in the 10% most deprived neighbourhoods in England, with Pakistani (31.1%) and Bangladeshi (19.3%) groups particularly affected. Black people also have a high likelihood (15.2%), while White British people are the least likely to live in these areas (9.1%) (Office for National Statistics, 2019). Living in deprived neighbourhoods represents a lack of opportunities linked to lower employment rates, income deprivation, lower education attainment, and higher crime rates. During the COVID-19 pandemic, evidence showed minoritised groups were more likely to have and die from the virus; however, experiencing socioeconomic deprivation exacerbated this risk (Magesh et al., 2021). Despite the overlap between deprivation and ethnicity, little research has explored the relationship between these two factors and the compounding impact on MLTC inequalities.

This chapter will delve into the intricate challenges and inequalities faced by people managing MLTC within the context of socioeconomic deprivation and ethnicity, looking at factors from an ecological perspective (i.e. at the individual, community, and societal level). We seek to highlight the common impact of living with MLTC whilst being from a minoritised ethnic group and experiencing deprivation, as well as offer solutions and directions for research and clinical practice. We draw upon our work, including systematic reviews exploring the international evidence base on MLTC and our UK-based interviews with 18 people experiencing socioeconomic deprivation from minoritised ethnic groups with MLTC, eight carers, and 18 healthcare professionals between 2021 and 2024 (Armstrong et al., 2025; Wyke et al., 2025; Okpako et al., 2023; Woodward et al., 2023, 2024).

All participants from our research were recruited across London and Sheffield. Locations were selected based on our local knowledge and networking opportunities within the research team which aided recruitment; both areas have clusters of deprivation and are ethnically diverse. Participants and their carers were from diverse ethnic backgrounds, including South Asian (n=12), Black British, African and Caribbean (n=11), and mixed ethnicity (n=3), and were aged between 20–90 years (mean age 55 years). Healthcare professionals were based in primary care and included general practitioners (GPs), nurses, and pharmacists. We will also draw upon two participatory workshops: one with eight people experiencing socioeconomic deprivation and one with eight voluntary and community sector organisations (VCSOs) that support people experiencing health inequalities . The participants were recruited from our previous qualitative studies, and VCSOs from London and Sheffield were contacted by our research team to invite them to our workshop. We chose to explore this work predominantly qualitatively to allow for an in-depth exploration of the experiences whilst applying an ecological lens. The case studies discussed throughout this chapter are an amalgamation of different people with pseudonyms to protect identities.

Individual factors in management of MLTC

Management of MLTC is a highly individualised process that must account for interactions between conditions, differing disease progressions, and personal preferences and circumstances. Some personal factors include, but are not limited to, the ability to understand medical information, cultural beliefs and practices, and psychological well-being. These individual factors are not often within the person's control and can lead two people from the same background on very different management paths, as demonstrated in case study one.

Case study one: Two individual approaches to MLTC management

Amina is a 58-year-old woman living with Type 2 diabetes, hypertension, and chronic obstructive pulmonary disease (COPD). Amina struggles to comprehend medical information as English is not her first language, leading to frequent hospital admissions due to poorly controlled diabetes and hypertension. Her well-being is also impacted by chronic stress related to financial instability and feelings of isolation, which result in depression. Additionally, her cultural beliefs discourage open discussion about illness, so she avoids seeking support from her community or family. Her well-being remains low, and her chronic conditions deteriorate due to non-adherence to treatment plans.

Ishitha is a 55-year-old woman managing Type 2 diabetes, osteoarthritis, and asthma. Unlike Amina, Ishitha's first language is English and finds the medical information understandable; therefore, Ishitha actively engages with her healthcare providers. She regularly attends education sessions on diabetes management and closely monitors her blood sugar levels. Ishitha's cultural beliefs emphasise the importance of holistic well-being, incorporating mental, physical, and spiritual health. Despite the challenges of living in a deprived area, Ishitha uses her cultural practices, such as cooking traditional, healthy meals and attending community health workshops, to stay engaged in her MLTC management. Her well-being is bolstered by her ability to find meaning and strength in her cultural identity, allowing her to navigate her conditions more effectively.

Health literacy, defined as 'the ability of an individual to obtain and translate knowledge and information in order to maintain and improve health in a way that is appropriate to the individual and system contexts' (Liu et al., 2020), is a critical factor in managing MLTC. Amina and Ishitha from the case study varied widely in their ability to understand medical information on their conditions; this is often due to language barriers or education level. People with higher health literacy levels are better equipped to understand their conditions and make informed decisions.

> *They gave me all these papers after my appointment, but I didn't really understand what any of it meant. It's all medical words. I just nodded, but I left more confused than when I came in.*
>
> *(Female, Black British, 68 years)*

Disparities in health literacy and accessibility of health information are a common barrier for ethnically minoritised and deprived populations, sometimes led by poor communication from healthcare professionals:

> *I don't think you're given enough information. You're just basically given 'This is the medication, whenever you're in pain, take this or whenever you feel this, do that.' But it doesn't – they don't really tell you the causes and what you can do so that you don't get the pain.*
>
> *(Male, South Asian, 37 years)*

Healthcare professionals have also described feeling powerless at not being able to access health information in a variety of languages or formats for their population:

> *And I've contacted the NHS, who provide information, they can't provide me a printed leaflet in any other languages other than English. We've got a big population of patients who are Slovakian – there isn't anything on whooping cough in Slovak that the NHS can provide. So, information is very hard to get. And also, it may not necessarily be in the format that people would be able to understand, anyway, because a lot of our Slovak patients only speak Roma, and Roma's not a written language. So it's challenging, as I say.*
>
> *(General Practice Nurse)*

Digital barriers further complicate this issue, with many individuals lacking access to reliable internet or digital health tools in part due to low income or living within rural areas where access to the internet can be limited. Evidence has shown that people from minoritised ethnic groups face digital barriers to self-managing their conditions (Nimmons et al., 2022). These challenges make it difficult for individuals to effectively manage MLTC, particularly when self-management interventions are not well-integrated into practice. Several older participants reported having limited or no digital skills, making access to online and/or electronic health services challenging:

> *I've got so many texts [from NHS] . . . and I haven't got a clue . . .*
>
> *(Male, Black Caribbean, 66 years)*

Younger generations may therefore be relied upon to assist older family members with technology.

For others, technological challenges were combined with financial barriers:

I do have problems, but then I can't afford to get the internet and plus I don't know how to do it.

(Female, Pakistani Muslim, 58 years)

If access and knowledge of how to use digital healthcare are increased across deprived, minoritised ethnic groups, it provides another incredibly vast resource for people to use. This can be particularly beneficial for people who may not feel they gained enough information in their healthcare appointments or need longer to digest information to allow them to make informed decisions. Many participants who were able to self-educate about their conditions through online resources displayed more proactive self-management behaviours:

when I experience an issue . . . the first thing I do is Google search, I try to see lots of YouTube videos and exercises, and eventually if you speak to the GP, or the GP refer you to another specialist, for example, physiotherapist, you would probably be able to do the same exercises but you have to wait two or three months just to get to see the physio, where you could find that information is a matter of seconds.

(Male, Bangladeshi, 30 years)

Cultural beliefs and practices also play an important role in the management of MLTC, by either enhancing or hindering care. Amina and Ishitha, in case study one, had different experiences of support from their families. Strong family support and communal caregiving traditions can enhance adherence to treatment plans, providing emotional and practical support for people managing chronic illnesses.

managing my conditions is hard . . . I have my friends because the carers have stopped coming now, I couldn't afford them anymore basically, so family and friends do all the running around at the moment. Especially as my mobility scooter is not working. My friend or my brothers, whoever, they do the shopping and anything like that .

(Male, Black Caribbean, 66 years)

Support within culturally diverse communities can be facilitated by the close proximity of family members and informal support within local communities. Strong family support and communal caregiving traditions can enhance adherence to treatment plans, providing emotional and practical support for people managing chronic illnesses:

Some of my family, they live quite close by, but sometimes I have to turn to them a lot, because of not having [external] support, like I can't manage, I can't do stuff, but I am lucky enough to have my family close by, otherwise who else would've supported me.

(Male, British South Asian, 26 years)

Some participants reported seeking alternatives (e.g. herbal remedies) to conventional medication or to use these alongside alternatives. However, this information was not always volunteered by patients during healthcare consultations unless specifically asked, which may in part be due to trust. In some cases, participants from minoritised ethnic groups made a connection between the use of alternative medicines and their cultural upbringing and background:

> *I think because of the kind of, the ethnic background that I've got, we already have our own type of herbal type cures and things that we can use. So I always feel as though I've got a little bit more of a toolkit in comparison to I think people who don't have a background with a different form of medicine.*
>
> *(Male, South Asian, 37 years)*

These cultural dynamics shape perceptions of illness, treatment acceptance, and overall healthcare engagement, influencing the efficacy of MLTC management. However, certain cultural beliefs may hinder management; for instance, some communities may favour alternatives (e.g. herbal remedies) over conventional medical treatment or delay seeking professional care due to stigmatisation of illness. Some cultural barriers were faced when there was a lack of culturally appropriate services to facilitate their health, which was highlighted by several minoritised ethnic participants:

> *to keep healthy, I wanted to . . . start swimming, but where our area is, it's terrible, right. Number one they don't have no facilities, right, for moral Asian women to swim. Because I don't like to go in mixed pools.*
>
> *(Female, Pakistani, 58 years)*

The last individual factor we will focus on is stress and well-being. People experiencing socioeconomic deprivation and from minoritised ethnic groups often face social and economic stressors such as poverty and discrimination, which exacerbate the challenges of managing MLTC. Poor well-being often leads to lower adherence to treatment plans, increased psychological distress, and reduced ability to engage with healthcare services and self-management strategies:

> *I've always been very active, always been very extrovert but my condition just changed me completely . . . If you're not well, you can't earn; if you can't earn, your standard of living goes down. If you can't see friends, you don't know what's happening in the outside world . . . You become isolated, you go deeper and deeper into black hole. So it's like a domino effect.*
>
> *(Female, British Pakistani, 54 years)*

Symptoms of depression and mental health problems were recognised as a catalyst for worsening other health conditions and impacted broadly on self-management practices:

> *[I]t'd be so much easier if I just had one health problem I could work on and not have multiple problems . . . I got really bad a few months ago . . . I just stopped taking everything . . . I went into a really deep depression and couldn't be bothered doing a thing.*
>
> *((Hardman et al., 2021) cited in (Woodward et al., 2023))*

The ability to self-manage conditions is a vicious cycle when well-being and mental health are impacted.

> *Sometimes I sit and cry. I do. I sit and cry 'cause I think 'God's sake you're only 50 years of age. How did it come to this that you're in so much pain? That you've got all these things you've got to do? And you've got all these illnesses. Just one after the other', you know, 'everything seems to be happening'. I can't make sense of it.*
> *(O'Brien et al., 2014) cited in (Woodward et al., 2023)*

We saw in case study one, that although Amina and Ishitha share similar socioeconomic challenges and ethnic backgrounds, their individual differences in health literacy, cultural beliefs and support, and well-being shaped their approaches to MLTC management. Enhancing well-being through culturally sensitive, equitable care, providing accessible health information, and addressing social determinants of health can improve people's ability to manage MLTC effectively, ultimately leading to better health outcomes and reduced health disparities.

Local community factors

In this section, we will consider the role of community support networks, focusing on faith-based groups, peer support and social prescribing, and the local environment in managing MLTC. Social capital, or the networks and relationships that provide social support, varies widely among different communities. Disparities in social capital can impact the availability and effectiveness of support for managing MLTC. In case study two, we explore two contrasting experiences highlighting the role of social support and the local environment in managing MLTC.

Case study two: The impact of the local support and environment

Aliyah, 58, lives with Type 2 diabetes, arthritis, and hypertension. Aliyah's faith-based group plays a vital role in her life, offering both emotional and practical support, which is culturally relevant. Through this group, she attends regular health workshops that educate her on managing her diabetes and hypertension through diet and exercise. The emotional support she receives from this close-knit group reduces her stress levels and helps her maintain a positive outlook. Her home is near a reliable bus route that enables her to attend medical appointments regularly and participate in community activities, such as gardening and art therapy, which she pays for. By staying connected with her community, she maintains control over her health and feels empowered in managing her conditions.

Hassan, 59, also lives with Type 2 diabetes, arthritis, and hypertension. Hassan is unaware of social prescribing programmes in his area but knows of some local support groups. However, crime rates in his neighbourhood are high, and Hassan often feels unsafe leaving his home. On top of this, Hassan's local environment lacks accessible green spaces, which limits his physical activity. Unreliable public transport in his area and financial restrictions make it difficult for him to travel to medical appointments or support group meetings, leading to missed appointments and a lack of engagement with services that could help him manage his conditions more effectively.

As in case study two, a common source of support from the people we interviewed was faith-based groups that provided emotional and culturally appropriate care, fostering a sense of belonging and hope. These groups helped to strengthen and build strong community networks, which can alleviate isolation and offer practical help. By understanding the cultural and faith-based dimensions of health, these groups can offer holistic, culturally sensitive care that enhances treatment adherence and overall well-being:

> *Once a week, we have our classes, we have Islamic classes, like the Quran, the book, it's in Arabic, so it means gobbledygook because I can only read English. So we have classes where I can actually learn. I don't have to do anything, I just sit, there's a teacher, it's like a lecture, so I sit there and I just learn. So there's people there, afterwards we all talk, we have a chat. So it's like a learning-slash-social event so I need that, I need to have interaction with other people.*
>
> *(Female, British Pakistani, 54 years)*

Another source of support was groups or other people also living with similar conditions (often referred to as peer supporters). Peer supporters in controlled intervention studies showed potential in increasing effectiveness for people experiencing socioeconomic deprivation. Below, a person living with MLTC discusses why advice from peer support is held in a higher regard than medical advice:

> *Because you won't be judged, there's no prejudice. And sometimes, they'll be able to give you feedback or offer you good advice because doctors don't go through it. But people don't, they talk from their experiences, that's what you need. Yes, it comes from the heart, doesn't it? Because you can say, 'Look, I've tried this, it didn't work for me, but why don't you try that?*
>
> *(Male, British Pakistani, 66 years)*

Community health programmes, including social prescribing, have shown promise in supporting MLTC management (Wilson et al., 2025). These programmes connect individuals with community resources, promoting holistic health management practices such as community groups, exercise programmes, volunteering opportunities, and mental health support. This approach helps improve well-being by reducing social isolation, promoting physical activity, and enhancing mental health, all of which are key to managing MLTC. However, many people, like Hassan in case study two, do not access social prescribing or are unaware of these services. Ethnically diverse and deprived population groups in particular are shown to be underserved in social prescribing (McMullen et al., 2024; Melam et al., 2025), the very populations the UK Government claim social prescribing will help (Office for Health Improvement and Disparities, 2022). Barriers to accessing social prescribing include a lack of culturally relevant services, low levels of awareness within diverse communities of social prescribing, and structural challenges within referral pathways:

> *There [was no one] like putting me in touch with a social prescriber or anything like that . . . since I've learnt about a social prescriber, I'm very shocked that I*

> *wasn't [referred] . . . I think at the lowest point that I was, for the doctor to [not] do anything about it, I was quite shocked about that.*
>
> *(Female, Pakistani Muslim, 41 years)*

Some participants had little access to social support groups and were identified as being at the extreme end of social isolation with no positive relationships in their lives to help them manage:

> *[M]y family, my mum and dad aren't here. My brothers and sisters . . . they're not good, they're ignorant . . . they haven't helped me. Instead, they make me more upset, all of them . . . that makes me more, you know, worse, my health condition.*
>
> *(Female, Pakistani Muslim, 58 years)*

Community-level environmental factors, such as access to healthy food and safe spaces for exercise, also affect the management of MLTC and are particularly important in deprived areas, where resources are often limited. In case study two, we read how Hassan felt unsafe leaving his home. Some participants we interviewed discussed the disadvantage of not being able to access support or living in high-crime areas:

> *I know that I feel quite lonely and I'd probably say quite isolated because I can't really do some of the things that a few of my friends can do . . . . I don't feel safe in the evenings, so I'm not able to kind of meet up with people.*
>
> *(Male, South Asian, aged 37)*

Access to provision that could facilitate or assist with self-management was worsened by poor transport links. One participant, who was recommended to attend daily sessions at an NHS mental health facility, said:

> *Because I live quite far from them, you know, they sometimes say to me that you should come every day . . . to do sessions. But I can't because my mobility and plus I can't go there all the time . . . That's the problem because I don't live near, I have to get [two or three] buses and then it's quite a long way to walk there as well, it's not easy.*
>
> *(Female, Pakistani Muslim, aged 58)*

Like Aliyah and Hassan, many people's experiences of managing their MLTC differ due to variations in their access to social support groups, local infrastructure, and environmental stressors. There is an urgent need for accessible social support and safer, more connected environments to improve health outcomes for people living with MLTC, especially those from minoritised ethnic groups living in deprived areas.

Academic institutions, health and social care, and VCSOs

Healthcare provider practices and academic research play critical roles in shaping MLTC management strategies; this section will explore how both institutes have a key role in researching and developing MLTC management strategies for people experiencing socioeconomic deprivation and people from minoritised ethnic groups, and how healthcare professionals and services support delivery of these strategies. Alongside this, we will consider how healthcare professionals and academic institutes can work with VCSOs to improve their inclusive practices. Case study three describes two different approaches to collaboration with differing outcomes.

Case study three: The role of collaboration in managing MLTC

In an inner-city borough with high deprivation and a large Bangladeshi population, a collaborative project known as the Health Bridges Initiative brought together a local NHS Primary Care Network, a university public health department, and a VCSO called the Bangladeshi Health Network (BHN). This partnership worked effectively by co-designing culturally appropriate self-management workshops tailored to people living with MLTC. The university supported healthcare providers with professional development in cultural competence and trauma-informed care, while BHN trained bilingual community health advocates who helped bridge communication and trust gaps between patients and services. These advocates provided ongoing support, helping patients navigate appointments and health advice in a culturally and linguistically accessible way. The collaborative approach extended to shared evaluation methods, incorporating both clinical and community-informed indicators. As a result, the project saw a 30% increase in patient confidence around managing their conditions, a reduction in emergency admissions related to preventable exacerbations, and stronger community trust in NHS services.

By contrast, in another urban area with a large Black Caribbean population experiencing high rates of MLTC, an NHS Clinical Commissioning Group partnered with a local university to launch a digital self-management app. Although the intention was to support patients in managing their conditions, the collaboration lacked genuine engagement with the local community or with the Caribbean Elders Support Alliance (CESA), a well-established VCSO in the area. The app was developed and rolled out without consulting patients or CESA and failed to account for digital barriers and cultural differences. Despite promotion through local GP surgeries, a few patients used the app, and no training or support was offered to guide them through it. CESA's concerns were overlooked, and they were not included in the delivery or adaptation of the tool. As a result, the app saw minimal uptake and had no discernible impact on health outcomes. Worse still, the process reinforced existing distrust of statutory services and left patients feeling excluded and misunderstood.

Academic research drives our understanding of MLTC and informs evidence-based practice. For example, systematic reviews can highlight what is being done well and areas needing improvement. A systematic review of 53 randomised controlled trials (RCTs) exploring the role of behaviour change techniques for people with MLTC found that these interventions are moderately effective at improving health outcomes (Rookes et al., 2024). The review highlights that interventions tend to be more successful if they are tailored to individual needs, incorporating components like self-management education, goal-setting, and personalised feedback. Additionally, the findings underscore the importance of involving patients in their care plans to enhance engagement and adherence. Another systematic review, which included 51 RCTs evaluating self-management techniques among people experiencing socioeconomic deprivation with MLTC, found that tailoring interventions to address specific barriers faced by this population, such as low health literacy and limited access to resources, is critical for effectiveness (Okpako et al., 2023). The review emphasises the need for clinicians to use accessible, culturally sensitive, and flexible approaches to better support people experiencing socioeconomic deprivation with MLTC.

Engaging with communities in research is also vital to ensure that findings are relevant and applicable to those most affected by MLTC. It also ensures the needs and challenges faced by those most affected are addressed. Strategies have been discussed by researchers for fostering trust, building relationships, and overcoming barriers like mistrust in research and logistical challenges (Armstrong & Woodward, 2024). These include creating safe and inclusive spaces, using co-design approaches, using familiar communication methods and supporting flexible and accessible participation in research. By prioritising community voices, researchers can co-create interventions and insights that better reflect the lived experiences of those experiencing deprivation, ultimately leading to more effective, equitable healthcare solutions.

Healthcare providers' practices significantly impact patients' experiences and outcomes. Cultural competence and sensitivity in healthcare delivery are crucial for effectively managing MLTC in ethnically diverse and socioeconomically deprived populations. The differences in provider practices can lead to disparities in care and outcomes. Below, a GP partner discusses feeling disempowered by the health system and tries in their own way to adapt their advice to be culturally competent:

> *Yeah, I guess it's quite disempowering, isn't it? I mean, that's how we've set up our health system and so, my role is to give advice. I try to tailor it, so kind of, if it's a Bengali patient, if they're cooking curries, we tell them not to use ghee because that's kind of super fatty. I guess you have to talk to people within local communities and find out what. You know, because there's no point in me advising taking a Mediterranean diet when that's not part of your culture. And there's alternative things you could eat which are as healthy, it's about understanding people's contexts.*
>
> *(GP Partner)*

Another concern of healthcare professionals was the patients' living situations and how this could impact their lives and their health:

> *Have they got access to hot water? I mean, there's – where do they live? Are they living in a house that's with 30 other people in it? Because some of our patients are. So it's – there's just so many factors. It's just not straightforward.*
>
> *(General Practice Nurse)*

Communication, verbal and non-verbal, from healthcare professionals is important to ensure the patient feels comfortable and trusts the healthcare professional to talk honestly about their health conditions. A patient discusses below feeling that the appointments are lacking empathy:

> *So there's no like you're speaking to me, there's no one-to-one, there's no eye contact, there's no concern, it's just like mechanical, does that make sense?*
>
> *(Female, British Pakistani, 54 years)*

Some factors that may improve communication and build trust include translators, longer appointments, continuity of care and adequate resourcing (i.e. more GPs in areas of deprivation).

> *I know one thing the practice has done in the past year of them undergoing all of this drastic change, is trying to lengthen appointment times. That's come from an acknowledgement that our patients are complex. They have multiple things going on. They need a bit of extra time and care.*
>
> *(Salaried GP)*

VCSOs play a vital role in supporting MLTC management. These organisations often provide essential services and support that complement those offered by the NHS and other healthcare providers. VCSOs also invest more time in building trust with local communities.

> *Specific groups that are working with specific communities. I think that probably helps for me to sell the idea to them to say, 'Look, we have this. There are people from certain areas that go there. It might be worthwhile. We do have an interpreter so language wouldn't be a problem. It's a very safe group. There's no judgement. You just go there and talk – or if you don't want to talk, that's fine. There's no compulsion. You can come out of it any time you want.' I think those things help, so work that's being done in the community is great.*
>
> *(Physiotherapist)*

Collaboration and integration between the NHS, universities, and VCSOs is crucial for delivering comprehensive care and support. Case study 3 showed how meaningful, inclusive collaboration can lead to practical and culturally relevant support, while poor collaboration risks deepening health inequalities and wasting resources. Working in genuine partnership with communities and valuing the contributions of all sectors is essential to improving outcomes for those living with MLTC in marginalised settings.

Policy and resource allocation

So far in this chapter, we have considered individual, community, and institute-level factors that influence how equipped people experiencing socioeconomic deprivation from minoritised ethnic groups are at managing their MLTC. This last section will explore how government policies and resource allocation across communities impact the management of MLTC. We will not explore individual policies but an overview of the UK living situation following many years of austerity and a pandemic.

The 'cost-of-living crisis' in the UK has severely impacted people's lives, with rising inflation, energy prices, and food costs stretching household budgets to their limits. People from minoritised ethnic groups are 2.5 times more likely to be in poverty than White British people (Edminston et al., 2022) and have been disproportionately impacted by the cost-of-living crisis (Lewis et al., 2025). Our research shows families are struggling to afford necessities, leading to increased reliance on food banks and government support schemes. Rent and mortgage payments have risen sharply, putting pressure on housing affordability and causing financial anxiety. As wages lag behind inflation, some people face difficult choices, such as cutting back on essentials or foregoing leisure activities, leading to heightened stress, reduced quality of life, and growing concern about long-term financial stability. This situation has exacerbated the lives of people already experiencing socioeconomic deprivation:

> *We do struggle, especially – we do struggle on food because, you know, we should be eating lots of meat, like you know, chicken and fish, fish is really expensive, fish and chicken. And, you know, for the iron, steak or lamb, you know, and red meat is expensive. Chicken is expensive. Vegetables, you know, even fruit is expensive so sometimes I have to compromise.*
>
> *(Female, British Asian, 57 years)*

A healthcare professional reflects on primary care in the UK and discusses how inequitable and underfunded health services fail to meet patient needs:

> *Primary care in the UK is not equitable, and places like ours are under-funded for the ill health of the population, and that's been really well proven by lots of people. And we just can't offer the number of appointments that would be necessary. It's particularly impacted for us, because we do about a third to half our consultations in a foreign language, so inevitably, it takes twice as long. So even if you've got a 15-minute appointment, actually, realistically, it's probably 30 minutes by the time you've finished it, and that reduces the number of appointments we can offer.*
>
> *(Salaried GP)*

Trust in government health initiatives varies among different populations and influences their engagement with these programmes. Building trust is essential for the success of public health initiatives aimed at improving MLTC management. This involves transparent communication, community involvement, and addressing the specific needs and concerns of diverse populations.

> *In my experience, working in communities that have been disadvantaged compared to not, the trust is a much bigger issue. So, I've worked in areas that are a lot more affluent and people generally feel like society and the system is working for them that people who are in positions of responsibility have their best interests at heart. I do find working with more deprived communities, it takes a longer time to produce that trust.*
>
> *(GP Partner)*

Conclusion

This chapter has highlighted how the management of MLTC is deeply entangled with issues of socioeconomic deprivation and racial and ethnic inequality. Through qualitative interviews with individuals from ethnically minoritised and socioeconomically deprived backgrounds, we explored the uneven landscape of support, access, and experience in managing MLTC. These findings resonate strongly with a growing body of evidence that underscores the structural determinants of health inequalities in the UK (Eto et al., 2023; Hayanga et al., 2021). Our findings support the notion that MLTC do not exist in a vacuum; rather, they operate within a societal framework where conditions are exacerbated by and interact with broader social, economic, and political inequities (Bambra, 2016).

Ethnically minoritised people living in deprived areas often face an accumulation of disadvantage that compounds their health conditions (Knies & Kumari, 2022). Common themes in our interviews that exacerbated MLTC management were limited income, poor housing, unsafe neighbourhoods, poor transport links, and barriers to culturally appropriate healthcare. Individuals described not attending recommended support services due to safety concerns or a lack of mobility and transport, which is an embodiment of what Bambra (2016) calls the 'spatial injustice' of deprivation.

Participants not only experienced material deprivation but also highlighted barriers related to cultural misunderstanding, language, and racial exclusion in the healthcare system. Participants described feeling dismissed or judged in healthcare appointments, lacking access to translators, or receiving advice that was not culturally appropriate. These findings point to the need to go beyond 'cultural competence' and towards a deeper structural critique of racism in healthcare. As our interviews with healthcare professionals revealed, the structure of the NHS can perpetuate exclusion, such as under-resourced practices in high-deprivation areas, short appointment times, and language barriers. While there were examples of promising local practice, such as longer consultations or GP awareness of dietary practices, these were often ad hoc and dependent on individual practitioners rather than institutional commitment.

People from ethnically minoritised backgrounds are more likely to experience early-onset of MLTC, leading to greater long-term healthcare use, polypharmacy, and premature mortality (Eto et al., 2023). Our study captures the lived reality behind the statistics with participants aged in their 30s and 40s speaking of high levels of stress, poor housing, isolation, and food insecurity. These social conditions act not just as barriers to managing MLTC but also as drivers of their early onset, particularly in the absence of preventive and tailored health interventions. But despite structural barriers, the chapter also highlighted the resilience and resourcefulness of local communities. Faith-based organisations and peer support networks offer valuable spaces of belonging, emotional care, and practical help, often stepping in where state services fall short. However, these supports were not universally available, and those without access to such networks faced isolation.

MLTC among people from minoritised ethnic groups experiencing socioeconomic deprivation cannot be understood or addressed without confronting the structural forces that shape health: poverty, racism, exclusion, and systemic neglect. A whole-systems approach is needed where policy, healthcare, academia, and communities work together to dismantle the barriers to health inequalities. Marmot (2020) situates health inequality within broader patterns of social injustice, arguing that health is a mirror of the unequal society in which we live. To move forward, we must centre the voices and experiences of those living with MLTC in marginalised contexts, and build models of care that are structurally aware, culturally grounded, and socially just.

Discussion questions

1. What are the structural barriers in healthcare that prevent effective management of MLTC among socioeconomically deprived individuals?
2. What cultural challenges do ethnically diverse communities face when trying to manage MLTC?
3. How can future studies better explore the intersection of ethnicity, socioeconomic deprivation, and MLTC management to create more equitable healthcare solutions?

Further reading

Armstrong, M., & Woodward, A. (2024). Engaging people experiencing socioeconomic deprivation in qualitative research: Reflections. *Qualitative Research in Psychology*, 1–8.

Bartley, M. (2016). *Health Inequality: An Introduction to Concepts, Theories and Methods.* John Wiley & Sons.

Imison, C. (2021). *Multiple Long-Term Conditions (Multimorbidity): Making Sense of the Evidence.* National Institute for Health Research.

McMullen, S., Poduval, S., Armstrong, M., Davies, N., Dayson, C., Kharicha, K., Nair, P., Mistry, M., Sajid, M., Walters, K., & Woodward, A. (2024). A qualitative exploration of the role of culturally relevant social prescribing in supporting Pakistani carers living in the UK. *Health Expectations*, *27*(6), e70099.

Okpako, T., Woodward, A., Walters, K., Davies, N., Stevenson, F., Nimmons, D., et al. (2023). Effectiveness of self-management interventions for long-term conditions in people experiencing socio-economic deprivation in high-income countries: A systematic review and meta-analysis. *Journal of Public Health*, *45*(4), 970–1041.

Woodward, A., Davies, N., Walters, K., Nimmons, D., Stevenson, F., Protheroe, J., et al. (2023). Self-management of multiple long-term conditions: A systematic review of the barriers and facilitators amongst people experiencing socioeconomic deprivation. *Plos One*, *18*(2), e0282036.

Woodward, A., Nimmons, D., Davies, N., Walters, K., Stevenson, F. A., Protheroe, J., et al. (2024). A qualitative exploration of the barriers and facilitators to self-managing multiple long-term conditions amongst people experiencing socioeconomic deprivation. *Health Expectations*, 27(2), e14046.

References

Ara, D. (2024). *Independent Investigation of the NHS in England.* https://www.gov.uk/government/publications/independent-investigation-of-the-nhs-in-england

Armstrong, M., Aker, N., Nair, P., Walters, K., Barrado-Martin, Y., Kupeli, N., Sampson, E. L., Manthorpe, J., West, E., & Davies, N. (2022). Trust and inclusion during the Covid-19 pandemic: Perspectives from Black and South Asian people living with dementia and their carers in the UK. *International Journal of Geriatric Psychiatry*, *37*(3).

Armstrong, M., Jeri-Wahrhaftig, A., Woodward, A., Nimmons, D., Chew-Graham, C. A., Protheroe, J., Stevenson, F., Davies, N. and Walters, K., 2025. Experiencing socioeconomic deprivation as a carer in the United Kingdom: A qualitative study. *Health Expectations*, *28*(6), e70502.

Armstrong, M., & Woodward, A. (2024). Engaging people experiencing socioeconomic deprivation in qualitative research: Reflections. *Qualitative Research in Psychology*, 1–8.

Arpey, N. C., Gaglioti, A. H., & Rosenbaum, M. E. (2017). How socioeconomic status affects patient perceptions of health care: A qualitative study. *Journal of Primary Care & Community Health*, *8*(3), 169–175.

Bambra, C. (2016). *Health Divides: Where You Live Can Kill You*. Policy Press.

Barnett, K., Mercer, S. W., Norbury, M., Watt, G., Wyke, S., & Guthrie, B. (2012). Epidemiology of multimorbidity and implications for health care, research, and medical education: A cross-sectional study. *The Lancet*, *380*(9836), 37–43.

Brilleman, S. L., Purdy, S., Salisbury, C., Windmeijer, F., Gravelle, H., & Hollinghurst, S. (2013). Implications of comorbidity for primary care costs in the UK: A retrospective observational study. *British Journal of General Practice*, *63*(609), e274–e282.

Dixon-Woods, M., Cavers, D., Agarwal, S., Annandale, E., Arthur, A., Harvey, J., Hsu, R., Katbamna, S., Olsen, R., & Smith, L. (2006). Conducting a critical interpretive synthesis of the literature on access to healthcare by vulnerable groups. *BMC Medical Research Methodology*, *6*, 1–13.

Du Vaure, C. B., Dechartres, A., Battin, C., Ravaud, P., & Boutron, I. (2016). Exclusion of patients with concomitant chronic conditions in ongoing randomised controlled trials targeting 10 common chronic conditions and registered at ClinicalTrials.gov: A systematic review of registration details. *BMJ Open*, *6*(9), e012265.

Edminston, D., Begum, S., & Kataria, M. (2022). *Falling Faster Amidst a Cost-of-Living Crisis: Poverty, Inequality and Ethnicity in the UK*. R. Trust.

Eto, F., Samuel, M., Henkin, R., Mahesh, M., Ahmad, T., Angdembe, A., Hamish McAllister-Williams, R., Missier, P., Reynolds, N. J., & Barnes, M. R. (2023). Ethnic differences in early onset multimorbidity and associations with health service use, long-term prescribing, years of life lost, and mortality: A cross-sectional study using clustering in the UK Clinical Practice Research Datalink. *PLoS Medicine*, *20*(10), e1004300.

Hardman, R., Begg, S., & Spelten, E. (2021). Multimorbidity and its effect on perceived burden, capacity and the ability to self-manage in a low-income rural primary care population: A qualitative study. *Plos One*, *16*(8), e0255802.

Hayanga, B., Stafford, M., & Becares, L. (2021). Ethnic inequalities in healthcare use and care quality among people with multiple long-term health conditions living in the United Kingdom: A systematic review and narrative synthesis. *International Journal of Environmental Research and Public Health*, *18*(23), 12599.

Hayanga, B., Stafford, M., & Bécares, L. (2023). Ethnic inequalities in multiple long-term health conditions in the United Kingdom: A systematic review and narrative synthesis. *BMC Public Health*, *23*(1), 178.

Knies, G., & Kumari, M. (2022). Multimorbidity is associated with the income, education, employment and health domains of area-level deprivation in adult residents in the UK. *Scientific Reports*, *12*(1), 7280.

Lewis, C., Yarker, S., & Phillipson, C. (2025). Living with financial insecurity: Analysing the impact of the cost-of-living crisis on older ethnic minority people. *Social Policy & Administration*, *59*(2), 265–279.

Liu, C., Wang, D., Liu, C., Jiang, J., Wang, X., Chen, H., Ju, X., & Zhang, X. (2020). What is the meaning of health literacy? A systematic review and qualitative synthesis. *Family Medicine and Community Health*, *8*(2).

Magesh, S., John, D., Li, W. T., Li, Y., Mattingly-App, A., Jain, S., Chang, E. Y., & Ongkeko, W. M. (2021). Disparities in COVID-19 outcomes by race, ethnicity, and socioeconomic status: A systematic review and meta-analysis. *JAMA Network Open*, *4*(11), e2134147–e2134147.

Marmot, M. (2020). Society and the slow burn of inequality. *The Lancet*, *395*(10234), 1413–1414.

McMullen, S., Poduval, S., Armstrong, M., Davies, N., Dayson, C., Kharicha, K., Nair, P., Mistry, M., Sajid, M., & Walters, K. (2024). A qualitative exploration of the role of culturally relevant social prescribing in supporting Pakistani carers living in the UK. *Health Expectations*, *27*(6), e70099.

Melam, C., Dyson, J., & Thomson, K. (2025). The role of social prescribing interventions in addressing health inequalities in the United Kingdom: A narrative review. *Health & Social Care in the Community*, *2025*(1), 6613809.

Mitchell, C., Fryer, K., Guess, N., Aminu, H., Jackson, B., Gordon, A., Reynolds, J., Huang, Q., Jayasooriya, S., & Mawson, R. (2023). Underserved 'Deep End' populations: A critical analysis addressing the power imbalance in research. *British Journal of General Practice*, *73*(732), 326–329.

National Institute for Health and Care Research Evidence. (2023). *Multiple Long-Term Conditions (Multimorbidity) and Inequality-Addressing the Challenge: Insights from Research*. NIHR Evidence.

Nimmons, D., Armstrong, M., Pigott, J., Walters, K., Schrag, A., Ogunleye, D., Dowridge, W., Read, J., & Davies, N. (2022). Exploring the experiences of people and family carers from under-represented groups in self-managing Parkinson's disease and their use of digital health to do this. *Digital Health*, *8*, 20552076221102261.

O'Brien, R., Wyke, S., Watt, G. G., Guthrie, B., & Mercer, S. W. (2014). The 'everyday work' of living with multimorbidity in socioeconomically deprived areas of Scotland. *Journal of Comorbidity*, *4*(1), 1–10.

Office for Health Improvement and Disparities. (2022, January 27). *Social Prescribing: Applying All Our Health*. GOV.UK.

Office for National Statistics. (2019). People Living in Deprived Neighbourhoods. *Ethnicity Facts and Figures*. Retrieved September 4, 2025, from https://www.ethnicity-facts-figures.service.gov.uk/uk-population-by-ethnicity/demographics/people-living-in-deprived-neighbourhoods/latest

Okpako, T., Woodward, A., Walters, K., Davies, N., Stevenson, F., Nimmons, D., Chew-Graham, C. A., Protheroe, J., & Armstrong, M. (2023). Effectiveness of self-management interventions for long-term conditions in people experiencing socio-economic deprivation in high-income countries: A systematic review and meta-analysis. *Journal of Public Health*, *45*(4), 970–1041.

Pan, D., Sze, S., Minhas, J. S., Bangash, M. N., Pareek, N., Divall, P., Williams, C. M., Oggioni, M. R., Squire, I. B., & Nellums, L. B. (2020). The impact of ethnicity on clinical outcomes in COVID-19: A systematic review. *E Clinical Medicine*, *23*.

Rookes, T. A., Nimmons, D., Frost, R., Armstrong, M., Davies, L., Ross, J., Hopkins, J., Mistry, M., Taylor, S., & Walters, K. (2024). Effectiveness of complex behaviour change interventions tested in randomised controlled trials for people with multiple long-term conditions (M-LTCs): Systematic review with meta-analysis. *BMJ Open*, *14*(6), e081104.

Salisbury, C., Johnson, L., Purdy, S., Valderas, J. M., & Montgomery, A. A. (2010). Epidemiology and impact of multimorbidity in primary care: A retrospective cohort study. *The British Journal of General Practice*, *61*(582), e12.

Samuel, L. J., Gaskin, D. J., Trujillo, A. J., Szanton, S. L., Samuel, A., & Slade, E. (2021). Race, ethnicity, poverty and the social determinants of the coronavirus divide: US county-level disparities and risk factors. *BMC Public Health*, *21*, 1–11.

Stafford, M., Bécares, L., Hayanga, B., Ashworth, M., & Fisher, R. (2022). Continuity of care in diverse ethnic groups: A general practice record study in England. *British Journal of General Practice*, *73*(729), e257–e266.

Stafford, M., Knight, H., Hughes, J., Alarilla, A., Mondor, L., Pefoyo Kone, A., Wodchis, W. P., & Deeny, S. R. (2022). Associations between multiple long-term conditions and mortality in diverse ethnic groups. *Plos One*, *17*(4), e0266418.

Office for Health Improvement and Disparities. (2022, January 27). *Social Prescribing: Applying All Our Health*. GOV.UK.

Wilson, A., Noble, H., Galway, K., & Doherty, J. (2025). Social prescribing for people living with long-term health conditions: A scoping review. *Systematic Reviews*, *14*(1), 114.

Woodward, A., Davies, N., Walters, K., Nimmons, D., Stevenson, F., Protheroe, J., Chew-Graham, C. A., & Armstrong, M. (2023). Self-management of multiple long-term conditions:

A systematic review of the barriers and facilitators amongst people experiencing socioeconomic deprivation. *Plos One*, *18*(2), e0282036.

Woodward, A., Nimmons, D., Davies, N., Walters, K., Stevenson, F. A., Protheroe, J., Chew-Graham, C. A., & Armstrong, M. (2024). A qualitative exploration of the barriers and facilitators to self-managing multiple long-term conditions amongst people experiencing socioeconomic deprivation. *Health Expectations*, *27*(2), e14046.

Wyke, E. J., Baxter, E., Chew-Graham, C. A., Woodward, A., Walters, K., Davies, N., Taylor, S. J. C., Ross, J., Protheroe, J., Mitchell, C. and Armstrong, M., 2025. Managing multiple long-term conditions in people experiencing socioeconomic deprivation: Primary care perspectives. *British Journal of General Practice.*

SECTION 6

Beyond resilience

In this closing section of this volume, one final chapter, by Kumah, Tufte-Hewett, and Berrahou, consolidates both the injustices faced and the restorations required to remedy them, through attention to the term 'resilience'. Chapter 11 serves as the final clarion call to action, identifying the challenges that racialised communities face while also naming pathways for change.

In Chapter 11, Kumah and colleagues discuss resilience as both an asset and a hindrance to accessing appropriate and timely mental healthcare. They speak of 'Black resilience', a protective mechanism which developed in response to historical injustices affecting the Black community. In discussing this phenomenon, they distinguish Black resilience from emotional unresponsiveness, noting that this coping strategy commonly evolves as a means through which to deal with discrimination in a bid towards self-preservation. While seemingly a sign of strength, Kumah et al. argue that Black resilience may, in some circumstances, be a maladaptive means of dealing with psychological stress, particularly when facing microaggressive behaviours and overt racism. Drawing on Critical Race Theory, the authors advocate for the centring of marginalised voices within mental health spaces to understand how best to challenge the power structures that uphold inequalities. Finally, they emphasise the enduring need for outlets where individuals can share their experiences in safety, deconstruct their resilient identity, and account for the unique stressors they face as members of African and African-Caribbean communities.

DOI: 10.4324/9781003466093-17

CHAPTER 11

The intersection of resilience and systemic barriers in accessing mental health services among Black African and African Caribbean communities in the UK

Angela D. Kumah, Angela Tufte-Hewett, and Fouad Berrahou

Introduction: The injustice of health inequalities

A growing body of research has explored health inequalities in mental health service delivery for racialised communities in the UK, leading to calls for equitable approaches that improve access to support for Black African and African Caribbean communities. Throughout this chapter, the term 'Black African and Caribbean' encompasses individuals of African and Caribbean descent residing in the UK and is used interchangeably with 'Black communities' to acknowledge common experiences of systemic oppression while recognising the distinct cultural identities within these groups. This chapter examines the dual nature of Black resilience – as both a protective factor rooted in cultural strengths such as faith, family support, and cultural pride, and as a potential barrier to help-seeking shaped by experiences of systemic racism and discrimination. Drawing on literature and primary data from West Birmingham, it explores how resilience narratives, influenced by gender and intergenerational differences, can perpetuate a culture of silence around mental illness and impact help-seeking behaviour. Understanding this complexity is crucial for developing culturally sensitive interventions that leverage community strengths while addressing systemic barriers to mental healthcare access.

Health inequalities among minority ethnic groups have been a major public health concern for decades with much research evidence collected on the detrimental effects of these inequalities on their quality of life, especially for these communities living in the United Kingdom (UK) (Chouhan & Nazroo, 2020). The World Health Organization (WHO, 2016) has defined health inequalities as 'the apparent disparity in the distribution of and contribution to health and well-being between various groups'. The NHS (2020) further defines health inequalities as:

> preventable, unfair and unjust differences in health status between groups, populations or individuals that arise from the unequal distribution of social, environmental and economic conditions within societies, which determine the risk of

DOI: 10.4324/9781003466093-18

people getting ill, their ability to prevent sickness, or opportunities to take action and access treatment when ill health occurs.

Economic disparities, social status, race, ethnicity, and gender, among other factors, are major social determinants of the level of support different populations may receive around health and social care (Hill, 2016; Mirza & Warwick, 2024). Particularly, in the history of Black African and African-Caribbean communities in the UK, systemic racism, discrimination, stigma, and other social determinants have been found to contribute to poorer outcomes for mental health (Nazroo, 2003; Bignall et al., 2019; Devonport et al., 2022).

Records exist of the presence of Black people in the UK as early as the 12th century (Millard, 2016). However, since the influx of Black African-Caribbean and African immigrants into the UK in the 1940s and 1980s, respectively, the 2021 National census data showed that there are 2.4 million people (4.0%) from Black ethnic groups, 2.5% and 1.0% of whom identify as Black African and Black Caribbean, respectively. The percentage of Mixed or multiple ethnic, White/Black African and Mixed White/Black African/Caribbean stands at 0.4% and 0.9%, respectively. The percentage of those identified as Other Black stood at 0.5% (Office of National Statistics, 2021). Despite this historical presence of Black people (Black Africans and African-Caribbeans) in the UK, they constitute a population that has been subjected to significant discrimination and disproportionate treatment when it comes to accessing social, educational, economic, and healthcare needs (Devonport et al., 2022).

The racial categorisation of Black Africans and African-Caribbeans within the Black, Asian and Minority ethnic (BAME) group further perpetuates the lack of consideration for the differences in culture and values between these groups, fostering narratives which downplay each group's origin and history (Hall, 1988; Modood, 1994). Aspinall (2021) raised one argument against the use of the term 'BAME', stating that it is not an adequate reflection of the self-identity of the various ethnic groups. He further argues that the term ignores essential socio-cultural elements that differentiate multiple ethnic groups from each other by classifying different continents as one group of people. Nonetheless, all categories of 'Black people' living in the UK, regardless of the variances in culture and values, share experiences of discrimination and oppression in various facets of their lives. Inequalities within these communities are rife across economic and social levels, putting many Black African and African-Caribbean people in disadvantaged positions. Across the UK, the highest rates of poverty and unemployment, exclusion in the education system (3 times more than the general student population) and over-representation in the juvenile detention and prison system are seen within the Black community (Youth Justice Board for England and Wales, 2025).

Despite the UK's long-standing position as a global leader in health inequalities research and policy, there are continued discussions within the UK highlighting the ever-widening health inequalities gap among Black, Asian and Minority ethnic groups (Smith et al., 2016; Wenham, 2020; Nazroo, 2024). The long-standing presence of health inequalities in the UK was initially outlined in The Black Report (Gray, 1982), which demonstrated evidence of inequitable access to healthcare and treatment and higher mortality rates among minority ethnic groups. This report suggested that disparities in health and access to social care had not only existed since the formation of the National Health Service (NHS) in 1948 but increased over time. In this report, health inequalities were generally attributed to social inequalities, such as low income, lack of education, and lower employment levels prevalent among these minority populations, rather than the shortcomings of the delivery system of health and social care services (Gray, 1982). More than 40 years on, in the face of glaring evidence, clearly highlighted during the recent COVID-19 pandemic that racism is a driver of poor health outcomes, the 2021 Race Report (2021) still purported that racial discrimination was not the key factor in the unfair treatment Black, Asian, and Minority ethnic groups have historically received within the UK's the health and social care system. Certainly, ethnicity alone does not determine health outcomes; however, coupled with the higher rates of poverty and socioeconomic disadvantage, along with the deleterious effects of structural and institutional racism along with that greatly affect ethnic minority communities, these populations are more likely to experience poorer mental health outcomes (Grey et al., 2013; Bignall et al., 2019; Kapadia, 2023).

The issue of mental illness and modes of treatment for people of minority ethnic descent, especially for people of Black African and African-Caribbean backgrounds, has also received considerable attention. In line with previous studies (Kiev, 1965; Hemsi, 1967), Sharpley et al. (2001) described that, as early as the 1950s and 1960s, when large numbers of people from the Caribbean migrated to England (Windrush day), higher than normal incidences of schizophrenia were already being diagnosed among these groups. More recent studies comparing rates of severe mental illness among various ethnic populations also found that Black African and African-Caribbean people were two to eight times more likely to receive a diagnosis of psychosis as compared to White populations and Black men are more likely to be detained under the Mental Health Act (MHA) that men of any other ethnicity (Department of Health, 2003; Vernon, 2011; NHS Digital, 2025). Black people are also more likely to be subject to excessive force in psychiatric facilities and also more likely to be injured while being restrained by the police for detention under the MHA (Royal College of Nursing, 2025). The reasons for the difference in the rate of diagnosis between ethnic groups remain unclear, and Sharpley et al. (2001) and Morgan et al. (2005) identified complex factors, including the scope of political influences, cultural variation, prejudice, and other social disadvantages in the diagnosis and treatment of Black people.

Despite these findings, several studies have also shown that Black Africans and African-Caribbeans access mental health services less frequently than other ethnic groups (Grey et al., 2013; Nazroo et al., 2020). Fear, in various forms, has been said to be a major contributing factor to the poor access to support for people living with mental health problems within the Black community, as well as other marginalised communities such as Gypsy and Roma travellers (McFadden et al., 2018). The negative experiences and discrimination of members of the Black community by mental health services have been long-standing, with no significant improvement in the last few decades despite recognition of the issue (Rabiee-Khan & Smith, 2014; Nwokoroku et al., 2022). The combination of fear of people with mental illness, mostly due to social stigma and preconceived notions that mental illness equates to violence, and fear of contact with services feeds into the deleterious cycle of poor mental health within the Black community (Sweeney et al., 2015; HM Government, 2007, 2018; Kapadia et al., 2022). This, consequently, reduces the likelihood of Black people accessing mental health support until critical care is needed, often occurring after encounters with the criminal justice system (Barnett et al., 2019). These distresses, combined, further lead to a delay in help-seeking among Black communities and reinforce the culture of silence and stigma (self, social and structural) that exists around mental illness (Mantovani et al., 2017; Jensen et al., 2021). The repeated cycle of maladaptive pathways to accessing mental health services, either through involuntary psychiatric detention under the MHA, social services and court involvement, further contributes to the reduction in help-seeking behaviour within these communities (Keating & Robertson, 2004; Synergi, 2018).

Beyond the negative experiences of racism and other forms of discrimination, there are many cultural strengths, dispositions of resilience, and protective factors that contribute towards maintaining the mental health and well-being of Black African and African-Caribbean communities. Recognising and celebrating these positive aspects can help challenge stereotypes of negative attitudes towards mental health by promoting community empowerment and fostering a more holistic approach to mental healthcare. It is imperative to evaluate how these negative experiences impact perceptions and demonstrations of resilience (Woods-Giscombe et al., 2023), not only as a protective factor but also as an identity that may act as a barrier to supporting help-seeking behaviour. Given the deleterious effects of racism and discrimination, (Nazroo et al., 2020), compounded by the culture of silence and stigma around mental ill health in these communities, deconstructing Black resilience and its associated function towards self-preservation may seem complex. Nevertheless, understanding this complexity can help in developing interventions that promote resilience while also addressing the potential reluctance to seek help and balancing the recognition of strength with the acknowledgement of vulnerability.

Defining resilience

Resilience is defined as 'a positive adaptation, or the ability to maintain or regain mental health, despite experiencing adversity' (Herrman et al., 2011). It can also be considered as one's ability to *bounce back* and cope in a stressful situation without breaking down. It is conceptualised as an interactive process between one's environment and internal, psychological protective factors that help mitigate one's reaction to various stressors (Rutter, 1985; Lindström, 2001). Within communities, resilience describes the process by which a group of people capitalise on their capacity to access various resources to cope in the face of adversity. This dynamic process is evident in the way these communities make use of the social support systems and other assets to achieve positive outcomes, especially in the face of stressful environmental factors (Panter-Brick & Leckman, 2013). Powell et al. (2014) and Siller and Aydin (2022) offer contextual and socio-constructivist perspectives to understanding resilience, suggesting that the systems that support one's socioeconomic and health needs are key factors in the process of developing resilience. Thus, the distinct levels of access to these systems and resources, in alignment with the social determinants of health for different populations, are important in understanding the prevailing narratives on resilience.

Defining Black resilience

Several studies examining resilience in Black communities have proposed resilience as a fluid process that can be evaluated as an expression of one's behaviour or identity (Teti et al., 2012; Jones, 2023). Thus, resilience cannot be assessed accurately independent of a historical perspective (Payne, 2011) and should be analysed as a process of relational coping (Gladwell, 2008), which can be determined by understanding the interactions between complex interpersonal relationships and social backgrounds. Evaluating resilience from a cultural and historical standpoint, therefore, requires gaining insights into the impact of culture on resilience at individual, family, and community levels (Kirmayer et al., 2009; Frounfelker et al., 2019).

Defining Black resilience, therefore, requires careful attention to the influence of contextual factors in this interactive process. Woods-Giscombe et al. (2023) defined resilience among African American women within the context of their social support, community safety, spirituality, and access to healthcare and financial support. Simply put, Black resilience encompassed a multifaceted approach that recognised the value of internal resources (spirituality) and external supports (community safety) in fostering resilience. Sumbul et al. (2020) pointed out that some of these adversities may include systemic, institutional and historical violence and oppression influenced by race, gender, and class, specifically impacting marginalised groups, within which Black communities are classed.

For example, Black resilience can be defined as the interconnectedness of personal, social, and structural elements that contribute to an individual's ability to overcome adversity experienced by marginalised groups and to maintain health. Historically, racism, discrimination, and oppression of Black people have been evidenced to widen the inequality gap and left many vulnerable. This contextual vulnerability (Krishnan et al., 2020) is what leads to the development of resilience, in a bid to survive adversity (Siller & Aydin, 2022). This resilience, born out of necessity, has evolved into a complex set of coping strategies and cultural practices that not only aid in survival but also preserve the identity of these communities, while fostering community empowerment and transformation. Black resilience, in the UK, in this same vein, can be defined as an identity, rather than a choice.

There are a few erroneous theories and assumptions around Black resilience as a 'buffer' against mental illness, such as those propounded by Kessler (1979) and Neff (1985), in which it is claimed that Black people are less susceptible to risk factors of mental illness because they face more adversities throughout their lives. Williams and Harris-Reid (1999) also suggested that as a result of the presence of protective factors, such as family support and faith, Black people have 'super-coping ability' against various life stressors. Such oversimplified theories gloss over the external factors that necessitate such coping abilities and perpetuate the disparities that Black Africans and African-Caribbean communities face in accessing mental health support. Ignoring the multifactorial influences and the social realities surrounding health and well-being, these assumptions further justify the need to develop a 'thick skin', perpetuating the culture of silence and delayed help-seeking (Muaygil, 2018).

Black resilience has often been misinterpreted to mean Black Africans and African-Caribbeans are not sensitive or emotionally responsive and are able to deal with any form of mistreatment. Especially within the workplace, where many professionals face microaggressions (Rollock, 2019), workplace culture and the expectation to maintain professional decorum have led to a culture of silence in the face of such discrimination. Woods-Giscombe et al. (2023) refer to this concept of being emotionally unresponsive as 'skin-deep' resilience and consider this as both an asset and a stressor, a double-edged sword, which has the potential to negatively impact the physical and mental well-being of the one facing this stressor. While much of the research on Black resilience has been explored in the context of North America, there is still a wide gap in the literature that explores the meaning of Black resilience among Black British people, let alone its impact on access to various levels of support, especially mental healthcare. This knowledge gap highlights the need for a more nuanced and contextually relevant lens to understanding Black resilience. Critical Race Theory (CRT) offers a framework for understanding the impact of systemic racism and inequalities on shaping the experiences of Black communities living in the UK, especially where it pertains to accessing mental health services.

Critical Race Theory (CRT) and Black resilience

Taylor (1998) defined critical race theory as 'a theoretical framework that challenges racial narratives that posit the experiences of white populations as the standard for understanding and evaluating social reality'. This theory is grounded in acknowledging the unique perspectives and lived experiences of people of colour. Delgado and Stefancic (2001) maintain that the social construct of race has a wide-reaching influence on every society's makeup. As such, challenging racial hierarchies and systems that perpetuate historically oppressive power dynamics is crucial for promoting social justice and achieving equity. As an emerging transdisciplinary, race-equity methodology, critical race theory (CRT) has been used in conjunction with other frameworks to address the issue of health inequalities and the impact of race in the delivery of healthcare (Simien, 2005). By actively engaging the narratives of racialised and minoritised populations, CRT's theoretical stance challenges existing power structures and advocates for the inclusion of voices from marginalised communities as a central component of the knowledge-generation process that leads to sustainable change.

CRT helps centre the voices and experiences of marginalised Black African and African-Caribbean communities and, therefore, sheds light on the need to evaluate the social construct of race in matters of healthcare delivery and significantly limit its impact on the health and well-being of individuals. This framework allows us to recognise Black resilience as a powerful asset that has enabled communities to thrive, supporting collective well-being while driving innovative approaches to improve communal health and develop empowering, culturally relevant systems, in the face of historically perpetuated adversity.

Black resilience as an asset

The appreciation of Black identity is a complex and multifaceted aspect of the Black experience. There is a widespread sense of pride in the achievements of Black people despite centuries of oppression. This pride extends to physical characteristics such as skin colour and hair, as well as cultural elements like food and creativity, all of which are integral to Black identity. The influence of Black culture on other cultures, particularly in areas such as food, music, fashion, and lifestyle, is recognised as a significant contribution to global trends, and this artistic creativity serves as a powerful medium for preserving and transmitting cultural heritage and traditions. The sense of community, rich family dynamics, and deep historical heritage are also highly valued aspects of Black identity. Pitt (2017) and Lordi (2020) emphasise the significance of Black arts and soul music in shaping cultural sensibilities and supporting Black pride and resilience. The global popularity of genres such as Reggae and Afrobeat music exemplifies this cultural influence and resilience. Food plays a crucial role in promoting family and community cohesion within Black communities. Research by Theron (2016) and Navarro (2022) demonstrates a positive correlation between food and health, linking culinary traditions to generational resilience and the reduction of inequalities. This connection between food, culture, and well-being underscores the multifaceted nature of resilience in Black communities.

For many individuals of African-Caribbean origin, exploring the global journey of Black people serves as a powerful means of self-discovery. Despite the traumatic history of slavery and ongoing discrimination, resilience remains a defining characteristic of Black communities. This resilience was repeatedly tested through the exploitative mechanisms of the British Empire, which, even after its formal dissolution, transformed formerly colonised peoples into an economic underclass of minimum wage labourers in Britain itself, replacing colonial exploitation with domestic marginalisation observed during the Windrush era. Ancestral connections have been said to play a crucial role as a source of resilience for many Black individuals, especially those of African-Caribbean descent, and the process of learning about one's history often inspires courage and perseverance (Fitzgerald et al., 2021). The endurance and survival of ancestors, parents, and grandparents through various hardships are sources of pride and strength and embracing their rich cultural heritage fosters hope for the future. Scholars have theorised about these phenomena, developing concepts such as post-racial resilience and Black resilience neoliberalism. These theories explore and celebrate the exceptionalism and empowerment demonstrated by Black people in the UK and the US (Joseph-Salisbury, 2018; Clay, 2019). They provide frameworks for understanding how historical experiences shape contemporary resilience and identity in Black communities.

These theories highlight the power of positive narratives in shaping our understanding of how communities evolve and interact with the systems around them and are crucial in transforming our knowledge of how people connect with each other and navigate their social environments. This understanding is particularly valuable when evaluating the determinants of health among diverse populations. By recognising and valuing these cultural strengths and resilience factors, mental health professionals and policymakers can develop more effective, culturally sensitive approaches to mental healthcare for Black African and African-Caribbean communities. This approach not only honours the rich cultural heritage of these communities but also leverages existing strengths to promote mental well-being and resilience.

Black resilience as a potential barrier

It is important to note that the emphasis on values such as perseverance and hard work, while positive can sometimes perpetuate a narrative of resilience that may influence attitudes towards mental health and help-seeking behaviours within these communities. While these aspects of Black identity and resilience are largely positive, they also present a complex interplay with mental health attitudes and behaviours. The strong emphasis on resilience, while a source of strength, may inadvertently create barriers to seeking mental health support. These dynamics highlight the need for multifaceted approaches to mental healthcare that respect these cultural strengths and practices while also addressing potential barriers to help-seeking behaviour. It requires a delicate balance between celebrating the resilience and achievements of Black communities while also creating space for vulnerability and help-seeking, which can inform the design of effective strategies for promoting mental well-being within Black African and African-Caribbean communities, respecting their cultural heritage while addressing contemporary mental health needs.

In understanding the value of resilience as an asset to promoting individual and collective well-being within the community, the contextual influences of systemic racial oppression, discrimination, and inequities in access to socioeconomic and healthcare resources must also be considered in light of the barriers they pose to help-seeking behaviour, specifically around accessing mental health support. When resilience is considered an identity rather than a choice, it perpetuates the culture of silence around mental health and reinforces stigma, which hinders help-seeking behaviour in Black African and Caribbean communities.

Resilience, though an asset and protective factor within the Black community, also encourages a sense of self-preservation that acts as an obstacle to help-seeking behaviour, especially in accessing mental health services. The prevailing viewpoint here is that, in the face of racial discrimination, putting up a defensive, resilient front impacts the decision to seek help when experiencing any form of mental distress (unless the issue becomes life-threatening and calls for crisis intervention). Owing to some preconceived notions held by other races about Black people as an inferior race, there may be the perception that openness about their mental health may only validate such erroneous beliefs. Unpublished data from a qualitative study conducted by Kumah (2024) highlighted concerns within the Black community that encouraging open discussions about mental health could, paradoxically, cause more harm than good to the perceived strength and resilience of the community. The phrase 'if it's not broken, don't fix it' captured a prevailing sentiment that disclosure, unless circumstances became entirely unbearable, risked exposing individuals to the harms of systemic racism.

The implication of this resilient identity, as linked to the fear of loss of freedom and dignity in disclosing the mental health challenges and potentially accessing services, as evidenced by Keating and Robertson (2004), feeds into the cycle of fear, which obstructs willingness to seek help in times of crisis. Clay (2019) consequently refers to this resilient identity as an illusion of empowerment, where the ideas around being a 'strong Black man or woman' are the product of survival skills developed in the face of racial discrimination, which eventually feed into mental illness stigma, late help-seeking behaviour, and poor health outcomes. Taylor (1995), in exploring the relationship between the 'strong Black woman' stereotype and depression, highlighted the feelings of exhaustion and frustration described by many women in her study stemming from the need to stand behind an armour of strength. Beauboeuf-Lafontant (2007) further explicated how the strong Black woman narrative normalised negative coping strategies among Black women who tried to demonstrate selflessness in their relationships with others, which eventually adversely affected both their physical and mental health. The once coveted 'strong Black man/woman' label is slowly becoming less desirable, given its impact on the mental health of Black people and leads to the unrealistic expectations of individual resilience despite indications of suffering (Abrams et al., 2014).

In a society like the UK's, which some refer to as 'elegantly racist' (Kumah, 2024), asking for help is often regarded as the equivalent of showing weakness and reinforces the culture of silence and stigma around mental health. Wallace et al. (2016) and Spotforth et al. (2021) demonstrated in their research that the fear of racial discrimination alone was enough to have a cumulative effect on the mental health of people of minority ethnic background. Critically evaluating the impact of resilience as an identity within these communities is relevant for addressing other areas of healthcare delivery, such as maternal health where the mortality rates of Black women are recorded to be higher than other ethnicities, as service providers buy into theories on 'super-coping' and make assumptions that Black people have high pain thresholds (Golden, 2021; Onanuga et al., 2023). Allan and Phillipson (2017) also identified the need for researchers to further evaluate the role of social capital in perpetuating harmful societal norms around toxic resilience, highlighting the need to unpick how such notions of keeping a 'stiff upper lip' perpetuated within the Black community discourage help-seeking behaviour and access to mental health resources.

Fundamentally, the promotion of resilience is critical towards encouraging good mental health and coping in the face of adversity. As one research participant states: 'Resilience means just being very, very strong. It means really standing up for yourself. It means being rude. Even if you have to be rude, be rude; be rude and right rather than be submissive and have someone walk over you . . . you're either a resilient doormat or resilient fighter, it's one or the other' (Kumah, 2024, p. 142). Nevertheless, it is important to promote healthy resilience and coping mechanisms that reframe the narrative around resilience (Taylor et al., 2020) and encourage open dialogues beyond the idea of 'bounce-back-ability'. Rather, the promotion of resilience should also encompass the need to see resilience as being vulnerable enough to ask for help in the face of a crisis. Reshaping mental health promotion initiatives to promote such ideas may prove to be instrumental in addressing mental illness stigma and late access to services within these communities.

The call for alternative terms to address resilience and the recognition of such 'toxic resilience' narratives as barriers to seeking mental health support align with CRT's emphasis on challenging dominant narratives and centring the voices and experiences of marginalised communities in shaping discourse and practice. CRT primarily emphasises the centrality of race and racism in shaping the lived experiences and social outcomes of people of minority ethnic background (Crenshaw et al., 1995); therefore, the notion of resilience as a means protecting oneself from the negative impacts of racial discrimination aligns with CRT's focus on the ways people of minority ethnic background resist and challenge oppressive systemic structures (Collins, 2022). This further highlights the complex and multifaceted nature of resilience within Black African and African-Caribbean communities in the UK, highlighting the need for further research that applies a CRT lens to investigate the influence of acculturation, Black British culture, and intergenerational dynamics on resilience and mental health.

Intersection of resilience and systemic barriers in mental health services

Racial and systemic discrimination play a significant role in perpetuating the fear and stigma surrounding mental health within Black African and African-Caribbean communities. This stigma is often exacerbated by preconceived notions held by healthcare practitioners and further stresses the impact of stigma, discrimination, and systemic racism on mental health and help-seeking behaviour within these communities (Bhui et al., 2015; Memon et al., 2016). The implications of the nuances surrounding the resilience narrative within Black communities provide valuable insights into help-seeking behaviour, demonstrating the influence of systemic racism and the historical legacy of slavery and oppression in contributing to a 'super-coping' resilience narrative, which has detrimental effects on mental health (Bécares et al., 2009).

Both overt and covert racism in various settings, including schools, workplaces, and healthcare systems, foster the development of a resilient identity within the Black community. This identity, while protective in some ways, can negatively influence perceptions of vulnerability and mental illness, often leading to these being viewed as signs of weakness (Carr et al., 2017). Hammond (2012) argues that poor help-seeking behaviour among Black men is partly due to their past experiences of racism and resulting cultural distrust. These concerns are echoed in studies by Mantovani et al. (2017), Memon et al. (2016), and Toleikyte and Salway (2018), highlighting how these factors further impede access to mental health and well-being support. The fear of victimisation, stemming from experiences of racism, contributes significantly to the reluctance in seeking mental health support, which is not merely a matter of individual choice but a complex response to systemic inequalities and historical traumas. The resilient identity, while a source of strength, can inadvertently become a barrier to acknowledging mental health concerns and seeking professional help.

The pertinent need to address the impact of racial discrimination in the workplace is also important, particularly in line with narratives around deconstructing resilience and addressing the psychological distress resulting from racial microaggressions. Research conducted by Myrie and Gannon (2013) and Memon et al. (2016) draws attention to the relationship that exists between continuous exposure and racial microaggressions in the workplace and the negative effects on both physical and mental health among minority ethnic staff. Yet very few interventions are provided for what Smith et al. (2011) referred to as 'racial battle fatigue', where the risk of continuously expending energy on race-related stressors in toxic work environments led to burnout and increased risk of mental health problems. They called for provision of safe spaces for Black professionals within the community. Arday (2022), who evaluated the experiences of minority ethnic staff in higher education settings in the UK, advocated for systemic changes that tackle foundational institutionally racist practices which have contributed to poorer mental health outcomes for ethnic minority staff. The need for safe spaces and psychological interventions that support mental health and promote healthy work environments, fostering organisational and professional growth, cannot be emphasised enough. There is much value in creating an empowering environment that seeks to nurture growth and encourage positive outcomes for the health and well-being of diverse populations, and schools and workplaces offer many prospects for accomplishing this goal. The need for culturally sensitive and equitable approaches in addressing microaggressions and racism towards professionals of Black African and African-Caribbean background is paramount. One innovative suggestion is the provision of after-work safe spaces for Black professionals, modelled after school clubs. These safe spaces could offer a crucial outlet for individuals to share their experiences and thoughts on workplace difficulties, thereby promoting mental health and well-being. It is essential to re-evaluate the representations and expectations surrounding unhealthy coping strategies, particularly considering the complex relationship between resilience and early help-seeking behaviour in accessing mental health support. The interplay between resilience and racial microaggressions in the workplace and other healthcare settings underscores the importance of promoting workplace-based support specifically tailored for professionals of Black ethnic background.

By implementing these culturally sensitive and equitable approaches, organisations can create more inclusive environments that acknowledge and address the unique challenges faced by Black professionals. This not only supports individual mental health but also contributes to broader systemic change, fostering a more equitable and psychologically safe workplace for all.

The role of community, voluntary, and statutory services

Understanding the impact of these systemic barriers is critical for developing effective, culturally sensitive mental health services. It requires acknowledging the complex interplay between historical trauma, ongoing discrimination, and community resilience. Mental health professionals and policymakers must work to create services that recognise these factors, build trust, and provide support in ways that do not conflict with the valued aspects of Black identity and resilience. The ARISE project (Keating, 2021) aimed at raising mental health awareness among young Black men in a borough in London found that many Black men were of the view that their identities were based on the expectations of society to stay resilient and keep a 'stiff upper lip', even in the face of racial injustice. The perceived lack of room to demonstrate vulnerability led to an instinctive portrayal of defensiveness, which was often perceived as violent behaviour. The need to remain vigilant against any form of racial discrimination meant that mental health was put in the background. In an evaluation of campaigns undertaken in various parts of the UK, such as Black Men on the Couch (Akinsete, 2011) and the Count Me In campaign by Mind (2019), Meechan et al. (2021) addressed the need for more Black role models who could help to break the barriers around the culture of silence around mental health. Citing Dillman Carpentier and Parrott (2016) and Francis (2021), participants highlighted the need to implement ideas that raise aspirations of young Black people, encourage, and promote safe spaces for addressing mental health concerns and deconstructing the identity surrounding resilience.

At the core of any mental health promotion initiative should be the drive to empower various target populations to manage their own health and well-being by efficiently utilising resources at their disposal. Similarly, the need for empowerment of both communities and grassroots service providers is crucial, particularly the kind of inclusive empowerment geared more towards Black people taking advantage of motivating one another to promote the resources and systems already in place to support mental health and well-being. A particular focus on school-based education, mentoring, and engagement is essential, where the need to enrich and inspire young Black people to optimistically anticipate a future filled with better possibilities and prospects, beyond the stereotypes placed on young Black men and women, should be actively encouraged. Given the historical evidence of exclusion of children of Black African and African-Caribbean backgrounds within the educational system (Bourne et al., 1994; Christian,

2005; Graham et al., 2019), these recommendations are significant towards promoting inclusion and good mental health. The use of innovative and progressive initiatives as a means of education and engagement, including the arts, music, and sports, also needs to be emphasised within both the school and community contexts. Several studies provide evidence of the potential for school-based mental health promotion to reduce stigma and remove barriers to help-seeking behaviour, particularly in school settings with a high population of students of minority ethnic backgrounds (Barry et al., 2009; O'Reilly et al., 2018). Creating safe spaces within the community is key, particularly when encouraging Black youth to aim higher when it comes to career prospects. This is aimed at bridging the attainment gap evident and decolonising career guidance within this population (Haywood & Darko, 2021; Ranavaya, 2022). This adds to Byfield and Talburt's (2020) advocacy for the development of targeted interventions aimed at promoting social, educational, and professional aspirations, as well as improving emotional well-being, particularly among Black boys.

Empowering service users and those with lived experience of mental illness in contributing to the leadership structure and decision-making process of services is also important for improving cultural sensitivity in service delivery. Given the current NHS agenda (NHS England, 2021) to foster community engagement and promote patient involvement in service delivery, the timing is favourable for encouraging more inclusive discussions. The UK Health Security Agency (Stansfield et al., 2020) 'whole systems' approach to community development seeks to promote bold leadership, collective bravery, and a shift in mindset surrounding the co-design of services for communities. These recommendations for equitable partnerships are crucial for breaking the cycles of mistrust of statutory services that have often been implicated in the low levels of help-seeking behaviour within the Black community. A recent report by the NHS Race and Health Observatory (2022) recommended that statutory mental health services should strive to establish and sustain connections with minority ethnic third and voluntary sector organisations (charities and community groups, which operate independently of the Government) (Kapadia et al., 2022). These partnerships are key to improving cultural competence in mental health service delivery and would validate the NHS mandate to decrease inequalities in mental health services by improving access, encouraging timely utilisation of services, and improving the quality in delivery of mental health services. The invaluable contributions voluntary sector organisations make towards the promotion of mental health in minority ethnic communities highlight the need to capitalise on equitable partnerships in the delivery of holistic culturally sensitive mental health services (Baskin et al., 2021).

Despite these findings, Ocloo and Matthews (2016) caution that stakeholders must be wary of tokenism in co-production initiatives. True empowerment requires ensuring equity in the distribution of power and fostering healthcare models that promote equitable decision-making. The creation of such models is crucial for meaningful community engagement and sustainable improvements in mental healthcare delivery. The issue of tokenism in community partnerships extends beyond mere inclusion. Many service providers and community experts find their opinions are sought by policymakers and healthcare commissioners, but often on an unpaid, voluntary basis. This practice undervalues the time, knowledge, and experience contributed by these experts. There is a growing call for appropriate recognition and compensation for such expertise, particularly through inclusion in policy and decision-making processes. Furthermore, it is crucial that community experts are granted access to influence the allocation of resources towards the provision of equitable mental healthcare. This level of involvement ensures that the unique needs and perspectives of Black African and African-Caribbean communities are effectively represented in the development and implementation of mental health services.

By addressing these concerns and moving towards more equitable partnerships, there is potential to create mental healthcare systems that are truly responsive to the needs of Black African and African-Caribbean communities. This approach not only validates the expertise within these communities but also contributes to the development of more effective, culturally sensitive mental healthcare provision. Perhaps, this is where the conversation around cultural safety and cultural humility comes in to yield a more complete understanding of the role of tailoring health services to the needs of the populations they support. As proposed by Papps and Ramsden (1996, p. 493), cultural safety is defined as 'a component of healthcare practice that encourages reflections on the influence of a healthcare practitioner's cultural identity in relation to that of the patient, and how this affects power relations and the practitioner's ability to respect the patient's rights'. Subsequent definitions, such as the one provided by Downing et al. (2011), include cultural safety being 'a means of addressing the impact of entrenched colonial systems and institutional racism on healthcare delivery, and how these systems perpetuate health inequalities'. Comas-Diaz et al. (1998) and Tervalon and Murray-Garcia (1998) were of the view that to exemplify cultural safety and humility, it was important not to approach culture as a construct that can be analysed or learned, but rather as a reflective process of understanding how others approach life, through the lens of acceptance and respect. They further propose that cultural humility requires consciously seeking to understand the power relations and socio-political structures that play a significant role in perpetuating health inequalities. Rather than seeking to fix culture, they propose a system of change that promotes mutually beneficial collaborations that highlight and align with the values of the communities served, in a manner that demonstrates respect and dignity for cultural practices (Lee et al., 2014). Abe (2020) corroborates these suggestions, proposing cultural humility as a social practice that has the potential to promote sustainable and impactful change in healthcare service delivery, where power imbalances, exacerbated by structural and systemic influences, are prominent in shaping policy and practice. Ranjbar et al. (2020), consequently, support the idea of cultural humility as an essential guiding principle, suitable for encouraging critical self-reflection and institutional accountability, particularly in instances where power imbalances exist in inter-organisational collaborations, such as in the case of statutory-voluntary sector partnerships. Hui et al. (2020) are also of the view that culturally competent health interventions are those that actively address the impact of institutional injustice in a manner that reduces its impact on holistic, person-centred care. They further state that such services should seek to alleviate health inequalities by effectively evaluating the impact of biopsychosocial influences on a patient's health, respecting their views, while consistently reflecting on the interplay and effects of individual and institutional biases on patient care. As society continues to evolve, constant reflection on awareness of self and others is crucial to understanding those around us and fostering healthy relations, particularly within multicultural communities like those represented in the United Kingdom.

Conclusion and future directions

In every society, individuals tend to view the world through the lens of their cultural background, and their very identity, along with their interpretation of life goals and social expectations. In a multicultural society like the UK, the approaches taken to promoting cultural competence in service delivery should be aimed at understanding a community's view of, and interactions with, the world around them, as well as recognising and respecting their values and beliefs (Edge et al., 2018; Kirmayer & Jarvis, 2019).

The evidence that exists regarding the poor and disproportionate treatment of people of Black African and African-Caribbean backgrounds within the mental health system in the UK is reflective of the systemic structures that still influence the delivery of healthcare to this population. Despite efforts of policymakers and healthcare practitioners to bridge the gap in health inequalities, there still exists a wide disparity between white and minority ethnic populations, leading to poorer health outcomes and quality of life for Black African and African-Caribbean communities. The BAME (Black, Asian, and Minority Ethnic) term, under which minority ethnic groups in the UK are classified and referenced in much of the literature on mental health inequalities, homogenises the experiences of the distinctive ethnic groups represented and poses a challenge to addressing the specific needs that may hinder access to mental health services. Even though the evidence of stigma around mental illness still exists within the Black African and African-Caribbean communities, there is a need to adopt a critical lens to addressing health inequalities within this population, and to critically evaluate how protective factors embodied within culture support mental health within this population.

It is essential that we re-evaluate resilience narratives and their impact on help-seeking behaviour, by objectively addressing the aspects of culture that perpetuate stigma and limit access to early mental health support among Black communities. This is imperative in bridging the current gaps in the delivery of mental health services for Black communities in the UK. Challenging the systemic and institutional racism that influence the outcomes of healthcare delivery and quality of life within the Black African and African-Caribbean communities, as well as empowering members of these communities through innovative approaches to mental health promotion and capacity-building initiatives. is crucial in the drive to reduce health inequalities. By harnessing the social and cultural capital available within these communities, the potential to foster strategic and sustainable partnerships between statutory and voluntary services is possible in response to addressing the gaps that still exist in service delivery.

Discussion questions

1. In what ways could resilience narratives impact the help-seeking behaviours of Black individuals, and how might these narratives differ from traditional views on mental health within healthcare systems?
2. Consider the duality of resilience as both a survival strategy and a potential barrier to seeking help, especially in relation to mental health services. What role could safe spaces play in addressing the effects of impacts of systemic racism and discrimination? How might these spaces be integrated into community-based participatory research?

3. Reflect on the importance of culturally sensitive environments that allow individuals to engage with negative experiences in a way that promotes healing and supports research that respects their lived experiences.
4. How could the application of critical race theory (CRT) reshape research and practice around resilience and trauma among Black communities in the UK?

Further reading

Albert, A., Islam, S., Haklay, M., & McEachan, R. R. C. (2023). Nothing about us without us: A co-production strategy for communities, researchers and stakeholders to identify ways of improving health and reducing inequalities. *Health Expectations*, *26*(2), 836–846. https://doi.org/10.1111/hex.13709

Bansal, N., Karlsen, S., Sashidharan, S. P., Cohen, R., Chew-Graham, C. A., & Malpass, A. (2022). Understanding ethnic inequalities in mental healthcare in the UK: A meta-ethnography. *PLOS Medicine*, *19*(12), e1004139. https://doi.org/10.1371/journal.pmed.1004139

Campinha-Bacote, J. (2002). The process of cultural competence in the delivery of healthcare services: A model of care. *Journal of Transcultural Nursing*, *13*(3), 181–184. https://doi.org/10.1177/10459602013003003

Codjoe, L., Barber, S., Ahuja, S., Thornicroft, G., Henderson, C., Lempp, H., & N'Danga-Koroma, J. (2021). Evidence for interventions to promote mental health and reduce stigma in Black faith communities: Systematic review. *Social Psychiatry and Psychiatric Epidemiology*, *56*, 895–911. https://doi.org/10.1007/s00127-021-02068-y

Franceschelli, M., Schoon, I., & Evans, K. (2017). 'Your past makes you who you are': Retrospective parenting and relational resilience among Black Caribbean British young people. *Sociological Research Online*, *22*(4), 48–65. https://doi.org/10.1177/1360780417726957

Race Equality Foundation. (2022). *Better Practice in Mental Health for Black and Minority Ethnic Communities* (pp. 1–20). https://raceequalityfoundation.org.uk/wp-content/uploads/2022/10/Better-practice-in-mental-health.pdf

References

Abe, J. (2020). Beyond cultural competence, toward social transformation: Liberation psychologies and the practice of cultural humility. *Journal of Social Work Education*, *56*(4), 696–707.

Abrams, J. A., Maxwell, M., Pope, M., & Belgrave, F. Z. (2014). Carrying the world with the grace of a lady and the grit of a warrior: Deepening our understanding of the "strong Black woman" schema. *Psychology of Women Quarterly*, *38*(4), 503–518.

Akinsete, E. (2011). *'Men on the couch': A grounded theory study of Black men, talking therapy, and desistance.* Doctoral thesis, University of East London. https://doi.org/10.15123/PUB.1723

Allan, G., & Phillipson, C. (2017). *Social Networks and Social Exclusion: Sociological and Policy Perspectives.* Routledge.

Arday, J. (2022). No one can see me cry: Understanding mental health issues for Black and minority ethnic staff in higher education. *Higher Education*, *83*(1), 79–102.

Aspinall, P. J. (2021). BAME (black, Asian and minority ethnic): The 'new normal' in collective terminology. *Journal of Epidemiology Community Health*, *75*(2), 107–107.

Barnett, P., Mackay, E., Matthews, H., Gate, R., Greenwood, H., Ariyo, K., . . . Smith, S. (2019). Ethnic variations in compulsory detention under the Mental Health Act: A systematic review and meta-analysis of international data. *The Lancet Psychiatry*, *6*(4), 305–317.

Barry, M. M., Canavan, R., Clarke, A., Dempsey, C., & O'Sullivan, M. (2009). *Review of Evidence-Based Mental Health Promotion and Primary/Secondary Prevention.* Report to the Department of Health, London.

Baskin, C., Zijlstra, G., McGrath, M., Lee, C., Duncan, F. H., Oliver, E. J., . . . Gnani, S. (2021). Community-centred interventions for improving public mental health among adults from ethnic minority populations in the UK: A scoping review. *BMJ Open*, *11*(4), e041102.

Beauboeuf-Lafontant, T. (2007). You have to show strength: An exploration of gender, race, and depression. *Gender & Society*, *21*(1), 28–51.

Bécares, L., Nazroo, J., & Stafford, M. (2009). The buffering effects of ethnic density on experienced racism and health. *Health & Place, 15*(3), 700–708.

Bhui, K. S., Rabeea'h, W. A., Palinski, A., McCabe, R., Johnson, M. R., Weich, S., Singh, S. P., Knapp, M., Ardino, V., & Szczepura, A. (2015). Interventions to improve therapeutic communications between Black and minority ethnic patients and professionals in psychiatric services: A systematic review. *The British Journal of Psychiatry*, *207*(2), 95–103.

Bignall, T., Jeraj, S., Helsby, E., & Butt, J. (2019). *Racial Disparities in Mental Health*. Race Equality Foundation.

Bourne, J., Bridges, L., & Searle, C. (1994). *Outcast England: How Schools Exclude Black Children*. Institute of Race Relations.

Byfield, C., & Talburt, T. (2020). Targeted intervention in education and the empowerment and emotional well-being of Black boys. In R. Majors, K. Carberry, & T. S. Ransaw (Eds.), *The International Handbook of Black Community Mental Health* (pp. 293–306). Emerald Publishing Limited. https://doi.org/10.1108/978-1-83909-964-920201019

Carr, S., Holley, J., Hafford-Letchfield, T., Faulkner, A., Gould, D., Khisa, C., & Megele, C. (2017). Mental health service user experiences of targeted violence and hostility and help-seeking in the UK: A scoping review. *Global Mental Health*, *4*, e25.

Chouhan, K., & Nazroo, J. (2020). Health inequalities. In *Ethnicity, Race, and Inequality in the UK* (pp. 111–130). Policy Press.

Christian, M. (2005). The politics of Black presence in Britain and Black male exclusion in the British education system. *Journal of Black Studies*, *35*(3), 327–346.

Clay, K. L. (2019). "Despite the odds": Unpacking the politics of Black resilience neoliberalism. *American Educational Research Journal*, *56*(1), 75–110.

Collins, P. H. (2022). *Black Feminist Thought: Knowledge, Consciousness, and the Politics of Empowerment*. Routledge.

Comas-Diaz, L., & Grenier, J. R. (1998). Migration and acculturation. In *Handbook of Multicultural Perspectives on Stress and Coping* (pp. 121–140). Springer.

Commission on Race and Ethnic Disparities. (2021). *Commission on Race and Ethnic Disparities: The Report*. https://assets.publishing.service.gov.uk/government/uploads/system/uploads/attachment_data/file/974507/20210331_-_CRED_Report_-_FINAL_-_Web_Accessible.pdf

Commission on the Social Determinants of Health. (2008). *Closing the Gap in a Generation: Health Equity through Action on the Social Determinants of Health: Final Report of the Commission on Social Determinants of Health*. World Health Organization.

Crenshaw, K., Gotanda, N., Peller, G., & Thomas, K. (Eds.). (1995). *Critical Race Theory: The Key Writings That Formed the Movement*. The New Press.

Delgado, R., & Stefancic, J. (2001). *An Introduction to Critical Race Theory*. New York University Press.

Department of Health. (2003). *Inside Outside: Improving Mental Health Services for Black and Minority Ethnic Communities in England*. https://www.dh.gov.uk/prod_consum_dh/groups/dh_digitalassets/@dh/@en/documents/digitalasset/dh_4019452.pdf

Devonport, T. J., Ward, G., Morrissey, H., Burt, C., Harris, J., Burt, S., Patel, R., Manning, R., Paredes, R., & Nicholls, W. (2022). A systematic review of inequalities in the mental health experiences of Black African, Black Caribbean, and Black-mixed UK populations: Implications for action. *Journal of Racial and Ethnic Health Disparities*, 1–13. https://doi.org/10.1007/s40615-022-01047-0

Dillman Carpentier, F. R., & Parrott, M. S. (2016). Young adults' information seeking following celebrity suicide: Considering involvement with the celebrity and emotional distress in health communication strategies. *Health Communication*, *31*(10), 1263–1270. https://doi.org/10.1080/10410236.2015.1045313

Downing, R., Kowal, E., & Paradies, Y. (2011). Indigenous cultural training for health workers in Australia. *International Journal for Quality in Health Care*, *23*(3), 247–257. https://doi.org/10.1093/intqhc/mzr031

Edge, D., Degnan, A., Cotterill, S., Berry, K., Baker, J., Drake, R., & Abel, K. (2018). Culturally adapted family intervention (CaFI) for African-Caribbean people diagnosed with schizophrenia and their families: A mixed-methods feasibility study of development, implementation, and acceptability. In *NIHR Journals Library*. Southampton, UK: NIHR Journals Library. https://doi.org/10.3310/hta22590

Fitzgerald, H. E., Johnson, D. J., Allen, J., Villarruel, F. A., & Qin, D. B. (2021). Historical and race-based trauma: Resilience through family and community. *Adversity and Resilience Science*, *2*(3), 215–223. https://doi.org/10.1007/s42844-021-00010-z

Francis, D. B. (2021). "Twitter is really therapeutic at times": Examination of Black men's Twitter conversations following hip-hop artist Kid Cudi's depression disclosure. *Health Communication*, *36*(4), 448–456. https://doi.org/10.1080/10410236.2020.1742102

Frounfelker, R. L., Islam, N., Falcone, J., Farrar, J., Ra, C., Antonaccio, C. M., Enelamah, N., & Betancourt, T. S. (2019). Living through war: Mental health of children and youth in conflict affected areas. *International Review of the Red Cross, 101*(911), 481–506.

Gladwell, M. (2008). *Outliers: The Story of Success*. Little, Brown.

Golden, M. (2021). *The Strong Black Woman: How a Myth Endangers the Physical and Mental Health of Black Women*. Mango Media Inc.

Graham, B., White, C., Edwards, A., Potter, S., & Street, C. (2019). *School Exclusion: A Literature Review on the Continued Disproportionate Exclusion of Certain Groups*. Department for Education. https://assets.publishing.service.gov.uk/government/uploads/system/uploads/attachment_data/file/800028/Timpson_review_of_school_exclusion_literature_review.Pdf

Gray, A. M. (1982). Inequalities in health: The Black report: A summary and comment. *International Journal of Health Services*, *12*(3), 349–380. https://doi.org/10.2190/xxmm-jmqu-2a7y-hx1e

Grey, T., Sewell, H., Shapiro, G., & Ashraf, F. (2013). Mental health inequalities facing UK minority ethnic populations: Causal factors and solutions. *Journal of Psychological Issues in Organizational Culture*, *3*(S1), 146–157.

Hall, S. (1988). New ethnicities. In K. Mercer (Ed.), *Black Film/British Cinema* (ICA Document 7). Institute of Contemporary Arts.

Hammond, W. P. (2012). Taking it like a man: Masculine role norms as moderators of the racial discrimination–depressive symptoms association among African American men. *American Journal of Public Health*, *102*(S2), S232–S241. https://doi.org/10.2105/AJPH.2012.300690

Haywood, M. M., & Darko, A. (2021). Breaking barriers: Using mentoring to transform representation, identity, and marginalization in Black higher education students. *The Journal of Educational Innovation, Partnership and Change*, 7(1). https://doi.org/10.21100/jeipc.v7i1.985

Hemsi, L. K. (1967). Psychiatric morbidity of West Indian immigrants: A study of first admissions in London. *Social Psychiatry*, 2, 95–100.

Herrman, H., Stewart, D. E., Diaz-Granados, N., Berger, E. L., Jackson, B., Yuen, T. (2011, May). What is resilience? *The Canadian Journal of Psychiatry*, *56*(5), 258–265. https://doi.org/10.1177/070674371105600504. PMID: 21586191.

Hill, S. (2016). Axes of health inequality and intersectionality. In K. Smith, S. Hill, & C. McKinney (Eds.), *Health Inequality in the UK* (pp. 155–180). Palgrave Macmillan.

HM Government. (2007). *Mental Health Act*. London: Department of Health. https://d353ahjsg66ro4.cloudfront.net/ukpga/2007/12/pdfs/ukpga_20070012_en.pdf

HM Government. (2018). *Modernising the Mental Health Act: Increasing Choice, Reducing Compulsion*. London: Department of Health.

Hui, A., Latif, A., Hinsliff-Smith, K., & Chen, T. (2020). Exploring the impacts of organisational structure, policy, and practice on the health inequalities of marginalised communities: Illustrative cases from the UK healthcare system. *Health Policy*, *124*(3), 298–302. https://doi.org/10.1016/j.healthpol.2020.01.004

Jensen, E., Carr, R., Degnan, A., Berry, K., & Edge, D. (2021). Exploring service user and family perspectives of a culturally adapted family intervention (CaFI) for African-Caribbean people with psychosis: A qualitative study. *British Journal of Clinical Psychology, 60*(2), 270–289. https://doi.org/10.1111/BJC.12273

Jones, J. M. (2023). Surviving while Black: Systemic racism and psychological resilience. *Annual Review of Psychology*, *74*(1), 1–25. https://doi.org/10.1146/annurev-psych-031121-044439

Joseph-Salisbury, R. (2018). Confronting my duty as an academic of colour in times of explicit racial violence. In A. Johnson, R. Joseph-Salisbury, & E. Kamunge (Eds.), *The Fire Now: Anti-Racist Scholarship in Times of Explicit Racial Violence* (pp. 23–41). Zed Books.

Kapadia, D. (2023). Stigma, mental illness & ethnicity: Time to centre racism and structural stigma. *Sociology of Health & Illness*, *45*(2), 348–365. https://doi.org/10.1111/1467-9566.13459

Kapadia, D., Zhang, J., Salway, S., Nazroo, J., Booth, A., Villarroel-Williams, N., Bécares, L., & Esmail, A. (2022, February). *Ethnic Inequalities in Healthcare: A Rapid Evidence Review.* Technical Report.

Keating, F. (2021). Black men's conversations about mental health through photos. *Qualitative Social Work*, *20*(3), 755–772. https://doi.org/10.1177/1473325019828382

Keating, F., & Robertson, D. (2004). Fear, Black people and mental illness: A vicious circle? *Health and Social Care in the Community*, *12*(5), 439–447. https://doi.org/10.1111/j.1365-2524.2004.00506.x

Kessler, R. C. (1979). Stress, social status, and psychological distress. *Journal of Health and Social Behavior*, 259–272. https://doi.org/10.2307/2136407

Kiev, A. (1965). Psychiatric morbidity of West Indian immigrants in an urban group practice. *The British Journal of Psychiatry*, *111*(470), 51–56. https://doi.org/10.1192/bjp.111.470.51

Kirmayer, L. J., & Jarvis, G. E. (2019). Culturally responsive services as a path to equity in mental healthcare. *HealthcarePapers*, *18*(2), 11–23.

Kirmayer, L. J., Sehdev, M., Whitley, R., Dandeneau, S. F., & Isaac, C. (2009). Community resilience: Models, metaphors, and measures. *International Journal of Indigenous Health*, *5*(1), 62–117.

Krishnan, L., Ogunwole, S. M., & Cooper, L. A. (2020). Historical insights on coronavirus disease 2019 (COVID-19), the 1918 influenza pandemic, and racial disparities: Illuminating a path forward. *Annals of Internal Medicine*, *173*(6), 474–481. https://doi.org/10.7326/M20-2743

Kumah, A. (2024). *Adapting a salutogenic critical appreciative inquiry approach to the co-production of culturally sensitive mental health service delivery for Black African and African Caribbean communities in Birmingham, UK*. Unpublished Doctoral thesis, Birmingham City University. https://www.open-access.bcu.ac.uk/id/eprint/15766

Lee, H. I., Leung, A. K. Y., & Kim, Y. H. (2014). Unpacking East-West differences in the extent of self-enhancement from the perspective of face versus dignity culture. *Social and Personality Psychology Compass*, *8*(7), 314–327.

Lindström, B. (2001). The meaning of resilience. *International Journal of Adolescent Medicine and Health*, *13*(1), 7–12.

Lordi, E. J. (2020). *The Meaning of Soul: Black Music and Resilience Since the 1960s*. Duke University Press.

Mantovani, N., Pizzolati, M., & Edge, D. (2017). Exploring the relationship between stigma and help-seeking for mental illness in African-descended faith communities in the UK. *Health Expectations, 20*(3), 373–384.

McFadden, A., Siebelt, L., Gavine, A., Atkin, K., Bell, K., Innes, N., Jones, H., Jackson, C., Haggi, H., & MacGillivray, S. (2018). Gypsy, Roma, and Traveller access to and engagement with health services: A systematic review. *The European Journal of Public Health*, *28*(1), 74–81. https://doi.org/10.1093/eurpub/ckx231

Meechan, H., John, M., & Hanna, P. (2021). Understandings of mental health and support for Black male adolescents living in the UK. *Children and Youth Services Review*, *129*, 106192. https://doi.org/10.1016/j.childyouth.2021.106192

Memon, A., Taylor, K., Mohebati, L. M., Sundin, J., Cooper, M., Scanlon, T., & de Visser, R. (2016). Perceived barriers to accessing mental health services among Black and minority ethnic (BME) communities: A qualitative study in Southeast England. *BMJ Open*, *6*(11). https://doi.org/10.1136/bmjopen-2016-012337

Millard, S. (2016). World directory of minorities and indigenous peoples. *Reference Reviews*, *30*(3), 26–27.

Mirza, H. S., & Warwick, R. (2024). Race and ethnic inequalities. *Oxford Open Economics*, *3*(Supplement_1), i365–i452. https://doi.org/10.1093/ooecon/ooac010

Modood, T. (1994). Political Blackness and British Asians. *Sociology*, *28*(4), 493–510. https://doi.org/10.1177/0038038594028004004

Morgan, C., Mallett, R., Hutchinson, G., Bagalkote, H., Morgan, K., Fearon, P., Dazzan, P., Boydell, J., McKenzie, K., Harrison, G., Murray, R., Jones, P., Craig, T., & Leff, J. (2005). Pathways to care and ethnicity I: Sample characteristics and compulsory admission: Report from the ÆSOP study. *British Journal of Psychiatry*, *186*(4), 281–289. https://doi.org/10.1192/bjp.186.4.281

Muaygil, R. A. (2018). From paternalistic to patronizing: How cultural competence can be ethically problematic. *HEC Forum*, *30*, 13–29. https://doi.org/10.1007/s10730-017-9342-5

Myrie, C. V., & Gannon, K. (2013). "Should I really be here?" Exploring the relationship between Black men's conceptions of wellbeing, subject positions, and help-seeking behavior. *Diversity and Equality in Health and Care*, *10*(1), 1–22.

Navarro, M. C. (2022). Blackness and food resilience: Black culinary epistemologies, the slow food movement, and racial justice. *Food, Culture & Society*, *25*(2), 201–217. https://doi.org/10.1080/15528014.2021.1960609

Nazroo, J. Y. (2003). The structuring of ethnic inequalities in health: Economic position, racial discrimination, and racism. *American Journal of Public Health*, *93*(2), 277–284. https://doi.org/10.2105/AJPH.93.2.277

Nazroo, J. Y. (2024). Race/ethnic inequalities in health: Moving beyond confusion to focus on fundamental causes. *Oxford Open Economics*, *3*(Supplement_1), i563–i576. https://doi.org/10.1093/ooecon/ooac021

Nazroo, J. Y., Atkin, K., Aspinall, P. J., Bajekal, M., Chattoo, S., Erens, B., Grewal, I., Johnson, M. R. D., Karlsen, S., McManus, S., Oakley, A., Papadopoulos, I., Ritchie, J., & Scambler, G. (2020). Where next for understanding race/ethnic inequalities in severe mental illness? Structural, interpersonal, and institutional racism. *Sociology of Health & Illness*, *42*, 262–276. https://doi.org/10.1111/1467-9566.13100

Nazroo, J. Y., & Bécares, L. (2023). *Ethnicity, Inequality and Structural Racism.* UK Covid-19 Inquiry. https://covid19.public-inquiry.uk/documents/inq000280057-expert-report-titled-ethnicity-inequality-and-structural-racism-prepared-by-professor-james-nazroo-and-professor-laia-becares-dated-15-september-2023/

Neff, W. S. (1985). *Work and Human Behaviour.* New York: Aldine.

NHS England. (2020). *Advancing Mental Health Equalities Strategy.* London. Retrieved June 11, 2021, from https://www.england.nhs.uk/wp-content/uploads/2020/10/00159-advancing-mental-healthequalities-strategy.pdf

NHS England. (2021). *Working in Partnership with People and Communities: Statutory Guidance.* [Online]. https://www.england.nhs.uk/long-read/working-in-partnership-with-people-and-communities-statutory-guidance/

NHS Digital. (2025). *Mental Health Act Statistics, Annual Figures, 2024–25: Detentions – Differences Between Groups of People.* https://digital.nhs.uk/data-and-information/publications/

statistical/mental-health-act-statistics-annual-figures/2024-25-annual-figures/detentions-differences-between-groups-of-people

Nwokoroku, S. C., Neil, B., Dlamini, C., & Osuchukwu, V. C. (2022). A systematic review of the role of culture in mental health service utilization among ethnic minority groups in the United Kingdom. *Global Mental Health*, 1–10. https://doi.org/10.1017/gmh.2022.29

Ocloo, J., & Matthews, R. (2016). From tokenism to empowerment: Progressing patient and public involvement in healthcare improvement. *BMJ Quality & Safety*, *25*(8), 626–632. https://doi.org/10.1136/bmjqs-2015-004500

Office for National Statistics. (2021). *2021 Census Data*. Retrieved July 16, 2023, from https://www.ons.gov.uk/

Onanuga, S., Grace, B., Saraki, T., Dhanjal, M., & Pinder, R. (2023). P-440 Equity in reproductive health: A systematic review of factors influencing higher maternal mortality among Black women in the United Kingdom. *Human Reproduction*, *38*(Supplement_1), dead093–788.

O'Reilly, M., Svirydzenka, N., Adams, S., & Dogra, N. (2018). Review of mental health promotion interventions in schools. *Social Psychiatry and Psychiatric Epidemiology*. https://doi.org/10.1007/s00127-018-1530-1

Panter-Brick, C., & Leckman, J. F. (2013). Editorial commentary: Resilience in child development – Interconnected pathways to wellbeing. *Journal of Child Psychology and Psychiatry*, *54*, 333–336. http://dx.doi.org/10.1111/jcpp.12057

Papps, E., & Ramsden, I. (1996). Cultural safety in nursing: The New Zealand experience. *International Journal for Quality in Health Care*, *8*(5), 491–497. https://doi.org/10.1093/intqhc/8.5.491

Payne, Y. A. (2011). Site of resilience: A reconceptualization of resiliency and resilience in street life–oriented Black men. *Journal of Black Psychology*, *37*(4), 426–451. https://doi.org/10.1177/0095798410391441

Pitt, M. (2017). Rhythm and "Resilience": Black young adults and poetry. *Macsphere*. Retrieved August 30, 2023, from https://macsphere.mcmaster.ca/handle/11375/21955

Powell, N. S., Larsen, R. K., & van Bommel, S. (2014). Meeting the 'Anthropocene' in the context of intractability and complexity: Infusing resilience narratives with intersubjectivity. *Resilience*, *2*(3), 135–150. https://doi.org/10.1080/21693293.2014.908974

Rabiee-Khan, F., & Smith, P. (2014). Understanding mental health and experience of accessing services among African and African Caribbean service users and carers in Birmingham, UK. *Diversity and Equality in Health and Care*, *11*(2), 125–134.

Ranavaya, V. (2022). Decolonising career guidance: Experiences of female, BAME career guidance professionals through the lens of intersectionality theory. *Journal of the National Institute for Career Education and Counselling*, *48*(1), 40–47. https://doi.org/10.20856/jnicec.4808

Ranjbar, N., Erb, M., Mohammad, O., & Moreno, F. A. (2020). Trauma-informed care and cultural humility in the mental health care of people from minoritized communities. *Focus*, *18*(1), 8–15. https://doi.org/10.1176/appi.focus.20190016

Rollock, N. (2019). Staying power: The career experiences and strategies of UK Black female professors. *Sociology*, *53*(5), 968–984. https://doi.org/10.1177/0038038519827580

Royal College of Nursing. (2025). *Seni's Law: Preventing Deaths from Restraint in Mental Health Settings*. https://www.rcn.org.uk/magazines/People/2025/Apr/Mental-health-restraint-preventing-deaths-through-Senis-Law

Rutter, M. (1985). Resilience in the face of adversity: Protective factors and resistance to psychiatric disorder. *The British Journal of Psychiatry*, *147*(6), 598–611. https://doi.org/10.1192/bjp.147.6.598

Sharpley, M., Hutchinson, G., McKenzie, K., & Murray, R. M. (2001). Understanding the excess of psychosis among the African-Caribbean population in England: Review of current hypotheses. *The British Journal of Psychiatry*, *178*(40), 60–68. https://doi.org/10.1192/bjp.178.40.s60

Siller, H., & Aydin, N. (2022). Using an intersectional lens on vulnerability and resilience in minority and/or marginalized groups during the COVID-19 pandemic: A narrative review. *Frontiers in Psychology*, *13*, 894103. https://doi.org/10.3389/fpsyg.2022.894103

Simien, E. M. (2005). Race, gender, and linked fate. *Journal of Black Studies*, *35*(5), 529–550. https://doi.org/10.1177/0021934704264521

Smith, K., Bambra, C., & Hill, S. (2016). Background and introduction: UK experiences of health inequalities. In *Health Inequalities: Critical Perspectives* (pp. 1–21). Oxford University Press.

Smith, W. A., Hung, M., & Franklin, J. D. (2011). Racial battle fatigue and the miseducation of Black men: Racial microaggressions, societal problems, and environmental stress. *Journal of Negro Education*, *80*(1), 63–82. https://doi.org/10.7709/jnegroeducation.80.1.0063

Spotforth, R. J., Ellams, J., Motsi-Omoijiade, I., & Ireton, G. (2021). Racial discrimination in health and care: Exploring the lived experience of Black and South Asian people in England and Wales. *Journal of Health Services Research & Policy*, 26(3), 210–217. https://doi.org/10.1177/13558196211005744

Stansfield, J., South, J., & Mapplethorpe, T. (2020). What are the elements of a whole system approach to community-centred public health? A qualitative study with public health leaders in England's local authority areas. *BMJ Open*, *10*(8), Article e036044. https://doi.org/10.1136/bmjopen-2019-036044

Sumbul, T., Spellen, S., & McLemore, M. R. (2020). A transdisciplinary conceptual framework of contextualized resilience for reducing adverse birth outcomes. *Qualitative Health Research*, *30*(1), 105–118. https://doi.org/10.1177/1049732319892204

Sweeney, L., Owens, C., & Malone, K. (2015). Communication and interpretation of emotional distress within the friendships of young Irish men prior to suicide: A qualitative study. *Health and Social Care in the Community*, *23*(2), 150–158. https://doi.org/10.1111/hsc.12124

Synergi Collaborative Centre Report. (2018). *Briefing Paper: The Impact of Racism on Mental Health*, 1–14. www.synergicollaborativecentre.co.uk

Taylor, H. A., Jr., Washington-Plaskett, T., & Quyyumi, A. A. (2020). Black resilience – Broadening the narrative and the science on cardiovascular health and disease disparities. *Ethnicity & Disease*, *30*(2), 365.

Taylor, S. L. (1995). Lessons in living. *Essence*, *26*(8), 57–58, 104, 106.

Taylor, S. L. (1998). Taking back our power. *Essence*, *29*(1), 107.

Tervalon, M., & Murray-Garcia, J. (1998). Cultural humility versus cultural competence: A critical distinction in defining physician training outcomes in multicultural education. *Journal of Health Care for the Poor and Underserved*, *9*(2), 117–125. https://doi.org/10.1353/hpu.2010.0134

Teti, M., Martin, A. E., Ranade, R., Massie, J., Malebranche, D. J., Tschann, J. M., & Bowleg, L. (2012). "I'ma keep rising: I'ma keep going forward, regardless": Exploring Black men's resilience amid sociostructural challenges and stressors. *Qualitative Health Research*, *22*(4), 524–533. https://doi.org/10.1177/1049732311431487

Theron, L. C. (2016). Toward a culturally and contextually sensitive understanding of resilience: Privileging the voices of Black, South African young people. *Journal of Adolescent Research*, *31*(6), 635–670. https://doi.org/10.1177/0743558415614873

Toleikyte, L., & Salway, S. (2018). Local action on health inequalities: Understanding and reducing ethnic inequalities in health. *Public Health England*, 3.

Vernon, P. (2011). Put race equality in mental health back on the agenda. *The Guardian*. http://www.guardian.co.uk/society/joepublic/2011/mar/01/race-equality-mental-health

Wallace, S., Nazroo, J., & Bécares, L. (2016). Cumulative effect of racial discrimination on the mental health of ethnic minorities in the United Kingdom. *American Journal of Public Health*, *106*(7), 1294–1300. https://doi.org/10.2105/AJPH.2016.303141

Wenham, C. (2020). What is the future of UK leadership in global health security post COVID-19? *IPPR Progressive Review*, 27(2), 196–203. https://doi.org/10.1111/newe.12201

Williams, D. R., & Harris-Reid, M. (1999). Race and mental health: Emerging patterns and promising approaches. In A. V. Horwitz & T. L. Scheid (Eds.), *A Handbook for the Study of Mental Health: Social Contexts, Theories, and Systems* (pp 295–314). Cambridge University Press.

Woods-Giscombe, C. L., Williams, K. P., Conklin, J., Dodd, A., Bravo, L., Anderson, A. M., Frazier, T., Bey, G., Robinson, M. N., Warren, B. J., & Wight, K. D. (2023). A scoping review of the concept of resilience among African American women. *Archives of Psychiatric Nursing*, *46*, 107–120. https://doi.org/10.1016/j.apnu.2022.10.003

World Health Organization. (2016). *Glossary of Terms Used*. www.who.int/hia/about/glos/en/index1.html

Youth Justice Board for England and Wales. (2025). The Evolving Response to Ethnic Disproportionality in Youth Justice. Available at: https://www.gov.uk/government/news/the-evolving-response-to-ethnic-disproportionality-in-youth-justice

Conclusions

Melanie Etti and Julie Botticello

The chapters presented in this volume clearly reveal the gross and preventable disparities that significantly reduce both the quality and length of life for people from racialised communities in the UK. In 21st-century Britain, these injustices in life chances are not acceptable. Centuries of racial and ethnic inequity cannot be easily undone, for systems have been built by those in power, representative of and exclusive to their needs. Even when specific attention is paid to surmounting inbuilt ethnic and racial hierarchies, the epistemic and experiential divergence between racial and ethnic groups, historical encounters with the medical profession, distrust, fear, and exclusion continue to impinge on access, experiences, and outcomes.

The deconstruction of the current system through concepts employed by the contributors to this volume, including Critical Race Theory (Delgado et al., 2012), Intersectionality (Crenshaw, 1991), the Screaming Silences framework (Serrant-Green, 2010), and Cultural Humility (Tervalon & Murray-Garcia, 1998), are urgently needed to shift the narrative from one of universal provision to the particularism required to provide individualised and culturally sustaining (Paris, 2012) care for the diversity of racialised communities living across the UK. Whitehead (2007) promotes a theory-based approach to tackling health inequity, with the success of interventions measured through their ability to strengthen individuals and communities, improve living and working conditions, increase access to essential services, and promote healthy macro-policies. We hope that the notions of change presented in this volume have laid the foundation for renewed efforts in pursuit of these objectives.

Despite decades of mistrust, neglect, and outright harm, racialised communities are advocating to collaborate in healthcare provisioning, policy making and research direction, so that their needs are squarely on the table from agenda setting, to intervention implementation, to post-programme evaluation. Quick fixes and short-term interactions must yield to long-term sustainable engagement and interventions that are founded on respect, cultivate trust, and foster a welcoming and health-granting environment for minority ethnic groups. Racism across the three domains – interpersonal,

DOI: 10.4324/9781003466093-19

institution, and structural – must be consciously eradicated, through cultural sensitivity training of current and future workforce, but more so through partnering with the minority ethnic groups who understand both their needs and the need for the healthcare system to be mobilised, through equitable distribution of funding, research, and care provision to meet them.

In order to effect systemic change, however, we *must* move towards a consensus that racism is the central issue. The NHS RHO (2024) emphasised 'naming racism' as the first essential step towards dismantling structurally racist systems. The unfounded conclusions of the Sewell (2021) report highlight how those aptly positioned to challenge the system can further strengthen its failures through their unwillingness to acknowledge its inadequacies. Though disappointing, this further highlights the essential roles of coalition building and collective action in moving the needle towards systemic change.

To this end, in her summary of the collection of narratives recorded in *Inside the Ivory Tower* a volume documenting Black women's experience in British academia, Gabriel (2017, p. 1) underscores the importance of resisting the status quo to advance the equity agenda. As she states,

> We can choose to assimilate into an organisational structure and institutional space that was never created for us, and adopt the dominant social norms with the hope that our compliance will be rewarded – or we can choose . . . to resist.

She addresses academia, yet the intention carries to the healthcare sector, as education and health are interlinked (Botticello & West, 2021). Increased access to the current structures, whether in education or healthcare, cannot redress their inbuilt biases. Echoing Gabriel's sentiments, Sowemimo (2023, p. 331) states in the closing of her first book, *Divided: Racism, Medicine and Why We Need to Decolonise Healthcare*:

> Our health systems are working as they were intended to – built by and still serving the needs of white, wealthier individuals and leaving others behind. We must dismantle these systems and build new ones. Every small step towards change can save lives.

The healthcare system in the UK is in desperate need of radical reform; however, this must occur in the context of public policy revision, which seeks to redress inequities across society that contribute to the poor health of racialised communities. Machirori (2022) warns against the over-reliance on data to drive this change and recommends a 'people-centred approach', where the needs of disenfranchised communities form the focus of future action. The creation of Anti-Racism Model for Improvement (MFI-AR) quality improvement tool by the NHS RHO (2025) is just one development signalling an important move away from merely collecting data about health inequities towards implementing interventions that aim to change the healthcare system to reduce harm and promote good health for all.

As for academia, attempts at assimilation and adaptation into a racially unjust healthcare system that upholds inequitable norms are what have thus far determined the inequitable health outcomes presented in this volume. If fair process and fair outcomes are the goals for all those living within a just society, then accepting that the system does not currently work for each member and needs to change must be understood as resistance. Not just on the part of those affected but by everyone. As noted in our introduction, the inequitable distribution of the conditions for good health is a profound injustice (Marmot et al., 2024). Turning this around means ensuring that the diversity of need, across the spectrum of racialised communities, is not only met but exceeded through proactive, personalised, collaborative care built through relationships of trust so that all can flourish.

References

Botticello, J., & West, T. O. (2021). Ethnic minority students in the UK: Addressing inequalities in access, support, and wellbeing in higher education. In E. Guerrero (Ed.), *Effective Elimination of Structural Racism* (pp. 165–180). London: IntechOpen.

Crenshaw, K. (1991). Mapping the margins: Intersectionality, identity politics, and violence against women of color. *Stanford Law Review, 43*(6), 1241–1299. https://doi.org/10.2307/1229039

Delgado, R., Stefancic, J., & Harris, A. (2012). *Critical Race Theory: An Introduction* (2nd ed.). NYU Press. http://www.jstor.org/stable/j.ctt9qg9h2

Gabriel, D. (2017). Introduction. In D. Gabriel & S. Tate (Eds.), *Inside the Ivory Tower, Narratives of Women of Colour Surviving and Thriving in British Academia* (pp. 1–4). London: UCL Institute of Education Press.

Machirori, M. (2022). *Don't Start with the Data: A People-Centred Approach to Addressing Health Inequalities.* Ada Lovelace Institute. https://www.adalovelaceinstitute.org/blog/dont-start-with-the-data/

Marmot, M., Allen, J., Goldblatt, P., Willis, S., Noferini, J., & Callaghan, O. (2024). *Structural Racism, Ethnicity and Health Inequalities in London.* Institute of Health Equity. https://www.instituteofhealthequity.org/resources-reports/structural-racism-ethnicity-and-health-inequalities

NHS Race and Health Observatory. (2024). *Seven Anti-Racism Principles and Briefings.* NHS Race and Health Observatory. https://nhsrho.org/resources/seven-anti-racism-principles/

NHS Race and Health Observatory. (2025). *Model for Improvement: Anti-Racism Framework Guidance.* NHS – Race and Health Observatory. https://nhsrho.org/resources/mfi-ar-framework-guidance/

Paris, D. (2012). Culturally sustaining pedagogy, a needed change in stance, terminology, and practice. *Educational Researcher, 41*(3), 93–97. https://doi.org/10.3102/0013189X12441244

Serrant-Green, L. (2010). The sound of 'silence': A framework for researching sensitive issues or marginalised perspectives in health. *Journal of Research in Nursing, 16*(4), 347–360. https://doi.org/10.1177/1744987110387741

Sewell, T. (2021). *Commission on Race and Ethnic Disparities: The Report.* GOV.UK. https://www.gov.uk/government/publications/the-report-of-the-commission-on-race-and-ethnic-disparities

Sowemimo, A. (2023). Divided: Racism, Medicine and Why We Need to Decolonise Healthcare. Wellcome Collection.

Tervalon, M., & Murray-Garcia, J. (1998). Cultural humility versus cultural competence: A critical distinction in defining physician training outcomes in multicultural education. *Journal of Health Care for the Poor and Underserved, 9*(2), 117–125. https://doi.org/10.1353/hpu.2010.0233

Whitehead, M. (2007). A typology of actions to tackle social inequalities in health. *Journal of Epidemiology and Community Health, 61*(6), 473–478. https://doi.org/10.1136/jech.2005.037242

Index

Note: Numbers in **bold** indicate a table. Numbers in *italics* indicate a figure. Underlined numbers indicate a box.